PHYSICAL THERAPY
of the SHOULDER

CLINICS IN PHYSICAL THERAPY
VOLUME 11

Forthcoming Volumes in the Series

PHYSICAL THERAPY of the SHOULDER

Edited by
Robert Donatelli, M.A., P.T.

Assistant Professor
Graduate Program, Orthopedic and
 Sports Physical Therapy
Georgia State University
Co-Founder, Physical Therapy Associates
 of Metro Atlanta
Co-Founder, Clinical Education Associates
 of Atlanta
Atlanta, Georgia

CHURCHILL LIVINGSTONE
NEW YORK, EDINBURGH, LONDON, MELBOURNE
1987

Library of Congress Cataloging-in-Publication Data

Physical therapy of the shoulder.

(Clinics in physical therapy ; v. 11)
Includes bibliographies and index.
1. Shoulder—Wounds and injuries—Treatment.
2. Shoulder joint—Wounds and injuries—Treatment.
3. Shoulder—Diseases—Treatment. 4. Shoulder joint—
Diseases—Treatment. 5. Physical therapy.
I. Donatelli, Robert. II. Series. [DNLM: 1. Physical
Therapy—methods. 2. Shoulder—injuries. 3. Shoulder
Joint—injuries. W1 CL831CN v.11 / WE 810 P578]
RD557.5.P48 1987   617'.572062   86-20722
ISBN 0-443-08458-0

© **Churchill Livingstone Inc. 1987**

Distributed in the United Kingdom by Churchill Livingstone,
Robert Stevenson House, 1-3 Baxter's Place, Leith Walk,
Edinburgh EH1 3AF, and by associated companies, branches,
and representatives throughout the world.

Accurate indications, adverse reactions, and dosage schedules
for drugs are provided in this book, but it is possible that they
may change. The reader is urged to review the package
information data of the manufacturers of the medications
mentioned.

Acquisitions Editor: *Kim Loretucci*
Copy Editor: *Leslie Burgess*
Production Designer: *Charlie Lebeda*
Production Supervisor: *Jocelyn Eckstein*

Printed in the United States of America

Second printing in 1988

I would like to dedicate this book to my late father, Revy Donatelli, and to my mother, Rose Donatelli. They provided the guidance, motivation, and love to help me through my college years, enabling me to pursue a career in physical therapy.

Contributors

Larry F. Andrews, B.S., P.T.
Supervisor, Orthopedic Physical Therapy, Emory University Hospital and Emory Clinic, Atlanta, Georgia

Edward Ayub, M.S., P.T.
Private Practice, Orthopedic and Sports Physical Therapy Specialists, Inc., San Diego, California

Turner A. Blackburn, Jr., M.Ed., P.T., A.T.C.
Adjunct Assistant Professor, Columbus College, University of Georgia System; Chief, Sports Physical Therapy, Rehabilitation Services of Columbus, Columbus, Georgia

Robert Burnham, M.D.
Resident, Department of Physical Medicine and Rehabilitation, University of Alberta Faculty of Medicine, Edmonton, Alberta, Canada

Robert Donatelli, M.A., P.T.
Assistant Professor, Graduate Program, Orthopedic and Sports Physical Therapy, Georgia State University; Co-Founder, Physical Therapy Associates of Metro Atlanta; Co-Founder, Clinical Education Associates of Atlanta, Atlanta, Georgia

Robert E. DuVall, M.M.Sc., P.T.
President, Medical and Sports Rehabilitation Associates, Inc., President, Medical Wellness Associates, Inc., Smellville; Vice President, Rehabilitation Medicine Services, Inc., Kings Bay, Georgia

Sanford E. Gruskin, D.D.S., M.S.D.
Private Practice, Atlanta, Georgia

Carol Ann Gunnels, P.T.
Coordinator, Orthopedic Physical Therapy, Emory University Hospital and Emory Clinic, Atlanta, Georgia

Julianne Wright Howell, M.S., P.T.
Co-Director, Hand Management Specialists, Richmond, Virginia

Martha Kaput, M.S., P.T.
Instructor, Clinical Education Associates of Atlanta; Clinical Specialist in Orthopedics, Physical Therapy Associates of Metro Atlanta, Atlanta, Georgia

Kathryn Levit, M.Ed., O.T.R.
Private Practice, Washington, D.C.

Christine A. Moran, M.S., P.T.
Assistant Clinical Professor, Graduate Studies in Physical Therapy, Medical College of Virginia, Virginia Commonwealth University, Richmond; Adjunct Assistant Clinical Professor, Program in Physical Therapy, Old Dominion University, Norfolk; Director, The Richmond Upper Extremity Center, Richmond, Virginia

Helen Owens-Burkhart, M.S., P.T.
Private Practice, Orland Park, Illinois

David C. Reid, M.D., M.C.S.P., M.Ch.(orth), F.R.C.S.(C)
Professor of Physical Education and Professor of Orthopaedic Surgery and Rehabilitation, University of Alberta Faculty of Medicine; Consultant in Sports Medicine, Glen Sather Sports Medicine Clinic, University of Alberta, Edmonton, Alberta, Canada

Susan Ryerson, M.A., P.T.
Clinical Consultant and Lecturer, Private Practice, Washington, D.C.

Linda Saboe, M.C.P.A., B.P.T.
Research Assistant, Division of Orthopaedic Surgery, University of Alberta Faculty of Medicine, Edmonton, Alberta, Canada

Sandra Richards Saunders, P.T.
Graduate Student, Orthopedic Physical Therapy, Medical College of Virginia, Virginia Commonwealth University; Therapist, The Richmond Upper Extremity Center, Richmond, Virginia

Patricia Scagnelli, M.S., P.T.
Chief Physical Therapist, Joseph, Phillips and Green, Falls Church, Virginia

Michael J. Wooden, M.S., P.T.
Instructor, Advanced Masters Program in Orthopedic Physical Therapy, Emory University School of Medicine; Clinical Specialist, Orthopedics, Manual Therapy, and Sports Injury Rehabilitation, Physical Therapy Associates of Metro Atlanta; Co-Founder, Clinical Education Associates of Atlanta, Atlanta, Georgia

Preface

For the past quarter of a century physical therapists have been treating shoulder pain and dysfunction. In the past, treatments have been based on an empirical approach. The contributors' and my intent is not to present a "cookbook" on how to treat the shoulder joint, although numerous techniques and procedures are reviewed. Our conviction is that the therapist should pursue an understanding of the anatomy, biomechanics, histology, and pathology underlying shoulder function and dysfunction. The content encompasses the normal function of tissues within and surrounding the shoulder girdle and the changes that occur as a result of dysfunction.

The topics of the chapters were chosen in an attempt to make the book a comprehensive review of the shoulder. The information is a collection of new material and ideas on examination and treatment of shoulder dysfunction. The authors have also included an extensive review of the literature regarding normal function, dysfunction, and treatment. Each chapter begins with an understanding of the appropriate anatomy, biomechanics, histology, and tissue changes that are specific to the topic presented. The treatment rationale presented is based on clinical experience, the available research, and sound anatomic and biomechanical principles.

Further research is needed in the area of assessment and treatment of the shoulder joint. The authors recognize this need and hope that this text will motivate more physical therapists and physicians to work together in furthering the research in this area.

Robert Donatelli, M.A., P.T.

Acknowledgments

I would like to thank my wife, Joni, for her support, and my friend, Scott Irwin, for his continuing professional motivation.

Contents

1 Anatomy and Biomechanics of the Shoulder

Martha Kaput

One of the most common peripheral joints to be treated in the physical therapy clinic is the shoulder joint. The physical therapist must understand the anatomy and mechanics of this joint to evaluate and design most effectively a treatment program for patients with shoulder dysfunction. This chapter will describe the pertinent functional anatomy of the shoulder complex and relate this anatomy to mechanics of shoulder abduction, flexion, and rotation.

The shoulder joint is better termed the shoulder complex because a series of articulations are necessary to position the humerus in space (Fig. 1-1). Most authors, when describing the shoulder joint, discuss the acromioclavicular joint, the sternoclavicular joint, the scapulothoracic articulation and the glenohumeral joint.[1-4] Kapanji has expanded on this list, and also includes the functional subdeltoid joint.[5] Cailliet discusses the importance of considering movement at the costosternal and costovertebral joints when evaluating shoulder girdle motion.[6] Dempster relates all these areas by using a concept of links. The integrated and harmonious roles of all the links are necessary for full normal mobility.[7]

The shoulder complex is one of the most mobile joints in the body. This wide range of mobility helps position the arm and hand for the many prehensile activities a person may perform. The shoulder can move through nearly a full arc in both the frontal and sagittal planes. This entire range is used in many athletic endeavors such as performing in the gymnastic rings or swimming the backstroke. Most activities of daily living do not require this full range of mobility. The contribution of the shoulder to upper extremity function may be

1

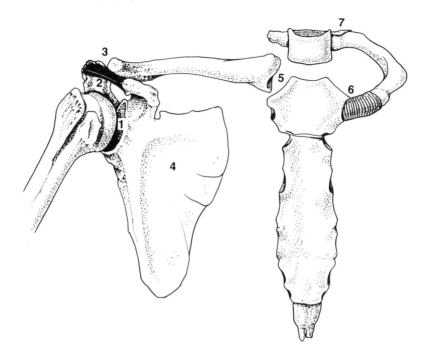

Fig. 1-1. The components of the shoulder joint complex: (1) glenohumeral joint; (2) subdeltoid joint; (3) acromioclavicular joint; (4) scapulothoracic joint; (5) sternoclavicular joint; (6) first costosternal joint; (7) first costovertebral joint.

small if the person can compensate with motion at the cervical spine and distal upper extremity joints. This contrast may explain the presence of shoulder dysfunction at both ends of the mobility spectrum—hypermobility associated with shoulder dislocations and hypomobility seen with adhesive capsulitis. Shoulder motion differs between individuals. Some of this variability is due to anatomical considerations.[8,9]

ANATOMY

Glenohumeral Joint

Osteology

The glenohumeral joint contributes the greatest amount of motion to the shoulder complex. This joint has been described as a ball and socket joint. Saha confirmed this description in 70 percent of his specimens. In the other 30 percent, the radius of curvature of the humeral head was greater than the radius of curvature of the glenoid. Thus the joint was not a true enarthrosis.[9] Saha

A

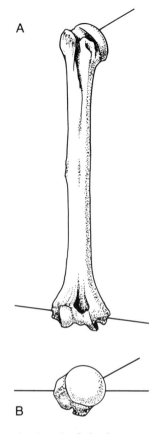

Fig. 1-2. (A) Humerus with marker through the head–neck axis and a second marker through the epicondyles. (B) Retrotorsion of the humerus as seen from above.

B

further described the joint surfaces, especially on the head of the humerus, as very irregular and having a great amount of individual variation.[9]

The head of the humerus is a hemispherical convex articular surface which faces superior, medial, and posterior. This articular surface is inclined 130 to 150° to the shaft of the humerus and is retroverted 20 to 30°[3] (Fig. 1-2). Only one-third of the humeral head can contact the glenoid fossa at a given time.[1] The glenoid fossa is a shallow structure deepened by the glenoid labrum. The labrum is wedge-shaped when the glenohumeral joint is in the resting position and changes shape with various movements.[10] The functional significance of the labrum is questionable. Most authors agree that the labrum is a weak supporting structure.[10,11] Moseley and Övergaard considered the labrum a redundant fold of the capsule composed of dense fibrous connective tissue but generally devoid of cartilage except in a small zone near its osseous attachment.[10]

The glenoid fossa faces laterally. There is some discrepancy regarding the superior or inferior tilt of the glenoid. Freedman and Munro found the glenoid faced downward in 80.8 percent of the shoulders they studied with roentgenograms.[12] Basmajian and Bazant described a superior tilt and hypothesized, that it aided in stability of the joint.[13] Another factor lending stability to this joint is a backward-facing glenoid. Saha found a 7.4° retrotilt of the glenoid in

73.5 percent of his normal subjects.[14] Both the humeral and glenoid articular surfaces are lined with articular cartilage. The cartilage is thickest at the periphery on the glenoid fossa and at the center of the humeral head.[9]

Periarticular Structures

The capsule and ligaments reinforce the glenohumeral joint. The capsule attaches around the glenoid rim and forms a sleeve around the head of the humerus, attaching on the anatomical neck, except medially where the capsule is reflected downward one half inch. The capsule is a lax structure; the head of the humerus can be distracted one half inch when the shoulder is in a relaxed position.[7] The capsule is reinforced anteriorly and posteriorly by ligaments and muscles. There is no additional support inferiorly, which causes weakness of this portion of the capsule.

The anterior capsule is reinforced by the glenohumeral ligaments. The support that these ligaments lend to the capsule is insignificant,[15] and they are not consistently present in each individual. Turkel et al described the inferior glenohumeral ligament as the thickest and most consistent structure.[16] Moseley and Övergaard found the inferior, as well as the superior, ligament consistent in their cadaver population.[10]

The coracohumeral ligaments are the strongest supporting ligaments of the glenohumeral joint. They are also thickenings of the capsule. These ligaments arise from the coracoid process and extend to the greater and lesser tuberosity.

In addition to ligamentous reinforcement, the capsule is also reinforced by muscles. The subscapularis muscle reinforces anteriorly, the supraspinatus reinforces superiorly, and the infraspinatus and teres minor lend support posteriorly. These rotator cuff muscles have been called the musculotendinous glenoid.[17]

Between the supporting ligaments and muscles lie synovial bursa or recesses. Anteriorly, there are three distinct recesses. The superior recess is the subscapular bursa. Separated from the subscapular bursa by the width of the subscapularis tendon is the axillary pouch or recess. The middle synovial recess lies posterior to the subscapularis tendon.[18]

Myology

The major muscles that act on the glenohumeral joint are the scapulohumeral and axiohumeral muscles. The muscles of the scapulohumeral group originate on the scapula and insert on the humerus. The rotator cuff muscles insert on the tuberosities and along the upper two-thirds of the anatomical neck.[19] The subscapularis has the largest amount of muscle mass of the four rotator cuff muscles.[4]

The deltoid comprises 41 percent of the scapulohumeral muscle mass.[4] This muscle, in addition to its proximal attachment on the acromion process

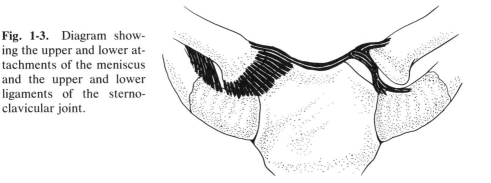

Fig. 1-3. Diagram showing the upper and lower attachments of the meniscus and the upper and lower ligaments of the sternoclavicular joint.

and the spine of the scapula, also arises from the clavicle. The distal insertion is on the shaft of the humerus at the deltoid tubercle. The mechanical advantage of the deltoid is enhanced by the distal insertion and the evolution of a larger acromion process.[4] The deltoid is a multipennate and fatigue-resistant muscle. This may explain the rare involvement of the deltoid in shoulder pathology.[20]

The next muscle group is the axiohumeral muscles. The pectoralis major, minor and latissimus dorsi form this group. Besides being prime movers of the arm, they can act on a fixed arm to move the trunk upward and forward, as in climbing.[19]

Sternoclavicular Joint

The sternoclavicular joint is the only articulation that binds the shoulder girdle to the axial skeleton. This joint is a sellar joint; the sternal articulating surface is greater than the clavicular surface, providing stability to the joint.[5] The joint is also stabilized by its articular disc, joint capsule, ligaments, and reinforcing muscles.[7,21] The articular disc attaches superiorly to the clavicle and inferiorly to the first costocartilage and rib[7,21] (Fig. 1-3). This disc binds the joint together and divides the joint into two cavities. The capsule surrounds the joint and is thickest on the anterior and posterior aspects. The section of the capsule from the disc to the clavicle is more lax, allowing more mobility here than between the disc, sternum, and first rib.[19] The interclavicular ligament reinforces the capsule anteriorly and superiorly. The rhomboid-shaped costoclavicular ligament connects the clavicle to the first rib.[19] Muscles, especially the sternocleidomastoid, sternohyoid, and sternothyroid, provide further support.[21] The clavicle itself forms a double curve, convex medially and concave laterally. This configuration allows increased mobility of this bone.[4]

Acromioclavicular Joint

At the other end of the clavicle is the acromioclavicular joint. This articulation is characterized by variability in size and shape of the clavicular facets and the presence of an intraarticular meniscus.[21] This joint's capsule is more lax than the sternoclavicular joint; thus, more motion occurs at the acromioclavicular joint and it is more prone to dislocations.[7] There are three major supporting ligaments. The conoid and trapezoid ligaments are collectively called the coracoclavicular ligament. It is through this ligament that scapula motion is translated to the clavicle.[7] The acromioclavicular ligament strengthens the superior aspect of the joint, along with the intertwined tendinous attachments of the trapezius and deltoid muscles.[21]

Scapulothoracic Joint

The scapulothoracic joint is not an anatomical joint but an important physiologic joint that adds considerably to the motion of the shoulder girdle. The scapula is concave, articulating with a convex thorax.[1] The scapula is without bony or ligamentous connections to the thorax, except from its attachments at the acromioclavicular joint and coracoclavicular ligament. The scapula is primarily stabilized by muscles. The axioscapula muscles include the trapezius, rhomboid major and minor, serratus anterior, and levator scapula. The tone in the upper trapezius is the chief mechanism for suspension of the entire shoulder girdle.[4]

BIOMECHANICS

Anatomical structures both promote and limit movement. The shoulder joint complex is designed for movement. Three important movements for function are shoulder abduction, flexion, and rotation. During each of these movements, synchronous motion is occurring at the four major component joints of the shoulder complex.

Abduction

Shoulder abduction is the most extensively studied shoulder motion.[4,8,12,22–25] Traditionally, abduction is movement in the coronal plane.[4,6,26] Therefore, this is movement of the humerus in relationship to the trunk. Abduction is also described utilizing the plane of the scapula. In this plane, the mechanical axis of the humerus approximates the mechanical axis of the scapula[22,24,27] (Fig. 1-4). This is not a fixed plane. The plane of the scapula is approximately 30 to 45° anterior to the coronal plane.[23,25] Movement in this

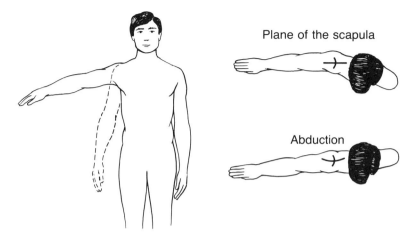

Fig. 1-4. Abduction in the plane of the scapula.

plane prevents twisting of the inferior capsular fibers. The surrounding muscles are parallel, maintaining an optimal length–tension relationship.[22]

Arthrokinematics

The amount of shoulder abduction varies between individuals with an average of 148 to 182° of osteokinematic motion.[12] Approximately 120 to 135° of this motion occurs at the glenohumeral joint.[4,9] The motion occurring at the joint surfaces is arthrokinematic motion, of which there are three types: rolling, gliding, and rotation (Fig. 1-5). Rolling occurs when various points on the moving surface contact various points on a stationary surface. Gliding occurs when one point on a moving surface contacts multiple points on a stationary surface. When rolling or gliding occurs, there is a significant change in the contact area between the two joint surfaces. The third type of arthrokinematic movement is rotation, which occurs when various points on a moving surface contact one point on a stationary surface. There is little displacement between the two joint surfaces in rotation.

All three arthrokinematic movements can occur at the glenohumeral joint, but they do not occur in equal proportions. These motions are necessary for the large humeral head to take advantage of the small glenoid articulating surface.[9] Saha investigated the contact area between the head of the humerus and the glenoid with abduction in the plane of the scapula[9] and found that the contact area on the head of the humerus shifted up and forward, indicating a rolling or gliding movement. Poppen and Walker measured the instant centers of rotation for the same movement.[24] They found that in the first 30° and often between 30 and 60°, the head of the humerus moved superiorly in the glenoid by 3 mm, indicating rolling or gliding. At >60°, there was minimal movement of the humerus, indicating almost pure rotation.[25]

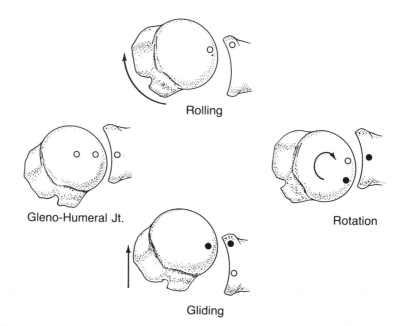

Fig. 1-5.   Arthrokinematic motion occurring at the glenohumeral joint: rolling, rotation, and gliding.

Concomitant external rotation of the humerus is necessary for abduction in the coronal plane.[4,9,26,28] Some authors have postulated that this motion is necessary for the greater tuberosity to clear the acromion and the coracoacromial ligament.[1,2,26] Although a decrease in the distance between the humeral head and the coracoacromial ligament has been associated with rotator cuff dysfunction,[29] there is sufficient room to prevent bone impingement.[9] External rotation also remains necessary for full coronal abduction even after the acromion and the coracoacromial ligament are surgically removed. Saha has reasoned that external rotation is necessary to prevent the humeral head from impinging on the glenoid rim.[9]

External rotation of the humerus is not necessary for full abduction in the plane of the scapula.[2,19] Poppen and Walker found that the humerus and scapula moved synchronously into external rotation at 90° of abduction so there was little relative rotation of the humerus on the glenoid with abduction in the plane of the scapula.[24]

Forces

A significant amount of force is generated at the glenohumeral joint during abduction.[4,23] In the early stages of abduction, the loading vector is beyond the upper edge of the glenoid.[17] During this stage of abduction, the pull of the deltoid produces an upward shear of the humeral head.[30] This shearing force

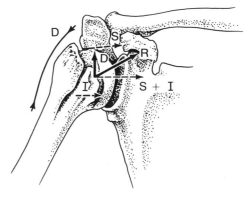

Fig. 1-6. In the early stages of glenohumeral abduction, the deltoid reactive force (D) is located outside the glenoid fossa. This force is counteracted by the transverse compressive forces of the supraspinatus (S) and infraspinatus (I) muscles. The resultant reactive force (R) is therefore more favorably placed within the glenoid fossa for joint stability.

peaks at 60° of abduction and is counteracted by the transverse compressive forces of the rotator cuff muscles.[23] (Fig. 1-6). At 90° of abduction, the loading vector is still eccentrically placed in the upper glenoid; however, at this range, the compressive forces are maximum, resulting in compressive stability.[17] Poppen and Walker estimated this compressive force at .89 times body weight.[23] Inman et al also describe a maximum compressive force at 90°, which is considerably less than Poppen and Walker's calculations.[4] At the end ranges of abduction, the loading vector is directed into the central axis of the glenoid, and the forces are equalized through all portions of the glenoid.[17]

Scapulohumeral Rhythm

Along with movement at the glenohumeral joint, synchronous movement also occurs at the adjacent articulations. Inman et al investigated scapulohumeral rhythm in subjects moving their shoulders in the coronal plane.[4] After the first 30° of motion, a fairly constant ratio of 2° humeral motion to every degree of scapula motion was present. Using x-ray studies, Freedman and Munro found a ratio of three to two in males.[12] Poppen and Walker, investigating abduction in the plane of the scapula, found a ratio of 5° to 4° after the first 30° of motion.[24] Doody et al, also investigating abduction in the plane of the scapula, found an average ratio of 1.74 to 1°, with a ratio of 7.240 to 1° early in the range to <1 to 1 later in the range.[8] The greatest amount of scapula movement occurred between 90 and 140°. When weight was added to the arm, the scapula moved sooner but contributed less to the overall range.[8]

Movement of the scapula is permitted by movement in the acromioclavicular and sternoclavicular joints. Shoulder abduction is accompanied by clavicular elevation. Sternoclavicular motion is most evident between 0 to 90°. For each 10° of shoulder abduction, there are 4° of sternoclavicular movement.[4] The acromioclavicular joint moves primarily before 30° and after 135°.[4] Motion can occur at the acromioclavicular joint with less movement occurring at the sternoclavicular joint because of clavicular rotation around its long axis. This allows the clavicle's curvature to act as a crankshaft[4] (Fig. 1-7).

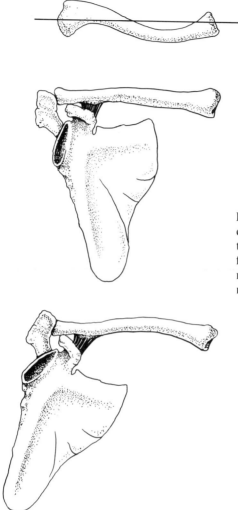

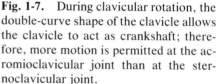

Fig. 1-7. During clavicular rotation, the double-curve shape of the clavicle allows the clavicle to act as crankshaft; therefore, more motion is permitted at the acromioclavicular joint than at the sternoclavicular joint.

Muscle Activity

Muscles are active to move the shoulder into abduction. Saha describes the rotator cuff muscles, active throughout the range of abduction, as steerers, because they are responsible for positioning the humeral head in the glenoid.[14,27] During abduction, the force vectors of the infraspinatus, teres minor, and subscapularis pass very close to the instant center of rotation. Therefore, these muscles cannot contribute significantly to abduction of the upper limb.[31]

The role of the supraspinatus and deltoid in shoulder abduction is controversial. Earlier literature indicated that the supraspinatus initiated abduction and the deltoid carried out the motion. Electromyogram (EMG) studies demonstrate that both muscles are active throughout the range of motion (ROM).[24]

However, there is an earlier rise in tension in the supraspinatus. This muscle activity helps to fixate the humeral head so that the deltoid works at an improved mechanical advantage.[2,4,15] With paralysis of either the supraspinatus or deltoid, the arm can be elevated but with a loss of power. Impairment of the supraspinatus results in a more significant loss of power.[32]

The axioscapula muscles fixate the scapula, allowing the scapulohumeral muscles to raise the arm.[4] The upper trapezius, levator scapula, serratus anterior, and rhomboids are aligned for power and are active throughout abduction. The serratus anterior is functionally the most significant of these muscles. Paralysis of this muscle limits elevation of the arm to 90°.[33]

Flexion

The movement of flexion has been less thoroughly investigated. Flexion is movement in the sagittal plane. Full flexion to 162 to 180° is possible only with synchronous motion in the glenohumeral, acromioclavicular, sternoclavicular, and scapulothoracic joints.[34] The movement is similiar to that of abduction.

Arthrokinematics

Saha has shown that during flexion the contact area on the head of the humerus moves upward and forward, though its change in the glenoid articular surface is negligible.[9] This indicates that primarily rotation has occurred. The scapula and clavicle move during flexion. Scapula movement occurs earlier in flexion than in abduction, to enhance muscle power.[4,9]

For full flexion in the sagittal plane, concomitant internal rotation is necessary.[34,35] Blakely and Palmer analyzed internal rotation with flexion and found that 94.9 ± 13.5° internal rotation accompanied full flexion. When the glenohumeral joint was held in full external rotation, flexion was limited to 30.2° ± 6.5°.[34]

Muscle Activity

Similiar muscle activity is present in the rotator cuff muscles during flexion and abduction.[4] However, the subscapularis is active earlier in the range from 30 to 120°. The anterior fibers of the deltoid and the clavicular portion of the pectoralis major are the most significant shoulder flexors.[15] These same muscles are also internal rotators; therefore, the motions of flexion and internal rotation are coupled together.[34]

Rotation

As described previously, rotation occurs concomitantly with both flexion in the sagittal plane and abduction in the coronal plane. Internal and external rotation can also occur in isolation. The amount of rotation depends on the position of the arm.[9,36] When subjects held their arms at their sides with their elbows flexed to 90°, Clarke et al measured 67° of external rotation. With a subject's arm was abducted to 90°, the amount of total internal and external rotation increased to 159°.[36] Although he did not measure the amount of rotation, Saha found that less motion was available when the subject's arm was raised overhead.[9]

Arthrokinematics

Saha describes posterior gliding of the humeral head with internal rotation and anterior gliding associated with external rotation.[9] Kummel demonstrated that the anterior capsule must be extensible for external rotation to occur.[18] Scapula movement is also important for full mobility into rotation. Scapula adduction is associated with external rotation, and scapula abduction is associated with internal rotation.[5]

Muscle Activity

Generally, more muscle force can be generated in internal rotation than in external rotation.[9] Scheving and Pauly describe the latissimus dorsi as the most important internal rotator.[37] Harms-Ringdahl et al investigated EMG activity of the internal rotators during resistive activity and found that the sternoclavicular portion of the pectoralis major was the most activated muscle.[38] The infraspinatus and teres minor muscles are the chief external rotators.[19]

Glenohumeral Stability

No single structure is responsible for glenohumeral stability as the shoulder is moved through its full ROM. Osseous, periarticular structures, and muscles are stabilizing structures.[9,13,15,16]

Osteology

The position and size of the glenoid fossa and humeral head will help determine stability of the glenohumeral joint. Saha found that if the ratio of the diameter of the glenoid to the diameter of the humeral head was <0.75 in the vertical direction and <0.57 in the transverse direction, the joint was inherently less stable.[14] He also found that a posterior tilting fossa and humeral head enhanced the stability of the joint.[14]

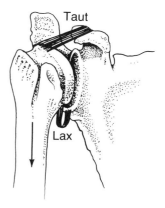

Fig. 1-8. With the arm resting at the side, gravity exerts a downward force on the humerus. This force is counteracted by tightening of the superior aspect of the glenohumeral joint capsule.

Periarticular Structures

Various periarticular structures support the glenohumeral joint as the shoulder moves through different ranges of motion. Dempster has shown that with various movements the capsule and ligaments become taut, binding the joint together and limiting further movement.[7] The structures opposite the side of movement become most tight (Fig. 1-8). For example, the superior aspect of the capsule prevents inferior movement of the humeral head when the arm is resting at the side.[13] Structures in the anterior aspect of the glenohumeral joint provide stability when the arm is moved into abduction and external rotation.[2] The supporting structures shift from superior to inferior as the angle of abduction increases. At 45° of abduction, the middle glenohumeral ligament and the anterior superior fibers of the inferior glenohumeral ligament stabilize against anterior dislocations of the humeral head. At 90° of motion, the inferior glenohumeral ligament or axillary pouch prevents dislocation, and this structure is an especially important stabilizer at end ranges of abduction.[16] The labrum may also provide a limited anterior buttressing effect.[39]

Muscles

The supraspinatus, deltoid, and subscapularis muscles are active stabilizers of the glenohumeral joint. When the arm rests at the side, the supraspinatus acts with the superior aspect of the joint capsule to support the joint.[13] If a load is carried in the hand, there is increased EMG activity in the supraspinatus and in the posterior fibers of the deltoid.[13] During abduction, the subscapularis tendon reinforces the anterior ligamentous stability.[16] This muscle and tendon is strongest up to the third decade of life and is a primary stabilizer in the young.[40] The subscapularis is most active up to 130° of abduction; therefore, this muscle provides the most support during the early and middle ranges of abduction.[3,4]

SUMMARY

Patients with shoulder dysfunctions are routinely treated in the physical therapy clinic. An understanding of the anatomy and biomechanics of this joint can help provide the physical therapist with a rationale for evaluation and treatment. Treatment may be directed toward restoring mobility, providing stability, or a combination of the two. The shoulder is an inherently mobile complex, with various joint surfaces adding to the freedom of movement. The shallow glenoid with its flexible labrum and large humeral head provides mobility. At times, this vast mobility occurs at the expense of stability. The shoulder relies on various stabilizing mechanisms, including shapes of joint surfaces, ligaments, and muscles to prevent excessive motion. Nearly 20 muscles act on this joint complex in some manner, and at various times can be both prime movers and stabilizers. Harmonious actions of these muscles are necessary for the full function of this joint.

REFERENCES

1. Kent BE: Functional anatomy of the shoulder complex. A review. Phys Ther 51:867, 1971
2. Lucas D: Biomechanics of the shoulder joint. Arch Surg 107:425, 1973
3. Sarrafian SK: Gross and functional anatomy of the shoulder. Clin Orthop Rel Res 173:11, 1983
4. Inman VT, Saunders M, Abbott LC: Observations on the function of the shoulder joint. J Bone Joint Surg 26A:1, 1944
5. Kapanji IA: The Physiology of the Joints—Upper Limb. Vol. 1. Churchill Livingstone, New York, 1970
6. Cailliet R: Shoulder Pain. FA Davis, Philadelphia, 1966
7. Dempster WT: Mechanism of shoulder movement. Arch Phys Med Rehabil 46A:49, 1965
8. Doody SG, Freedman L, Waterland JC: Shoulder movements during abduction in the scapular plane. Arch Phys Med Rehabil 51:595, 1970
9. Saha AK: Theory of Shoulder Mechanism: descriptive and applied. Charles C Thomas, Springfield, Ill, 1961
10. Moseley HP, Övergaard B: The anterior capsular mechanism in recurrent anterior dislocations of the shoulder: morphological and clinical studies with special reference to the glenoid labrum and glenohumeral ligaments. J Bone Joint Surg 44B:913, 1962
11. Reeves B: Experiments in the tensile strength of the anterior capsular structures of the shoulder in man. J Bone Joint Surg 50B:858, 1968
12. Freedman L, Munro RR: Abduction of the arm in the scapular plane: scapular and glenohumeral movements. A roentgenographic study. J Bone Joint Surg 48A:1503, 1966
13. Basmajian JV, Bazant FJ: Factors preventing downward dislocation of the adducted shoulder joint: an electromyographic and morphological study. J Bone Joint Surg 41A:1182, 1959

14. Saha AK: Dynamic stability of the glenohumeral joint. Acta Orthop Scand 42:491, 1971

15. Basmajian J: The surgical anatomy and function of the arm–trunk mechanism. Surg Clin North Am 43:1475, 1963

16. Turkel SJ, Panio MW, Marshall JL, Girgis FG: Stabilizing mechanisms preventing anterior dislocation of the glenohumeral joint. J Bone Joint Surg 63A:1208, 1981

17. Himeno S, Tsumura H: The role of the rotator cuff as a stabilizing mechanism of the shoulder. p. 17. In Bateman S, Welsh P (eds): Surgery of the Shoulder. CV Mosby Co, Saint Louis, 1984

18. Kummel BM: Spectrum of lesions of the anterior capsular mechanism of the shoulder. Am J Sports Med 7:111, 1979

19. Warwick R, Williams P (eds): Gray's Anatomy, 35th British Ed. WB Saunders Co, Philadelphia, 1973

20. Hagberg M: Electromyographic signs of shoulder muscular fatigue in two elevated arm positions. Am J Phys Med 60:111, 1981

21. Moseley HF: The clavicle: its anatomy and function. Clin Orthop Rel Res 58:17, 1968

22. Johnston TB: Movements of the shoulder joint—Plea for use of "plane of the scapula" as plane of reference for movements occurring at humero-scapula joint. Br J Surg 25:252, 1937

23. Poppen NK, Walker PS: Forces at the glenohumeral joint in abduction. Clin Orthop Rel Res 135:165, 1978

24. Poppen NK, Walker PS: Normal and abnormal motion of the shoulder. J Bone Joint Surg 58A:195, 1976

25. Saha AK: Mechanism of shoulder movements and a plea for the recognition of "zero position" of glenohumeral joint. Clin Orthop Rel Res 173:3, 1983

26. Codman EA: The Shoulder. Thomas Dodd Co, Boston, 1934

27. Saha AK: Mechanics of elevation of glenohumeral joint. Acta Orthop Scand 44:668, 1973

28. Sohier R: Kinesitherapy of the Shoulder. John Wright and Sons, Bristol, 1967

29. Werner DS: Superior migration of the humeral head: a radiological aid in the diagnosis of tears of the rotator cuff. J Bone Joint Surg 52B:524, 1970

30. Cliftman H: Biomechanics of muscle with particular application to studies of gait. J Bone Joint Surg 48A:368, 1966

31. De Duca CS, Forrest WJ: Force analysis of individual muscles acting simultaneously on the shoulder joint during isometric abduction. J Biomechanics 6:385, 1973

32. Bechtol C: Biomechanics of the shoulder. Clin Orthop Rel Res 146:37, 1980

33. Brunstrom S: Muscle testing around the shoulder girdle. J Bone Joint Surg 23A:263, 1941

34. Blakely RL, Palmer ML: Analysis of rotation accompanying shoulder flexion. Phys Ther 64(8):1214, 1984

35. Steindler A: Kinesiology of the Human Body. Charles C Thomas, Springfield, Ill, 1966

36. Clarke GR, Willis LA, Fish WW, Nichols PJR: Assessment of movement at the glenohumeral joint. Orthopaedics 7:55, 1974

37. Scheving L, Pauly J: An electromyographic study of some muscles acting on the upper extremity of man. Anat Rec 135:239, 1959

38. Harms-Ringdahl K, Ekholm J, Arborelius UP, et al: Load moment, muscle strength

and level of muscular activity during internal rotation training of the shoulder. Scand J Rehabil Med, Suppl., 9:125, 1983

39. Townley C: The capsular mechanism in recurrent dislocations of the shoulder. J Bone Joint Surg 32A:370, 1950
40. Reeves B: Experiments in the tensile strength of the anterior capsular structures of the shoulder in man. J Bone Joint Surg 50B:858, 1968

2 | Evaluation of the Shoulder: A Sequential Approach

Christine A. Moran
Sandra Richards Saunders

The shoulder patient can be regarded either as a challenge or as drudgery. The evaluation of such a patient is often clouded by the multiple joints and muscles involved. Frequently, the therapist becomes frustrated. The final degree of motion achieved by the patient is usually less than satisfactory.

The sequential approach to shoulder girdle evaluation described in this chapter is designed to clarify the picture. Each step of the evaluation as outlined in Figure 2-1 aids the therapist in obtaining specific information. Based on a diagnosis of the patient, the therapist may choose to bypass one or more steps. But, at the completion of this sequential evaluation, the therapist will have much more information than is provided by the traditional evaluation and will be able to establish a more specific treatment program. Each limiting factor is identified and can then be treated.

HISTORY TAKING

The initial step in evaluation is history taking. (Fig. 2-1) Questions regarding injury, surgery, pain, etc, are asked, but in more specific detail. By taking time for a detailed history, the therapist determines the direction of the remaining evaluation. The initial diagnosis should not limit the fact-finding nature of the history. If the patient describes pain and limited motion prior to the recent surgical procedure, the therapist will be alerted to examine more carefully for pain, soft tissue limitation through range of motion (ROM) and

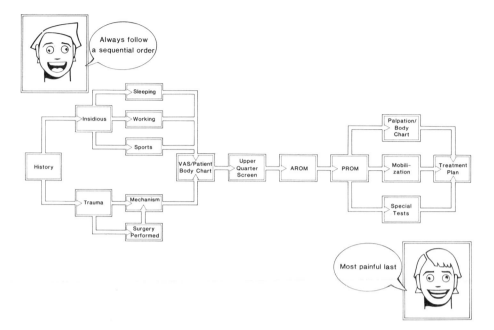

Fig. 2-1.   Sequential shoulder girdle evaluation.

joint mobilization examination, and abnormal posturing. The subsequent evaluation sequence is then determined from the history information.

Insidious Onset

Initially, examination of the patient with shoulder pathology of unknown etiology requires a knowledge of microtrauma vs. macrotrauma. Insidious pain can develop from sleep, work, and sport postures or from an acute episode. As discussed by Jobe and Moynes, macrotrauma can be easily identified as some sort of frank trauma such as a rotator cuff rupture or humeral neck fracture.[1] Microtrauma, on the other hand, is the persistent irritation of periarticular tissues which provokes local inflammatory response. Continued irritation causes scarring, tendinitis, muscular trigger points, and progressive shoulder limitation. This form of trauma develops over periods of weeks and months, and the patient often describes the pain and limitation as "coming on gradually."[2-4] Travell and Simons define idiopathic frozen shoulder as the activation of trigger points in the subscapularis muscle with subsequent sensitization of surrounding shoulder girdle muscles and progressive motion restrictions.[2] Evaluation of insidious shoulder pain also requires knowledge of referred pain and trigger points. Studies by Kellgren and Inman and Saunders identified specific reproducible patterns of pain activated when selective connective tissue and

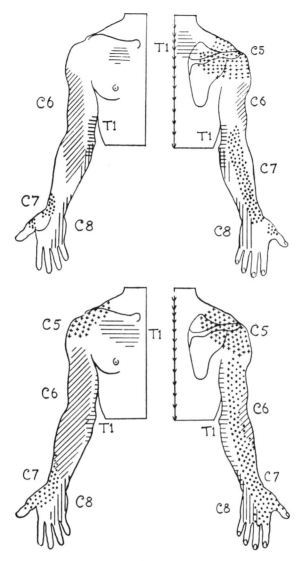

Fig. 2-2. Mappings of referred pain from local irritation of rhomboids (crosses); flexer carpiradialis (oblique hatching); abductor pollicis longus (stippling) third dorsal interosseus (vertical hatching); first intercostal space (horizontal hatching). (Reprinted by permission from Kellgren JH, Observations on referred pain arising from muscles. Clin Sci 3:175 © 1938 The Biochemical Society, London.)

muscle structures were irritated.[5,6] (Figs. 2-2 and 2-3) They have also mapped specific patterns of referred pain at a site distal to the irritated muscle, tendon, or ligament. When compared with Forester's dermotomal and myotomal charts, the areas of referred pain sometimes correspond, although not specifically.[7]

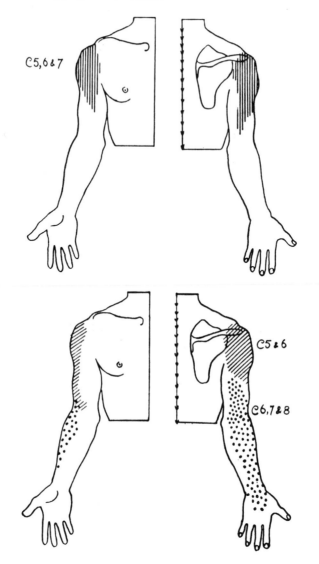

Fig. 2-3. Mappings of referred pain from local irritation of serratus anterior (vertical hatching); latissimus dorsi (stippling). (Reprinted by permission from Kellgren JH, Observations on referred pain arising from muscle. Clin Sci 3:175 © 1938 The Biochemical Society, London.)

(Figs. 2-4 and 2-5) Many authors have observed that the key factors in identification are (1) constant locus of referred pain and (2) the ability to reproduce the pain consistently.[2,5,6,8]

Several mappings are characteristic of shoulder pain.[2] The first is the referral pattern for the anterior glenohumeral (GH) capsule, which is identified

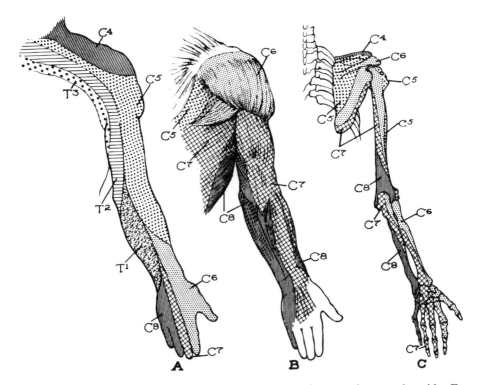

Fig. 2-4. Dermatome, myotome, and scleratome posterior mappings produced by Forester. (Inman VT, Saunders JBdeCM: Referred pain from skeletal structures. J Nerv Ment Dis 99:660, © 1944, The Williams & Wilkins Co., Baltimore.)

at the deltoid insertion. Next is the referral pain area for the subscapularis muscle (Fig. 2-6), followed by the mapping of infraspinatus muscle (Fig. 2-7), and teres minor muscle (Fig. 2-8). Very often, these muscles not only have become sensitized and have developed trigger points, but also have shortened adaptively due to lack of motion. Using only the limited available motion, the patient provokes further irritation to the shortened muscles. Again, the key factors in identification are consistent reproduction of the patient's pain and a characteristic pattern of presentation. The reproduction technique is described in more detail later in the chapter.

In summary, history taking from the patient with insidious onset of shoulder pain or frozen shoulder requires a careful review of pain/limitation onset. Although initially the patient may not recall the cause, a careful discussion of customary day and night postures usually reveals it. Careful notation of the patient's referred pain will indicate the focus of pain. Thus, the patient with a diagnosis of deltoid tendinitis can be identified instead as having anterior capsule pain/restriction.

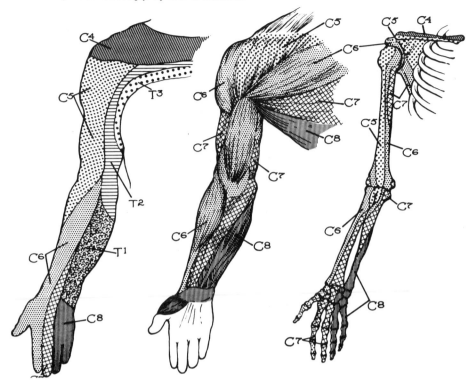

Fig. 2-5.   Dermatome, myotome, and scleratome anterior mappings produced by Forester. (Inman VT, Saunders JBdeCM: Referred pain from skeletal structures. J Nerv Ment Dis 99:660, © 1944, The Williams & Wilkins Co., Baltimore.)

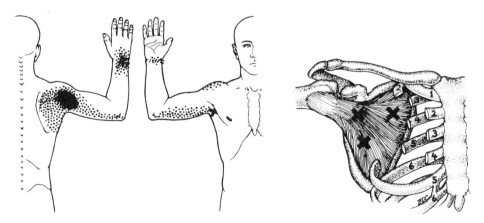

Fig. 2-6.   Location of trigger points and areas of referred pain for the subscapularis muscle. (Reprinted from Travell J, Simon DG: Myofascial Genesis of Referred Pain: The Trigger Point Manual, © 1984, The Williams & Wilkins Co., Baltimore.)

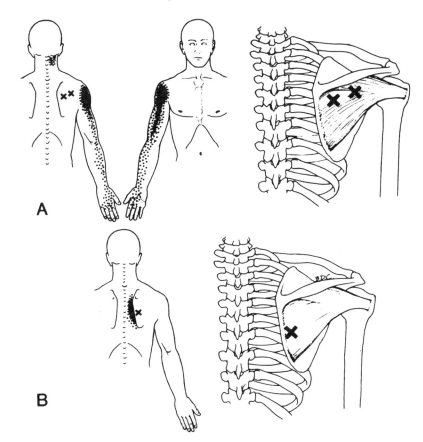

Fig. 2-7. Location of trigger points and areas of referred pain for the infraspinatus muscle.

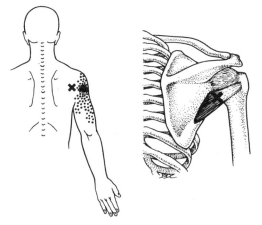

Fig. 2-8. Location of trigger points and corresponding referred pain area of the teres minor muscle. (Reprinted from Travell J, Simon DG: Myofascial Genesis of Referred Pain: The Trigger Point Manual, © 1984, The Williams & Wilkins Co., Baltimore.)

Shoulder Pain and Sleeping Postures

Characteristically, the patient with shoulder pain caused by abnormal sleeping postures describes morning pain or being awakened during the night by pain. Much information can be gathered by having the patient demonstrate his or her usual sleeping positions.[1] If the patient sleeps on one side with the shoulder joint protracted, the pain may be caused by an overstretched infraspinatus muscle and adaptive shortening of the subscapularus muscle, the pectoralis major muscle, and the anterior shoulder capsule. A patient who sleeps with an arm under the head may have impingement syndrome, because this sleeping posture forces the humeral head against the acromion, impinging upon the supraspinatus tendon and subdeltoid bursa. A patient should be asked how many pillows he or she uses when sleeping. Although this question seems more appropriate in the case of a patient with neck pain, overstretching of the levator scapulae muscle through improper head and neck alignment can provoke shoulder problems. A sensitized levator scapulae muscle protectively shortens, causing a downward tilt of the glenoid fossa. Because the glenoid fossa is normally positioned in an upward tilt and is 30° retroverted, such rotational shifting of the scapula prevents pain-free elevation. When a patient with a painful shoulder sleeps supine, the GH joint is unsupported. During the patient's sleep, the shoulder slowly falls toward the bed, stressing painful anterior structures. This is especially true of postsurgical patients who complain of pain during the night. The following case study describes a patient with insidious shoulder pain, who described her pain as one of gradual onset which began as an inability to sleep comfortably through the night. Finally, the patient was referred with a diagnosis of thoracic outlet syndrome; later, the diagnosis was changed to frozen shoulder.

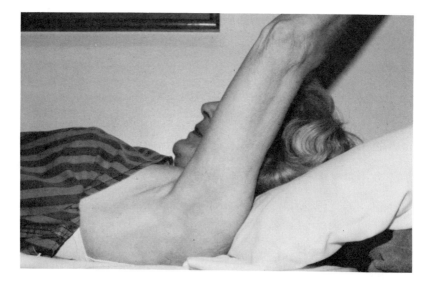

Fig. 2-9.   Patient (L.S.) demonstrates initial active shoulder flexion (supine).

CASE STUDY 1

A 52-year-old, right-dominant woman noticed a gradual onset of left shoulder pain during the summer of 1984. She could not associate any

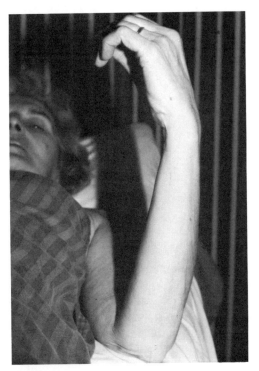

Fig. 2-10. Patient (L.S.) demonstrates initial external rotation.

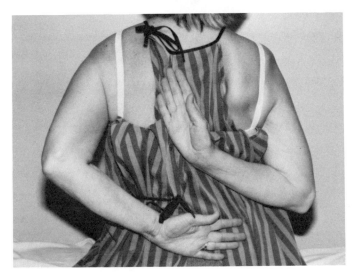

Fig. 2-11. Patient (L.S.) demonstrates initial active internal rotation; note lack of scapular mobility.

particular event or posture with her shoulder complaint. In November 1984, the pain was severe enough to cause her to seek medical attention, and she was referred for physical therapy with a diagnosis of thoracic outlet syndrome. Initial findings indicated that she was unable to sleep supine or on her left shoulder, had pain during the day with constant use, and was unable to dress or comb her hair. Active range of motion (AROM) was limited except in forward flexion, (Figs. 2-9 through 2-11) and passive range of motion (PROM) was limited and painful in all shoulder motions.

Pain diagram: Figure 2-12
Upper quarter screen: Limited cervical rotation but nonpainful.

AROM:		Supine	Sitting
Flexion		135°	115°
Extension		90°	50°
Abduction		90°	80°
Internal rotation		45°	45°
External rotation at	0° abduction	25°	—
	45° abduction	—	—
	90° abduction	—	—

PROM:	Not Tested
Mobilization:	Anterior glide—limited and extremely painful; posterior glide—mildly painful; distraction—painful.
Special tests:	Supraclavicular Tinel's sign—negative; costoclavicular manuever—negative.
Palpation:	Trigger point in infraspinatus.
Initial thoughts:	As revealed by the initial evaluation, the patient's chief complaint is that of a painful shoulder, not tho-

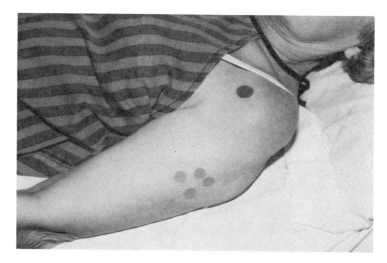

Fig. 2-12. Patient (L.S.) reproduces referred pain (small dots) from the anterior capsule (large dot).

racic outlet symptoms. The cervical restriction was long-standing and did not affect her activities. The most painful area elicited in the examination was the anterior capsule, identified in the active/passive motion testing of external rotation and anterior glide mobilization testing. This information was confirmed in the history by her description of functional level and sleeping postures. Treatment was directed toward relieving the anterior capsule pain and the secondary trigger point in the infraspinatus muscle. All stretching and mobilization was then directed toward the capsule. The patient was discharged with pain-free full shoulder mobility.

SHOULDER PAIN IN WORKERS

An article from Sweden has brought to light the need for careful examination of the painful shoulder brought on by work-related motion. Herberts et al noted a 30 to 40 percent incidence of industrial shoulder pain, and the percentage is increasing.[9] In Sweden, the problem characteristically arises in light-assembly factories, a pattern similar to that found in light industry in the United States. In their study, they observed that arm elevation and hand load had the greatest affect on muscle involvement and strain. Specifically, they observed that the infraspinatus muscle showed the greatest dependence on hand load and was strained in an arm position of forward flexion; the supraspinatus muscle was more often involved when the arm was abducted. They also identified an earlier onset of supraspinatus tendinitis in workers who performed static work and later onset in workers who performed dynamic work.

A study by Delacerda outlined the development of myofascial shoulder girdle syndrome in assembly line workers,[10] who developed trigger points in the muscles stabilizing the scapula. Shoulder girdle posture of worker patients requires complete evaluation because the mechanics of the complex can become altered by constant muscular and tendon irritation from sustained work postures.

SHOULDER PROBLEMS IN ATHLETES

The onset of shoulder pain in athletes is well documented.[11–17] Repetitive overuse of the shoulder in swimmers and baseball players evidences the cumulative effect of microtrauma, but is often overlooked in the athlete who plays only occasionally. Intensive weekend play or improper shoulder postures can contribute to muscular, tendinous, and capsular complaints. Characteristically, such patients display the same referred pain patterns shown by the insidious shoulder pain patient. Examination of the athlete must include a careful evaluation of the sport movement. How is the shoulder held? What is the relationship of the arm and hand during the movement? This topic is discussed further in Chapters 9 and 10.

Traumatic Onset of Shoulder Pain

Traumatic onset of shoulder pain and instability can range from a simple contusion to a fracture or dislocation. Although the latter is a surgical challenge for the physician, the physical therapist must manage the persistent soft tissue pain which may result from the contusion. Four concepts must be considered: (1) secondary soft tissue damage, (2) preinjury lifestyle, (3) a series of microtrauma or macrotrauma events, and (4) altered biomechanics leading to secondary and primary tigger points. Even if the mechanism and pathology seem very straightforward, these concepts should be addressed, as should specific questions that indicate specific pathology. Here, for clarification, we review a case study.

CASE STUDY 2

S.P., a 34-year-old man, sustained a clavicular fracture and acromioclavicular AC separation on January 9, 1984. Treatment consisted of immobilization with velcro straps for 6 to 7 weeks. The patient reported much discoloration and edema in the area of the teres major, subscapularis, and infraspinatus muscles. He was allowed to exercise independently for 1 week and was then referred to a physical therapist. At that time, active flexion was ~60°. The treatment consisted of heat, joint mobilization, and exercise. No soft tissue mobilization was reported. The patient obtained

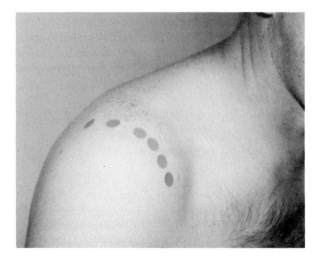

Fig. 2-13. Pain produced with active elevation (patient S.P.).

functional ROM in 1 month, but continued to experience pain. He received cortisone injections two or three times, but obtained no permanent pain relief. In February 1985, he was given a 10 percent disability settlement and was discharged from the attending physician's care. The patient refused settlement and sought care from another physician, who performed arthroscopic surgery after noting a necrotic spot on the humeral head and scar tissue that was limiting the patient's motion. Surgical release of the scar tissue adhesions afforded the patient increased ROM, especially into horizontal adduction. The patient was sent to our clinic for the goals of increasing ROM, decreasing pain and increasing strength. His functional complaint, apart from pain, was an inability to throw a ball. Initial evaluation revealed:

Visual Analogue Scale: 7
Pain diagram: Figures 2-13 through 2-15
Upper quarter screen: Normal.

AROM:		Supine	Sitting
Flexion		150°	140°
Internal rotation at	90° abduction	60°	—
External rotation at	0° abduction	85°	—
	45° abduction	85°	—
	90° abduction	85°	—
Abduction		160°	132°

Mobilization: Inferior glide—painful and limited; scapular distraction—limited; posterior glide—painful.

Special tests: Negative.

Palpation: Local tenderness—pectoralis major muscle, teres minor muscle, long head triceps tendon insertion, subscapularis muscle.

Initial thoughts: This was a patient whose history revealed soft tissue injury (discoloration and edema in the area of the teres major, subscapularis, and infraspinatus muscles) as well as a clavicular fracture and AC separation. Initially, the fracture was treated. The resulting frozen shoulder was then treated, but the original soft tissue damage was never addressed; thus, the patient had continuing pain from his teres minor, long tendon of the triceps, and subscapularis muscles. We believe that if the secondary soft tissue damage had been addressed initially, the rehabilitation period would have been shortened. His inability to throw a ball was the result of an abnormal scapulohumeral rhythm demonstrated in active and passive flexion (scapula protrusion); that is, the scapula was excessively protracted and upwardly rotated during flexion, a movement that places the ro-

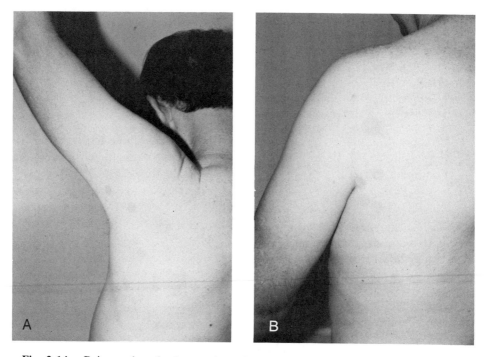

Fig. 2-14.   Pain produced when patient (S.P.) abducts (A) and extends elbow (B).

tator cuff muscles at a mechanical disadvantage. Continued attempts to throw would lead only to compensation by other muscles, development of secondary trigger points, and further pain. Prior to injury, the patient had led an active life. Further questioning revealed no previous recurrent shoulder pain during or after activities, which allowed the evaluator to assume that the patient had no preexisting microtrauma and treatment can be vigorous.

Treatment plan: The patient's treatment consisted of soft tissue mobilization treatment of trigger point with transcutaneous electrical nerve stimulation (TENS), phonophoresis, scapular isometrics, and resistive exercise/stretching with scapular stabilization.

The history should elucidate the four concepts mentioned above: (1) secondary soft tissue damage, (2) preexisting lifestyle, (3) previous microtrauma, and (4) altered biomechanisms leading to secondary and primary trigger points. With this accomplished, the following traumatic injuries commonly seen can be evaluated in a new light.

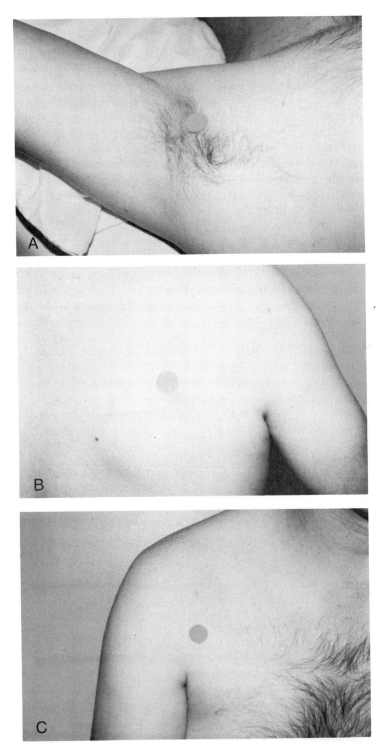

Fig. 2-15. Latent trigger points of patient (S.P.) in the subscapularis muscle (A), infraspinatus muscle (B), and pectoralis major muscle (C).

ACROMIOPLASTIES AND ROTATOR CUFF REPAIR

Acromioplasties and rotator cuff repairs are two commonly encountered surgical procedures. The various methods of surgery are not within the scope of this chapter to review. Numerous articles have been written on surgical techniques, and techniques will continue to change due to the frequency of unsatisfactory results, especially in the throwing athlete.[18,19] The references offer the reader more complete information. The procedure used should be reviewed prior to treatment to allow safe, early mobilization and avoid undue stress on operated tissues. Chapter 10 discusses an innovative rehabilitation program following rotator cuff repair in the athlete.

Several authors have tried to classify rotator cuff injuries.[18,20] Neer described impingement of the supraspinatus tendon and, to a lesser extent, the infraspinatus and long head of the biceps tendon on the anterior edge of the coracoacromial ligament and the anterior one-third of the acromium.[20] He described three stages: (1) edema and hemorrhage, (2) thickening and fibrosis, and (3) tearing of the rotator cuff and bicep tendon. The first stages have been recognized in athletes but also occur in those who are not athletes and in workers. The patient initially reports anterior shoulder pain after use, then during use; by stage 3, the patient reports almost constant pain.[11] In stages 1 and 2 conservative measures geared toward protecting the involved structures and decreasing inflammation are effective. By stage 3, surgery is recommended.[15]

In the history, information should be obtained to enable the therapist to determine if the pain is primarily after use (stage 1), during use (stage 2), or almost constant (stage 3). Even if a single incident is reported as having caused the patient to seek medical care, a history of recurrent pain should alert the therapist to microtrauma and resultant weakened tissue. An exercise program must be developed to protect the injured tissue. Special tests and palpation will direct the therapist to the injured tissue. Sports medicine literature will aid the therapist in selecting proper activity to stress different structures. It is also important that the therapist learn what kind of life the patient leads. A sedentary patient will not have the same tensile strength in the injured structure and surrounding tissue that an active or athletic person has.

The history should clarify the patient's condition and determine the treatment. Finally, the evaluator should consider the possibility that the patient is compensating for local trauma. Such compensation can lead to altered biomechanics, which in turn can lead to trigger point activation, which refers pain that mimics the primary pathology. The upper extremity activity may produce muscle microtrauma in the infraspinatus which then develops into a trigger point. The infraspinatus muscle can refer pain to the anterior shoulder; this may be confused with a local pathology. Palpation performed during evaluation of the patient will help distinguish between a local or a referred problem.

Trigger points can also occur secondarily from the altered biomechanics of the postsurgical recovery period. Comparison of preinjury and postsurgery pain diagrams can shed light on this subject. The pain may be the same or different. More often, it is not exactly the same, implying a different source of pain than the site of surgery. The following case study is an example of a postsurgical patient with trigger points. Were the trigger points preexisting or secondary to immobilization?

CASE STUDY 3

A. B. was an avid golfer who complained of persistent left shoulder pain of 2 years duration that occurred between 60° and 120° of shoulder elevation and at night. She underwent an arthrogram which revealed no significant rotator cuff tear. On November 20, 1984, she underwent an acromioplasty that included a release of the coracoacromial ligament. She was seen in our clinic on December 11, 1984, with complaints of decreased shoulder motion (Fig. 2-16) and severe shoulder pain.

Visual Analogue Scale: 3
Pain diagram: Pain over incision, deltoid insertion, and anterior shoulder.
Upper quarter screen: Normal.

AROM:	Supine	Sitting
Flexion	20°	45°
Extension	68°	60°
Internal rotation	30°	50°
External rotation	45°	30°
Abduction	Not Tested	45°
Elevation	Not Tested	35°

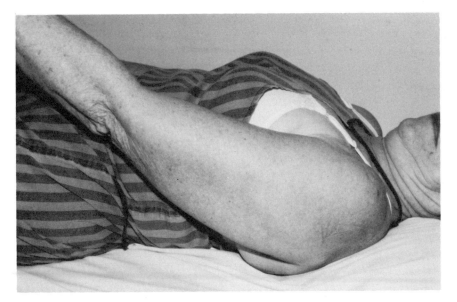

Fig. 2-16. Patient's (A. B.) initial supine flexion.

PROM:

Flexion		50°
Extension		60°
Internal rotation	30° abduction	55°
External rotation	0° abduction	45°
	45° abduction	35°
	90° abduction	Not Tested

Mobilization: Limited inferior glide, external rotation, distraction, anterior glide, scapular distraction.

Special tests: Not applicable.

Palpation: Trigger points in the infraspinatus, subscapularis, and teres minor muscles. (Fig. 2-17A and B).

Initial thoughts: Initially, we thought that the patient had a dual problem: the acromioplasty and trigger points that limited motion and caused her pain. Her inability to sleep at night preoperatively was thought to be caused by the trigger points, probably preexisting and brought on by the repetitive motion of golf. We therefore chose to treat her soft tissue pain first by use of soft tissue stretching techniques, pain-relieving modalities over the trigger points,

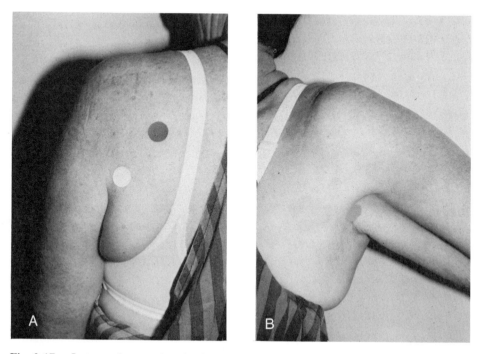

Fig. 2-17.   Latent trigger points in the teres minor muscle (A, light dots); infraspinatus muscle (A, dark dots); and subscapularis muscle (B). (Patient A. B.)

and grade I and II mobilization techniques. Her pain was under control after the first week, at which time more vigorous mobilization techniques were used. The patient led a very active life prior to her injury, and we felt that she could tolerate such vigorous treatment. The trigger points were reevaluated throughout treatment. Results: Full ROM, no pain while playing golf (18 holes) at least three times a week.

ACROMIOCLAVICULAR JOINT PATHOLOGY

Acromioclavicular joint pathology is generally local. The patient points to the local area when describing the pain, and may have edema and local tenderness. Because the clavicle rotates during elevation, reaching maximum rotation with maximum elevation, the painful arc of AC joint occurs during the final 30° of elevation, in contrast to subacromial pathology, in which the painful arc is between 60 and 120°.[21] The mechanism of injury is either direct trauma to the posterosuperior aspect of the shoulder or a fall on the outstretched arm. Separations are graded in three categories[22]:

Grade I

In grade I, pain occurs with elevation; there is marked edema and local tenderness but no instability. The coronoid and trapezoid ligament are intact, with loss of some integrity of the acrominoclavicular ligament. Edema resolves quickly, but pain remains for 7 to 10 days. The throwing athlete may take 3 to 5 weeks to return to preinjury level.

Grade II

In grade II, there is tearing of the acromioclavicular ligaments with incomplete tearing of the coronoid and trapezoid ligaments. Pain and edema is similar to that of grade I, but stress x-ray views may show separation.

Grade III

In grade III, the coronoid, trapezoid, and acromioclavicular ligaments are disrupted. The outer edge of the clavicle usually rides high, although initially edema and muscle spasm may mask this. Examination reveals marked instability. Stress (traction) x-rays show displacement; but this can be negated by acute muscle spasm.

Treatment of grade II can be operative with K-wiring, screws, and joint debridement; immobilization of 0 to 6 weeks may be required.[22] Conservative immobilization techniques have also been proposed (over-the-shoulder clavicle holder).[23] There are more than 70 different methods of treatment, both operative and nonoperative.[24] The goal of all treatment is normalization of the biomechanics of the joint to avoid later degenerative changes. The grade of injury determines the pace of rehabilitation; therefore, this information must be obtained from the physician.

As illustrated by case study 2 (S. P.), secondary soft tissue trauma must be addressed. Evaluation of trigger points, (preexisting, secondary to the trauma or secondary to altered biomechanics during the recovery period) must be performed to speed treatment and a return to a pain-free lifestyle. Soft tissue trauma can lead to persistent pain or even frozen shoulder.

FRACTURES

Fractures of the humerus and clavicle must be immobilized or surgically stabilized to allow bone healing. The position of immobilization is a large factor in predicting the type of soft tissue tightness that will be evinced by the patient. The shoulder is most often immobilized in a sling, although at times a wedge is used to position the arm in 45° abduction. Rarely, an airplane splint is used to immobilize the arm in 90° elevation. A capsular pattern will be seen when the arm is immobilized in a sling that provides restricted elevation and external rotation is greater than internal rotation limitation. If the arm is positioned into more abduction/elevation, the anterior and inferior capsule are in a more elongated position, resulting in a less severe capsular pattern.

For treatment of patients who have soft tissue restriction secondary to immobilization of a fracture, the concepts of secondary soft tissue injury, altered biomechanics that produce trigger points, and preexisting lifestyle are important. The earlier the first two concepts can be addressed, the better. Early identification of trigger points, secondary soft tissue injury, and review of sleeping postures can prevent later problems. Many of these problems can be addressed before bone healing is complete and motion is allowed.

Once the fracture has healed, evaluation can be extended to ROM and joint mobility. Close attention should be paid to palpation of muscle at this point. Even though the bone cannot withstand force, soft tissue mobilization techniques can be administered to muscles that are limited and/or contain trigger points.

The patient's past lifestyle in conjunction with the physician's communication of the x-ray findings dictate the pace of rehabilitation. If the patient has been an active person and has no previous history of microtrauma, the rehabilitation pace can be quickened. If the patient has a history of microtrauma, the rehabilitation pace is slowed and the traumatized area should be scrutinized initially and throughout the treatment.

GLENOHUMERAL DISLOCATIONS

There are two major categories of shoulder dislocation: the primary GH dislocation and the recurrent GH dislocation. Many authors believe that primary dislocation will recur and therefore will need immediate attention. Many authors also report a higher incidence of recurrence in younger patients, although the actual percentages of recurrence differ. This information is important in evaluating the younger patient for whom recurrence is high. A physician may immobilize the patient for as long as 6 weeks. Some authors support the concept that immobilization reduces recurrence,[14,25–27] but other authors state that it makes no difference.[28,29] Better results were reported when immobilization was followed by a strengthening program for 6 weeks with abduction not allowed past 90°.[14,28]

Dislocations can be further divided into directions of dislocations. By far the most common dislocation is anterior. The mechanisms by which it is caused are many hyperextensions of the abducted arm, excessive external rotation of the abducted arm, a direct posterior blow on the humeral head which forces the head anterior, and a fall on the abducted arm.[12] There may be associated injuries, such as fractures of the greater trochanter, rotator cuff injuries, and brachial plexus damage. These injuries are more commonly found in patients ≥ 45 years of age.[30]

Posterior dislocations are rare, although we have seen two in our clinic in the past year. Both persons were injured while playing football. The injury may occur as a result of an anterior blow to the humeral head which forces the humerus posteriorly; with our patients, the upper extremity was supported by the ground and other players fell on the backs of our patients.

As with surgical repair of other injuries in the shoulder area, many techniques are used for stabilization of the GH joint; many of them sacrifice external rotation for stability, leading to the popularity of the modified Bristow procedure which allows more external rotation. Such surgery is appropriate for the patient who needs external rotation of the shoulder for work or participation in sports.

It is important to know the different procedures for GH dislocations and whether they allow full rotation. All information regarding the mechanism of injury, the extent of injury, and surgical or conservation treatment already rendered should be obtained during the history so that the shoulder can be appropriately managed. Not all shoulder injuries can be treated in a similar manner owing to the various mechanisms, pathologies, and treatments in use today. Thus, one must use the information obtained not only to determine treatment but also the extent and vigor of the evaluation. During immobilization, all structures of the shoulder girdle receive minimal to no stress. Because stress is the stimulus for tissue strengthening, all structures should be considered weak. If the patient was a sedentary individual prior to injury, the shoulder girdle structures should be considered weaker, and the pace of the rehabilitation should be slowed accordingly. For further discussion on subluxations, the reader is referred to Chapter 9.

PATIENT PAIN DIAGRAM AND VISUAL ANALOGUE SCALE

Pain mapping, an accurate way to localize the patient's pain, is the next step in the evaluation sequence. Figure 2-18 is an example of the body diagram which is used in our clinic. The patient places marks on the body diagram

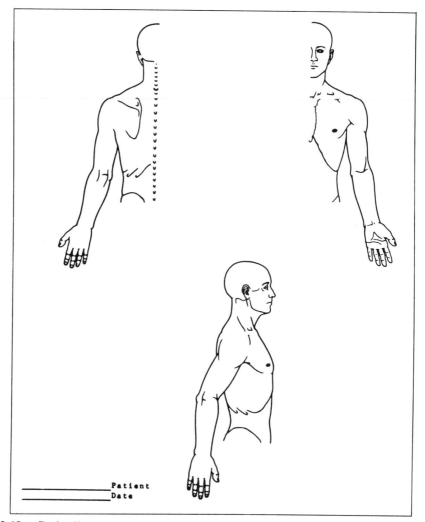

Patient _____

Date _____

Fig. 2-18. Body diagram used for patient's and therapist's identification of local and referred pain.

exactly where the pain is located. When the diagram is complete, the therapist reviews it with the patient, making sure that nothing has been overlooked and that it contains information regarding the quality of their patient's pain. Is the pain constant or intermittent? Often the patient will first claim that the pain is constant, but questioning by the therapist may reveal that it is intermittent. If pain occurs while the patient assumes stationary positions, the therapist should seek a muscular component. Constant pain is less common and occurs with serious pathology that is beyond the scope of physical therapy treatment or is caused by a complex soft tissue problem with severely altered biomechanics which do not allow structures to rest. Is the pain sharp or diffuse? A sharp pain on movement may indicate an instability or abutment of structures in which the diffuse pain is the result of either a chronic situation of multiple trigger points, cervical involvement, or thoracic outlet syndrome. Such answers allow the therapist insight into the patient's problems but are not diagnostic.

The therapist should note any skin changes (as identified is case study 2), scars, surgical procedures, and edema. The progression of pain with respect to microtrauma and macrotrauma should also be noted. It may be enlightening for the therapist if surgical patients fill out two pain diagrams—one representing the pain that existed prior to surgery, and the second representing postsurgical pain. This can help the therapist determine whether there is an irritated surgical area, whether preexisting trigger points are still producing pain, or whether new pain is being produced by immobilization or surgery.

When all information regarding location, quality, and precipitating factors has been collected, the quantitative aspect of the patient's pain must be assessed. The use of a visual analogue scale (VAS) serves this purpose. (Fig. 2-19) The VAS, as described by Price, is a 15-cm line.[31] One end is designated as "the most intense sensation imaginable"; the other end is designated "no sensation." It is important for the purpose of validity that these exact words be used because this analogue scale has been proven experimentally using ratio data.

Unpleasantness of pain can also be assessed with the VAS. The ends of the 15-cm line are then designated respectively as "the most intense bad feeling for me" and "not bad at all." This second aspect represents the degree of disturbance the pain causes the patient. In evaluating the chronic pain patient, both of these scales are helpful. We have encountered patients who say they are still hurting but are improving functionally. By using both scales—pain intensity and unpleasantness—both aspects of pain are evaluated. Other professionals have used similar VASs to rate function, anxiety, etc. These scales are acceptable for the therapist's own knowledge but have not yet been deemed valid.

The body diagram and VAS produce a clear picture of the patient's complaints and relevant history. Much information has been obtained before a hand has been placed on the patient. At this point, and with this information, the therapist determines irritability, limitations and precautions that determine which manual tests should be included. Progression of evaluation should always proceed from the most benign tests to the most provoking so that the picture

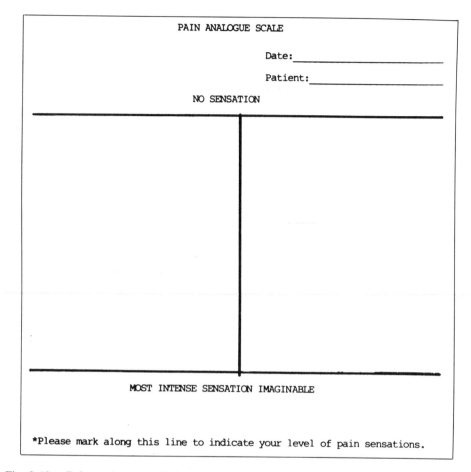

Fig. 2-19. Pain analogue scale is used to quantify the patient's complaint of pain. The patient marks on the line the level of painful sensation that is experienced. The scale is a 15-cm line. The "X" on the scale corresponds to a numerical value.

of the pain and mechanics is not clouded. Certain evaluation steps may be postponed until an appropriate time.

UPPER-QUARTER SCREEN

In keeping with the philosophy of evaluating the most benign condition first and ruling out concomitant pathology, an upper-quarter evaluation is used next. This is a systematic way of evaluating all structures that could contribute to or be the sole cause of the patient's chief complaint. It is designed to be quick yet comprehensive. The following screen was developed by Personius at the Medical College of Virginia (Fig. 2-20).

It is advisable to evaluate even postoperative patients with a modified screen, the obvious rationale being a search for secondary limitations due to

Patient _____

Date _____

Observation and Inspection
1. Body build: endo _____ , ecto _____ , meso _____ ; ht _____ ; wt _____
   Unusual features _____
2. Assistive devices _____
3. Skin _____
4. Upper Quarter Functions
   Position _____
   Use _____
5. Posture
   Lateral _____
   Posterior _____
   Anterior _____

Function Tests

1. Cx ROM   active   OP
   FB   ____ M ____ ; ____ P _____ ____ P_____
   BB   ____ M ____ ; ____ P _____ ____ P_____
   LRot   ____ M ____ ; ____ P _____ ____ P_____
   RRot   ____ M ____ ; ____ P _____ ____ P_____
   LSB   ____ M ____ ; ____ P _____ ____ P_____
   RSB   ____ M ____ ; ____ P _____ ____ P_____
   Comp   ____ M ____   ____ P_____
   Trac   ____ M ____   ____ P_____

2. Neuro
   Motor
           C1   ____
           C2,3   ____
           C3,4   ____
           C5   R ____ = L ____
           C6   ____ =   ____
           C7   ____ =   ____
           C8   ____ =   ____
           T1   ____ =   ____

   Sensory
           Dizziness: ☐ yes   ☐ no
           Tinnitus: ☐ yes   ☐ no
           Light Touch & Pinprick   R   LT   L   R   PP   L
                 C4   ____ = ____   ____ = ____
                 C5   ____ = ____   ____ = ____
                 C6   ____ = ____   ____ = ____
                 C7   ____ = ____   ____ = ____
                 C8   ____ = ____   ____ = ____
                 T1   ____ = ____   ____ = ____

   Reflex   R   L
                 C5,6   ____   =   ____
                 C7   ____   =   ____

3. Vascular
   Radial Pulse
   Thoracic Outlet

4. Peripheral Joints
   Shoulder
        UE Elevation   ____ M ____ ; ____ P _____ (OP)_____
        Locking Position   ____ M ____ ; ____ P _____
        Quadrant Position ____ M ____ ; ____ P _____
   Elbow   (OP)
        Flex RL   ____ M ____ ; ____ P _____ ____ P_____
        Ext   ____ M ____ ; ____ P _____ ____ P_____
   Forearm
        Sup   ____ M ____ ; ____ P _____ ____ P_____
        Pro   ____ M ____ ; ____ P _____ ____ P_____
   Wrist
        Flex   ____ M ____ ; ____ P _____ ____ P_____
        Ext   ____ M ____ ; ____ P _____ ____ P_____
        RD   ____ M ____ ; ____ P _____ ____ P_____
        UD   ____ M ____ ; ____ P _____ ____ P_____

Fig. 2-20. Upper quarter scanning examination. (Walter J. Personius, Ph.D., P.T., Fall 1980. Medical College of Virginia Department of Physical Therapy.)

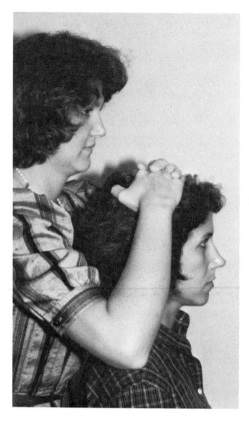

Fig. 2-21. Axial compression maneuver as part of upper-quarter screen.

immobilization. Less obvious conditions may be discovered—subtle irritations or abnormalities that either add to the present problem or that may be aggravated during the rehabiliation of the primary problem. If such conditions are not treated initially, the patient's recovery is hampered.

The first three steps are self-explanatory and require only a few seconds. Step four requires a short description of the position in which the arm is held and used. With regard to the patient's posture, the therapist should look for scapular position (protraction/retraction/elevation), and head position, all of which may signal abnormal biomechanics. Under functional tests, the cervical (CX) region is examined first by the active cervical motion of forward bend (FB), back bend (BB), left rotation (LROT), right rotation (RROT), left side bend (LSB), right side bend (RSB), axial compression (COMP) (Fig. 2-21), and axial distraction (TRAC) (Fig. 2-22). The later two are manually administered. Both the mechanics (M) (degree and quality of motion) and the pain (P) location and severity, are recorded. After each active motion, overpressure (OP) is applied while pain is located and severity is assessed. Many therapists refuse to apply OP if pain is present on active motion. The decision is made by the therapist with regard to the particular patient. The CX motion and M evaluation is made to identify or exclude pathology originating in the CX region. The

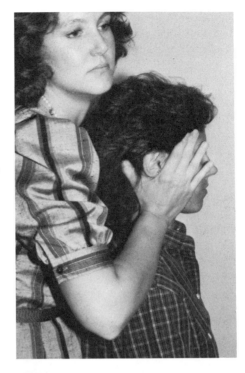

Fig. 2-22. Cervical distraction as part of upper-quarter screen.

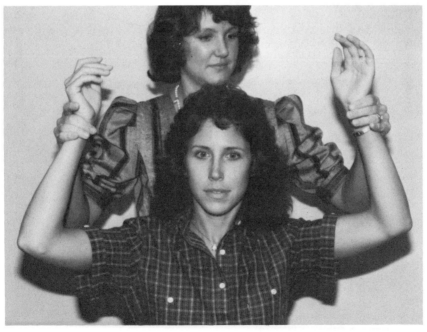

Fig. 2-23. Therapist stands behind the patient, giving bilateral resistance to elbow extension as part of upper-quarter screen.

neurological exam is a quick manual muscle test which checks for weakness. The therapist stands behind the patient (Fig. 2-23) and gives resistance bilaterally to the following movements, evaluating motor functions at that level:

C2	Axial flexion
C3–C4	Shoulder shrug
C5	Shoulder abduction at 90°
C6	Elbow flexion
C7	Elbow extension
C8	Wrist extension
T1	Finger abduction

The sensory component involves looking for and asking about dizziness and tinnitus to rule out vascular problems. The therapist tests sensation by running the fingers and a pin over all dermatome areas of the patient bilaterally, looking for difference in sensation in the patient's right side as compared to the left. The dermatomes are represented as follows:

C4	Top of the shoulder
C5	Deltoid area
C6	Lateral arm to thumb
C7	Middle finger
C8	Ulnar aspect of hand
T1	Medial upper arm

The reflexes of the biceps (C5,C6) and triceps (C7) are tested with a reflex hammer. Results are compared right to left. The radial pulse is palpated in the

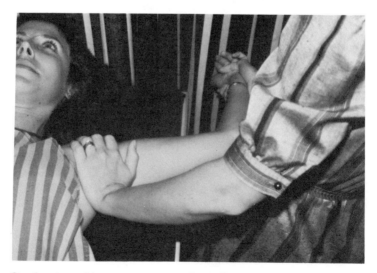

Fig. 2-24. Quadrant position manuever performed as part of upper-quarter screen; patient's arm is placed in abduction and external rotation.

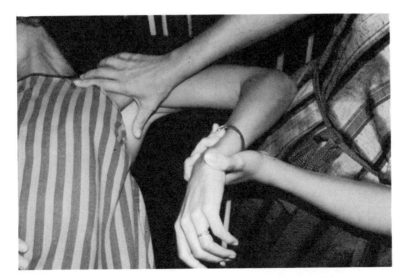

Fig. 2-25. Locking position manuever performed as part of upper-quarter screen.

resting position and in the elevated position to determine strength and regularity.

Finally, each peripheral joint is examined for M and P. Overpressure is applied where appropriate, to discover pain. The locking position and quadrant position are evaluated with the patient supine. The shoulder is abducted to 90° and is then externally rotated (quadrant position) (Fig. 2-24) and then internally rotated and placed in abduction (locking position) (Fig. 2-25).

It is obvious that, for most postsurgical patients, tests such as the quadrant position, locking position, and thoracic outlet (radial pulse in elevation) cannot be performed. They should be omitted initially and be evaluated at the appropriate time. In other patients, it may be that only at these extreme positions—where the capsule is taut and maximal stress is placed on the ligaments—that pain will be reproduced or abnormal mechanics observed.

The screening exam is just that, a scan of the total upper quadrant to rule out problems and note areas that need more specific testing. For example, a thoracic outlet test that shows diminished radial pulse in elevation is a red flag to the therapist to pursue this area in more detail and with more reliable tests. The whole procedure should take no more than 5 minutes, producing a volume of information.

ACTIVE RANGE OF MOTION

Traditionally, AROM provided the most information in the shoulder evaluation.[32–35] Measurements are taken with the patient in the sitting and supine positions as a dual assessment of functional joint motion and muscle strength. As shown noted in Figure 2-1, it is only one part of the complete shoulder

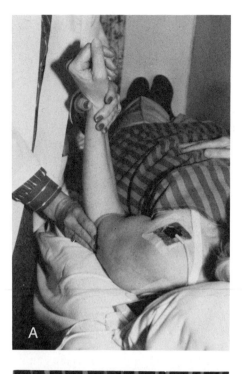
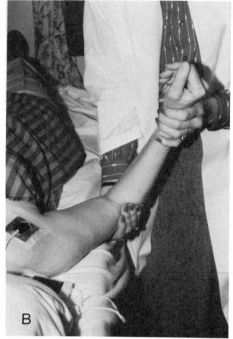
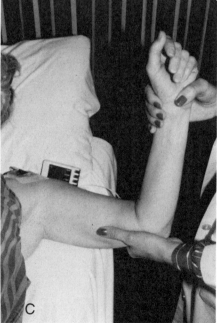

Fig. 2-26. Identification of external rotation/elevation limitation by test position: (A) 0° abduction (anterior capsule, superior/middle glenohumeral ligaments), (B) 45° abduction (middle/inferior glenohumeral ligaments, inferior capsule), and (C) 90° abduction (inferior capsule, scapular musculature).

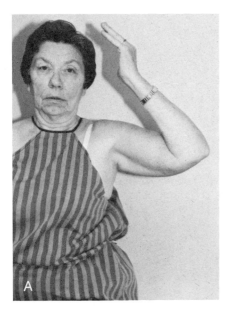

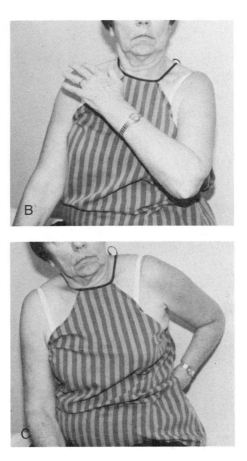

Fig. 2-27. Patient is asked to (A) reach up actively (elevation); (B) touch opposite shoulder (internal rotation, adduction); and (C) touch behind the back (internal rotation, extension).

evaluation. Two additions to this part of the evaluation are recommended. As noted by several authors, the plane of the scapula lies 30° to 45° in the horizontal plane.[36–38] Therefore, a true measure of functional shoulder elevation should occur in this position, and abduction and flexion do not represent true shoulder motion, which should be performed in the plane of the scapula. As noted in the two case studies, AROM and PROM should include the measurements of elevation. Flexion and abduction are then component movements to this functional shoulder motion—elevation. If the therapist asks the patient to raise the arm over the head, the patient does not flex or abduct the shoulder but elevates it instead (30° to 45° from the horizontal axis). Second, much information about periarticular structure limitation can be obtained by measuring external rotation from three positions of abduction in the supine position.[38,39] (Fig. 2-26A through C). As shown in Figure 2-25, selective stressing of the structures is identified and provides a more realistic measure of external rotation than does the classic position of 90° abduction. Again, notations are made on the body diagram of limitations, local vs. referred pain, and scapular winging as the patient performs the requested motion (Fig. 2-27 A through C). Scapular winging is indicative

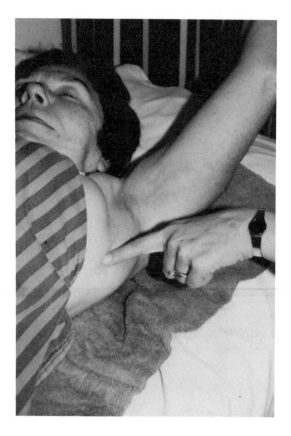

Fig. 2-28. In active elevation, the scapula "wings" or glides laterally, indicating shortening of the posterior shoulder girdle muscles.

of posterior shoulder girdle musculature restriction not rhomboid muscle or serratus anterior muscle weakness. This is illustrated with the patient supine (Fig. 2-28) and prone (Fig. 2-29).

PASSIVE RANGE OF MOTION

Passive joint motion notes the available joint motion as well as any painful restricting tissues. Painful muscles can limit active motion while passive motion remains good. Again, notations are made as to what shoulder motions produce local pain as opposed to referred pain and whether the scapula is detected protruding laterally.

MOBILIZATION EVALUATION

Mobilization techniques for the shoulder girdle can provide very specific evaluation information to enhance your findings from active motion and passive motion testing.[40-42] Active and passive motion tests provide general infor-

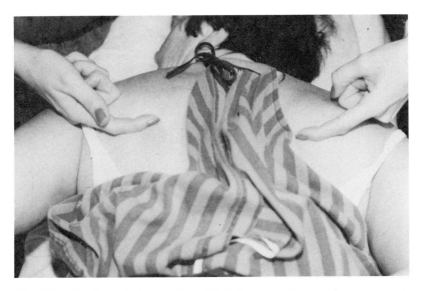

Fig. 2-29. Examination of the heights of inferior scapular angles to assess levator scapulae muscle irritation, which provokes elevation and downward rotation of the scapula.

mation on how the muscle functions in the shoulder girdle area and about the general available joint motion of the girdle. The mobilization techniques specify periarticular structures that are causing pain and limiting motion. Second, they recreate arthrokinematic motions necessary for the proper osteokinematics of the shoulder girdle. For example, shoulder elevation occurs when the humeral head glides inferiorly and concomitant rotation occurs. All treatment techniques outlined in Chapter 11 can be used as evaluation techniques. Notations are made on the body diagram as to what mobilization manuevers are limited or provoke local symptoms or referred pain. Next, necessary special tests are determined based on information already obtained in the evaluation sequence (Fig. 2-1).

SPECIAL TESTS

Various special tests described is this chapter have been developed to test specific lesions in the shoulder girdle area. The examiner must remember that these are called special tests because they test special conditions, not because they are particularly reliable. Much controversy exists as to the value of certain tests. The examiner must acknowledge each test as only a small piece of the total picture and not predictive in itself.

Impingement Syndromes

Impingement syndrome tests have been described by Neer[20] and Hawkins and Kennedy.[11] The tests are similar but each author believes his or her variation has a better predictive value. Neer and Welsh produce impingement pain by forceful elevation (flexion) of the humerus, which forces the abutment of the rotator cuff tissues into the anterior third of the acromion.[14] If pain is eliminated during this procedure by injection of 10 mL of 1 percent Xylocaine into the subacromial space, the test is positive. Hawkins and Kennedy believe that the pain is better reproduced by 90° of humeral flexion with forceful internal rotation, which drives the rotator cuff tissue under the coracoacromial ligament.[11]

If complete rupture of the supraspinatus tendon exists, the therapist should perform a positive "drop arm test." That is, if the arm is placed in 90° of abduction, the patient is unable to lower the arm slowly and smoothly.

Bicipital Tendinitis

Another condition with symptoms similar to those of rotator cuff pathology is tendinitis of the biceps long head. Many authors have described test variations for this condition. Yergason's test, based on one case study in 1931, is still widely used, but its reliability is being questioned.[43] The test is performed by having the patient to supinate actively against the examiner's resistance with the patient's elbow flexed 90° and forearm pronated. The patient will experience pain in the anterior, inner aspect of the shoulder. Lippman's test, on the other hand, relies on palpation of the tendon. Unfortunately, the tendon is difficult to palpate in the muscular shoulder of an athlete. In this test, the examiner displaces the patient's tendon from the side, producing a sharp pain.[44] The reverse of Lippman's test was described by deAnquin: in this test, the examiner rotates the patient's shoulder internally and externally while palpating the anterior portion of the shoulder.[32] The test is positive if the most tender spot occurs as the biceps tendon passes under the examiner's fingers. In Ludington's test, a patient grasps the top of his or her head, and then actively flexes the affected elbow, producing sharp pain.[45] Hawkins and Kennedy elicit pain by having the patient resist humeral flexion with an extended elbow; thus, their test is called the straight arm test.[11]

Transverse Humeral Ligament Rupture

To test for rupture of the transverse humeral ligament, the therapist positions the patient's arm in shoulder abduction and external rotation. The arm should be internally rotated while the examiner palpates over the bicipital groove. If the transverse ligament holding the tendon of the biceps long head is ruptured, the tendon can be felt snapping in and out of the groove.[32]

Thoracic Outlet Syndrome

Although numerous thoracic outlet syndrome tests exist, their relationship to the pathology is questionable. Most tests rely on the vascular component of the entrapment, which is discussed, in more detail in Chapter 7. However, the pathology does not have a vascular component.[46] Adson's sign, most commonly used, consists of palpating for the loss of the radial pulse while the patient extends the affected arm and rotates the head to the opposite side and simultaneously takes a deep breath.[47] Wright's test adds abduction of the shoulder to 90° and full external rotation to Adson's test manuever.[46] In the costoclavicular compression maneuver, both neurological (tingling) or vascular (decreased radial pulse) components are evaluated. While the patient allows shoulder slumping, traction is added inferiorly to the arm. The 3-minute abduction stress test and the supraclavicular Tinel's sign test use neurological indicators and are reported to be positive in 80 percent of cases.[48] The patient's arms are in 90° of abduction and external rotation while the patient flexes and extends the fingers for 3 minutes. The examiner elicits a positive supraclavicular Tinel sign by tapping on the patient's brachial plexus in the supraclavicular area. The special tests listed are indicated by the upper quarter examination, history, and general shoulder evaluation.

PALPATION

Because palpation can be a strong stimulus for pain, it must be performed at the end of the evaluation. If palpation is performed early in the evaluation, it may produce persistent pain, clouding the remainder of the evaluation and rendering further information useless. The examiner must choose, based on the information from the evaluation sequence, the least painful area to examine first (local vs. referred pain). If the patient reports a history of a "snap" in the shoulder and now complains of anterior shoulder pain, palpation of the tendon of the long head of the biceps should be done last. Remote trigger points should be evaluated first. Last, it is important to make sure that the pain produced by palpation is the patient's chief complaint and not a new pain produced by the examiner. By pressing hard enough, the examiner can produce pain in many structures of the shoulder. In the shoulders of many persons who are not muscularly overdeveloped, the rotator cuff tendons, biceps tendon (long head), transverse humeral ligament, acromioclavicular joint, and sternoclavicular joint can be palpated.

The rotator cuff and biceps tendon are best palpated with the patient seated and the examiner standing behind the patient. As the examiner's finger drops off the patient's acromion anteriorly, it should palpate the bicipital groove. This can be confirmed by having the subject rotate the shoulder internally and externally. The examiner feels for elevation on each side of the depression or groove, which contains the tendon of the long head of the biceps. Medial to the groove is the lesser tuberosity with the insertion of the subscapularis. Lateral to the groove (greater tuberosity) is the tendinous insert of the supraspinatus, the most commonly afflicted tendon. If the subject's shoulder is internally rotated and adducted behind the patient's back, the cuff insertions of the supraspinatus, infraspinatus, and teres minor muscles become more anterior. They can be palpated from the anterior to posterior as the supraspinatus, infraspinatus, and teres minor muscles. In persons who are less muscular, a firm roundness can be felt at the supraspinatus and infraspinatus tendons. These tendons should be palpated for pain, but the edema, increased temperature, or crepitus should also be sought by using palpation in the same manner. The examiner palpates from the prominant anterior curve of the clavicle laterally to find the AC joint. The clavicle sits superiorly to the acromion and can be distinguished from the flat acromion by its roundness. Bilateral symmetry, crepitus with flexion and extension of the shoulder, as well as local pain, should be noted. The sternoclavicular joint is found at the medial end of the clavicle, immediately lateral to the sternal notch. Again, symmetry, crepitus, and pain should be noted.

All muscles innervated by the same segmental level as the area of chief complaint (dermatone) must be evaluated by palpation. If the patient reports pain on palpation, the examiner must ask if it is the original pain or a new pain. Designation must be made between active and latent trigger points. The trigger

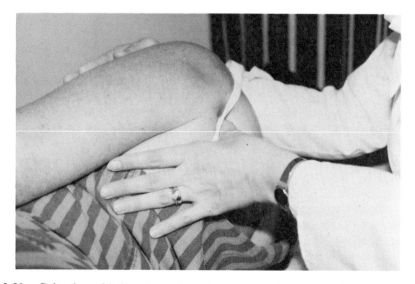

Fig. 2-30. Palpation of infraspinatus/muscle/tendon to identify a trigger point and referred pain.

point should be marked by an "X" on the pain diagram, and the area of referral pain should be designated by dots or slashes. For referral patterns, those of Travell and Simon, Reeves, and Kellgren are suggested.[2-5] Although these authors differ on the segmental relationship between trigger point and referral area, the clinical importance of the two symptoms is clear. If the patient complains of anterior shoulder pain and the history suggests referred pain, the palpation examination should first rule out a local problem and then proceed to the more pain-producing trigger point palpation. Because the anterior shoulder is C5 dermatome, all muscles innervated by C5 should be evaluated. They include the subscapularis, infraspinatus, teres minor, teres major, supraspinatus, serratus, anterior, latissimus dorsi pectoralis major, pectoralis minor, deltoid, and biceps muscles. We have found that the infraspinatus muscle most commonly refers pain to the anterior shoulder area. (Fig. 2-30).

SUMMARY

Evaluation of the shoulder girdle complex requires examination of all soft tissue structures and involved synovial joints that comprise this mobile unit. Traditionally, gonimetric measurements, muscle testing, and special tests were performed. However, as we learn more about the effects of connective tissue immobilization and the synovial joint biomechanics needed for functional movement, these traditional means of assessment do not provide a complete picture. As a consequence, our results are not optimal, and both patient and therapist are dissatisfied. Use of new evaluation techniques as well as resurrection of older techniques yields more specific information that better directs our treatment efforts. Our treatment goals become more specific. New parameters of the shoulder girdle evaluation will permit specific identification of symptoms and limitations that will help direct a more exact course of treatment.

REFERENCES

1. Jobe FW, Moynes RD: Delineation of diagnostic criteria and a rehabilitation program for rotator cuff injuries. Am J Sports Med 10:336, 1982
2. Travell JG, Simons DG: Myofascial Pain and Dysfunction. The Trigger Point Manual. Williams & Wilkins, Baltimore, 1983
3. Reeves B: Arthographic changes in frozen and post-traumatic shoulders. Proc R Soc Med 59:827, 1966
4. Reeves B: The natural history of frozen shoulder syndrome. Scand J Rheumatol 4:193, 1976
5. Kellgren J: Observations of referred pain arising from muscle. Clin Sci 3:175, 1938
6. Inman VT, Saunders JB: Referred pain from skeletal structures. J Nerv Ment Dis 99:660, 1944
7. Forester O: The dermatomes in man. Brain 56:1, 1938
8. Cyriax J: Textbook of Orthopaedic Medicine—Volume I: Diagnosis of Soft Tissue Lesions. 2nd Ed. Williams & Wilkins, Baltimore, 1975

9. Herberts P, et al: Shoulder pain and heavy manual labor. Clin Orthop Rel Res 191:166, 1984
10. Delacerda F: A comparative study of three methods of treatment for shoulder girdle myofascial syndrome. J Orthop Sports Phys Ther 4:51–54, 1982
11. Hawkins RJ, Kennedy JC: Impingement syndromes in athletes. Am J Sports Med 8:151, 1980
12. Collins RH, Wilde AH: Shoulder instability in athletics. Orthop Clin North Am 4:759, 1973
13. Jobe FW, Jobe CM: Painful athletic injuries of the shoulder. Clinic Ortho 173:124, 1983
14. Neer CS, Welsh RP: The shoulder in sports. Orthop Clin North Am 8:583, 1977
15. Cofield RH, Simonet WT: The shoulder in sports. Symposium on sports medicine: part 2. Mayo Clin Proc 59:157, 1984
16. Penny JN, Welsh RP: Shoulder impingement syndromes in athletes and their surgical management. Am J Sports Med 9:11, 1981
17. Watson M: The impingement syndrome in sportsmen. In Bayley I, Kessel L (eds): Shoulder Surgery. Springer-Verlag, Berlin, 1982
18. Warren RF: Surgical considerations for rotator cuff tears in athletes. p. 73. In Jackson DW (ed:) Shoulder Surgery in the Athlete. Aspen Systems Corp., Rockville, Maryland, 1985
19. Norwood L, Del Pizzo W, Jobe FW, Kerlan RK: Anterior shoulder pain in baseball pitchers. Am J Sports Med 6:103, 1978
20. Neer CS II: Anterior acromioplasty for the chronic impingement syndrome in the shoulder: a preliminary report. J Bone Joint Surg 54:41, 1972
21. Kussel L, Watson M: The painful arc syndrome: clinical classification as a guide to management. J Bone Joint Surg 59:166, 1977
22. Behling F: Treatment of acromioclavicular separations. Orthop Clin North Am 11:727, 1980
23. Darrow JC, Smith JA, Lockwood RC: A new conservative method for treatment of type III acromioclavicular separations. Orthop Clin North Am 11:727, 1980
24. Rockwood CA Jr, Green DP (eds): Fracture. JB Lippincott, Philadelphia, 1975
25. Rowe CR, Sakellarides HT: Factors related to recurrence of anterior dislocation of shoulder. Clin Orthop 20:40, 1961
26. Kazar B, Belowszky E: Prognosis of primary dislocation of the shoulder. Acta Orthop Scand 40:216, 1969
27. Yoneda B, Welsh P, Macintosh DL: Conservative treatment of shoulder dislocation in young males. p. 76. In Bayley I, Kessel L, (eds): Shoulder Surgery. Springer-Verlag, Berlin, 1982
28. Hovelious L, Ericksson K, Fredin H, et al: Incidence and prognosis of shoulder dislocation: a preliminary communication. p. 73. In Bayley I, Kessel L (eds): Shoulder Surgery. Springer-Verlag, Berlin, 1982
29. McLaughlin HL, McLellan DI: Recurrent anterior dislocation of the shoulder. A comparative study. J Trauma 7:191, 1967
30. Johnson JR, Bayler JIL: The early complications of anterior dislocation in the middle-aged and elderly patient. p. 79. In Bayley I, Kessel L (eds): Shoulder Surgery. Springer-Verlag, Berlin, 1982
31. Price DD, McGrath PA, Rafi A, Buckingham B: The validation of visual analogue scales as ratio scale measures for chronic and experimental pain. Pain 17:45, 1983
32. Booth RE, Marvel JP: Differential diagnosis of shoulder pain. Orthop Clin North Am 6:353, 1975

33. Moore M: Clinical assessment of joint motion. p. 192. In Basmajian J (ed): Therapeutic Exercises, 4th Ed. Williams & Wilkins, Baltimore 1984

34. Mosley HF: Examination of the shoulder. In Mosley HF (ed): Shoulder Lesions. Williams & Wilkins, Baltimore, 1969

35. Neviaser RJ: Anatomic considerations and examination of the shoulder. Orthop Clin North Am 11:187, 1980

36. Poppen N, Walker P: Normal and abnormal motion of the shoulder. J Bone Joint Surg 58A: 195, 1976

37. Saha AK: Dynamic stability of the glenohumeral joint. Acta Ortho Scand 42:491, 1971

38. Kapanjdi I: The Physiology of the Joints. Upper Limbs. Vol. 1. Churchill Livingstone, New York, 1970

39. Matsen F: Biomechanics of the shoulder. p. 221. In Frankel V, Nordin M (eds): Basic Biomechanics of the Skeletal System. Lea and Febiger, Philadelphia, 1980

40. Brodin H: Principles of examination and treatment in manual medicine. Scand J Rehab Med 11:181, 1979

41. Moritz U: Evaluation of manipulation and other manual therapy. Scand J Rehab Med 11:173, 1979

42. Nicholson G: The effects of passive joint mobiliation on pain and hypomobility associated with adhesive capsulites of the shoulder. J Orthop Sports Phys Ther 6:238, 1985

43. Yergason RM: Supination sign. J Bone Joint Surg 13:160, 1931

44. Lippman RK: Frozen shoulder: periarthritis, bicipital tenosynovitis. Arch Surg 47:283, 1943

45. Ludington NA: Rupture of the long head of biceps flexer cubiti muscle. Ann Surg 77:358, 1923

46. Wright JS: The neurovascular syndrome produced by hyperabduction of the arm. Am Heart J 29:1, 1945

47. Adson AW, Coffey JR: Cervical rib: a method of anterior approach for relief of symptoms by division of the scalenus anticus. Ann Surg 85:839, 1927

48. Jaeger SH, Read R, Smullens SN, Breme P: Thoracic outlet syndrome: diagnosis and treatment. p. 378. In Hunter J, Mackin E, Bell J, Callahan A (eds): Rehabilitation of the Hand. C. V. Mosby, St. Louis, 1984

3 | Isokinetic Evaluation and Treatment of the Shoulder

Michael J. Wooden

Isokinetic exercise has become a popular form of resistive exercise in the physical therapy clinic. Since the late 1960s, the literature has consisted primarily of research data and clinical information relating to the knee. However, recent advances in equipment have made it possible to use positioning to apply isokinetics effectively to most other extremity joints, including the shoulder complex. The purposes of this chapter are to list some advantages of isokinetics in shoulder evaluation and treatment and to describe the adaptability of the Cybex II dynamometer to shoulder diagonal patterns.

PRACTICAL ADVANTAGES OF ISOKINETICS

Isokinetic exercise, unlike isotonic, offers totally accommodating resistance to a muscular contraction.[1-3] Because the speed of movement is constant, resistance to the movement varies according to the amount of force applied to the resistance arm. Therefore, in a maximum-effort isokinetic contraction, the muscle is loaded maximally at each point in the range of motion (ROM).[1-3]

With isotonic equipment or free weights, because the speed of movement is not pre-set, resistance to muscle contraction will vary due to gravity, positioning, lever arm lengths (in the equipment and in the patient's limbs), and cam sizes.[3] If, owing to these factors, effective resistance occurs only at a certain point in the range, it is possible that the muscle is being exercised only at that point.

The primary advantage to isokinetic exercise, then, is the ability to load a muscle effectively throughout its ROM by fixing the speed of movement.

The Cybex II offers several other clinical advantages. One of these is the capability of using a wide range of speeds, both for testing muscle function and for rehabilitation or strength training.[4] This allows the clinician to determine at what velocities muscle torque deficits occur: at low speeds (so-called "strength" deficits), or high speeds ("power" and "endurance" deficits).[2] Testing and training at higher speed attempts to simulate normal activities in which angular velocities (as in walking, running, swimming, throwing, and other activities) are far in excess of most isotonic speeds.[3] Even the highest speed of the Cybex II, at 360° per second, is not fast enough to match all activities. Exercising at different speeds may cause quantitative and qualitative recruitment of different muscle fiber types, however; therefore, most or all of the muscle can be loaded.[5–8]

Studies have shown that an increase in speed of isokinetic contraction decreases both torque output and electromyographic (EMG) activity of the muscle.[1,5–8] Therefore, compressive reaction forces at the joint should also decrease. In joints that exhibit an inflamed or painful response to exercise, increasing the speed may temporarily "spare the joint" by reducing joint reaction forces. Whether training solely at high speeds contributes to an increase of strength at low speeds is controversial, however.[4,5] Nevertheless, the use of higher speeds is an important safety factor in reactive joint conditions.

Whether at fast or slow speeds, isokinetic resistance will accommodate to pain levels, further insuring safety because if the patient needs to decrease or stop the contraction suddenly because of pain, the resistance will decrease immediately, since resistance will never exceed the amount of force applied.[3] Unlike in isotonic exercise, little momentum factor is involved. In cases of pain or suspected joint reaction problems, another safe means of isokinetic exercise is submaximal effort, whereby the patient is instructed to reduce the contractile effort purposely. Again, decreasing the force will decrease the resistance, theoretically reducing joint reaction forces.

In addition to the advantages already discussed, Davies[3] cites many other physiologic and clinical advantages of isokinetics. Also listed are a few disadvantages, some of which should be mentioned here.

A major physiological limitation of the Cybex II is its inability to exercise muscle eccentrically. Because muscle generates the most amount of tension eccentrically[9] and because much of functional movement requires eccentric contraction, rehabilitation in an eccentric mode seems important. Only isontonic exercise can load a muscle eccentrically; however, for reasons already stated, it does not fully accommodate to the contractile force applied. Another consideration is that the resistance mechanism, at least on Cybex equipment, is uniaxial. Extremity joints, of course, are multiaxial, as their instantaneous centers of rotation change constantly through movement.[10]

Some practical disadvantages of isokinetics in the clinic include the high cost of the equipment, the amount of floor space required, and the time required to change positions and attachments to test the different movements. The latter is a particular problem with shoulder evaluation, since so many positions and motions are recommended in the Cybex II manual.[4] One can deal with the time factor by modifying positioning to test diagonal patterns in the shoulder.

EVALUATION OF SHOULDER DIAGONALS

The Cybex II manual contains detailed information on testing all the cardinal plane movements of the shoulder.[4] Photographs and descriptions of positioning and machine settings allow for isolated testing of abduction, adduction, flexion, extension, internal, and external rotation. These procedures provide excellent information on specific muscles or muscle groups and are indicated for certain pathologies. The process of testing all of these movements as part of a comprehensive shoulder evaluation is quite time-consuming, however, and can be clinically unmanageable. The time management problem can be solved by evaluating overall muscle function with two diagonal movements, thus eliminating several lengthy steps.

In addition to its practical benefits, diagonal movement testing may also be more functional than cardinal plane movements, which fail to isolate and measure motion of the acromioclavicular, sternoclavicular, and scapulothoracic joints.[4] Of course, movement of these joints occurs throughout the range of glenohumeral motion. Resisted diagonal movement will load muscles which effect movement at all joints in the shoulder girdle. Knott and Voss,[11] pioneers in proprioceptive neuromuscular facilitation (PNF), first described "mass movement patterns" as being inherently diagonal in nature. These diagonals are dictated by anatomy—shapes of joints, lines of muscle pull, and soft tissue restrictions—and are those movements observed to be most used in everyday activities.[11] The movements to be described in this chapter are similar to the classic upper extremity PNF patterns.

TESTING PROCEDURE

The first diagonal movement described is the combination of extension, abduction, internal rotation (Ext/Abd/IR); and flexion, adduction, external rotation (Flex/Add/ER). Figure 3-1A shows the initiation of the Ext/Abd/IR movement; Fig. 3-1B shows the end of that same diagonal, here blocked manually to prevent hyperextension. Figure 3-1C illustrates the end positions for the Flex/Add/ER movement.

For both movements, the patient is instructed to try to keep the elbow straight, and to rotate the arm internally or externally depending on which movement is being performed. To allow for rotation, a swivel handle is used. It should be pointed out, however, that the rotational component cannot be resisted by the apparatus, as would be the case if manual resistance were used in PNF.[11] The dynamometer is tipped forward 15° to account for trunk movement and the forward-inclined plane of the scapula.[12,13]

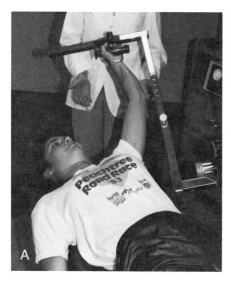

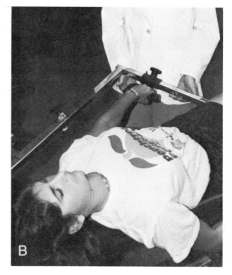

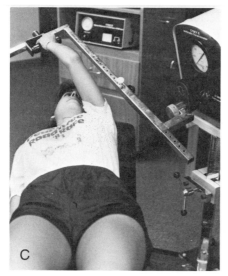

Fig. 3-1. (A) Initiation of the diagonal movement Ext/Abd/IR. (B) End of diagonal movement Ext/Abd/IR. (C) End of diagonal movement Flex/Add/ER.

In most extremity joints, including the shoulder, there are little or no normative data regarding expected peak torques. Therefore, until more research is done, the clinician must rely on bilateral comparison testing, in which peak torque at the injured joint is expressed as a percentage of deficit as compared with the uninvolved ("normal") side. Unfortunately, this method fails to consider natural side-to-side differences in strength which might be owing, for example, to hand domination, occupation, sports activity, or preexisting injuries.

Figure 3-2A is the normal torque curve for the diagonal Ext/Abd/IR and Flex/Add/ER in a post–anterior-dislocation patient who has recovered most of her ROM. The shoulder is tested at 60° per second (low speed) and 180° per

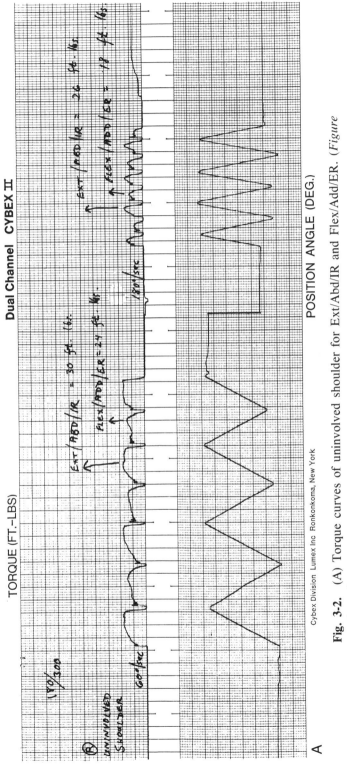

Fig. 3-2. (A) Torque curves of uninvolved shoulder for Ext/Abd/IR and Flex/Add/ER. (*Figure continues.*)

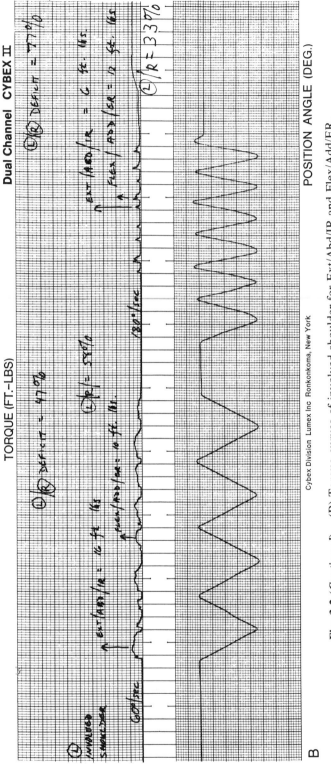

Fig. 3-2 (*Continued*). (B) Torque curves of involved shoulder for Ext/Abd/IR and Flex/Add/ER.

Table 3-1. Summary of Peak Torque Deficits

Diagonal	Speed	Right Uninvolved (ft-lb)	Left Uninvolved (ft-lb)	Deficit (%)
Ext/Abd/IR	60°/s	30	16	47
	180°/s	26	6	77
Flex/Add/ER	60°/s	24	10	58
	180°/s	18	12	33

Data from Figure 3-2A and B.

second (high speed), the speeds recommended by Cybex for flexion and extension.[4] An athlete or unusually strong person can also be tested at higher speeds as long as measurable torque is being produced. Figure 3-2B represents the torque curve for the injured side in the same patient. The lower foot-pound readings for the "left involved shoulder" indicate strength deficits, at low and high speeds, ranging from 33 to 77 percent. Table 3-1 is a summary of the torque measurements taken from Figure 3-2A and B.

Not only can strength deficits be computed, but the shapes of the torque curves in Fig. 3-2A and B can also be compared. The low speed (60° per second) curves for the involved shoulder show a slower "rate of rise" than for the normal side. That is, the weaker side took longer to reach its peak torque. In addition, the duration of each Ext/Abd/IR and Flex/Add/ER contraction at low and high speed is shorter, as compared with the opposite side, indicating inability to sustain tension. These variations in curve shape are further indications of muscle weakness which should improve after appropriate isokinetic training. Last, a comparison of the lower "position angle" scale, indicates limitations at the extremes of ROM, although in this case the differences are slight.

This evaluation procedure can also be done for a second diagonal, the combination of Ext/Add/IR, and Flex/Abd/ER. The sequence of these movements is illustrated in Figure 3-3A through C. The start and finish positions for Ext/Add/IR are shown in Fig. 3-3A and B, respectively, and initiation of Flex/Abd/ER is shown in Fig. 3-3C. In this diagonal, the extreme of the flexion movement was blocked either manually or, as shown, using UBXT attachments. Torque deficit computation and shape of curve comparisons were done as previously described.

TREATMENT PROTOCOLS

In general, when a shoulder is deemed ready for progressive resistive exercise (PRE) through its available ROM, it is ready for isokinetic rehabilitation. Fractures, dislocations, muscle tears, and other soft tissue injuries should be well-healed, stable, and past the acute stage. Although ROM need not be full, it should be relatively painless at the extremes. In postoperative cases, knowledge of the surgical approach is essential in determining direction of resisted movement. In all cases of painful restriction or possible instability at end-range, appropriate blocking of movement is necessary, especially when using faster speeds.

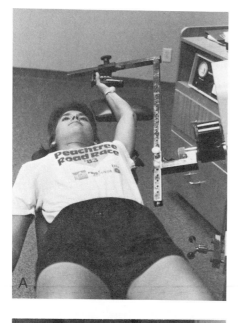

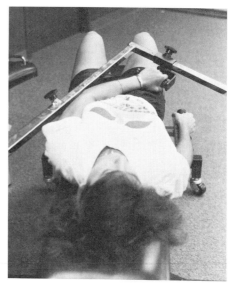

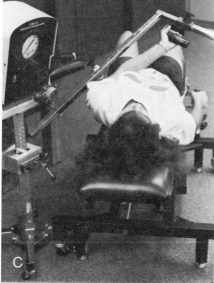

Fig. 3-3. (A) Initiation of diagonal movement Ext/Add/IR. (B) End of diagonal movement Ext/Add/IR. (C) Initiation of diagonal movement Flex/Abd/ER.

In choosing which speed to use in isokinetic rehabilitation, several criteria are used. The most simple determination is based on the evaluation. For the most part, low-speed torque deficits require low-speed training, whereas faster speeds are used for high-speed deficits. Often, however, deficits occur at both testing speeds as the curves in Fig. 3-2A and B indicate. In this case, a helpful guideline is the "25 percent rule." That is, if the strength deficit at the 60° per second testing speed is >25 percent, rehabilitation at that speed is indicated.

Table 3-2. Guidelines for Isokinetic Speed and Protocol Selection in Shoulder Rehabilitation

Isokinetic Speed	Protocol
60°/s	1. Strength deficit >25% 2. Patient too weak to generate torque at higher speeds 3. High-speed movement too painful
180°/s	1. Stength deficit <25% 2. Low-speed contraction too painful 3. Decrease joint reaction forces
Velocity spectrum protocol	Train at several speeds; simulate speeds used in normal activities
Short-arc contraction	To avoid painful ranges; possible instability at end-range
Sub-maximum effort contraction	1. Not ready for maximum effort at any speed due to pain, inflammation, incomplete healing, etc. 2. Poor tolerance to initial test done at maximum effort

If the deficit is <25 percent at the lower testing speed, training should be at 180° per second or faster.

There are several exceptions to this rule. As mentioned previously, the need to reduce joint reaction forces may necessitate high-speed training even though major deficits at the low testing speed are found. The same is true for a painful joint when the patient will not tolerate movement at the indicated speed. Contractile pain is usually less at faster speeds, although occasionally slow-speed exercise is tolerated better. Other ways of lessening pain include submaximum effort and short-arc contraction which avoids pain localized to a portion of the range of movement. Some general guidelines for selecting speeds and pain reducing protocols are listed in Table 3-2. Submaximum effort training is sometimes done for a few treatment sessions prior to actual testing of a patient who is not yet ready for the maximum effort contractions that are necessary for bilateral strength comparisons.

Questions regarding numbers of repetitions and frequency of training sessions are difficult to answer since there is great variability among patients and the conditions requiring rehabilitation. A recommended starting protocol for low-speed diagonal training is 100 repetitions (e.g., 10 sets of 10 repetitions) at 60° per second. To avoid overuse, patients work out no more than three times a week at regular intervals, with 50 to 100 repetitions added at each session depending on tolerance, until several hundred are performed. Patients are routinely retested after each six sessions to determine when workouts can be advanced to higher speeds.

Table 3-3. Velocity Spectrum Rehabilitation Protocol

Repetitions per Speed	Velocities in Degrees per Second
10	60–90–120–150–180–210–210–180–150–120–90–60 Add 5 to 10 repetitions each session.

(Modified from Davies G: A Compendium of Isokinetics in Clinical Usage: Workshop and Clinical Notes. S&S Publishers. La Crosse, Wis., 1984.)

High-speed training can be progressed in a similar way at 180° per second, although Davies[3] recommends the use of several speeds at each session, using the velocity spectrum rehabilitation protocol (VSRP).[3] Again, patients build up to hundreds of repetitions which are divided among many speeds of movement. Table 3-3 is an example of VSRP.

In general, when retesting shows strength deficits to be reduced to ≤10 percent, Cybex II training is discontinued.

SUMMARY

A method of evaluating and treating shoulder girdle muscle weakness has been described. Diagonal movements relate closely to normal activity and provide time-saving and practical means of applying isokinetics to the shoulder. For specific weakness of a muscle or small muscle group (e.g., in rotator cuff tears), the isolated movements described in the Cybex manual may be more helpful. Similarly, certain injuries or surgical repairs may necessitate isolation of movement to a cardinal plane.

Continued research into isokinetics is needed, especially for the shoulder, for which no normative data are available. The clinician would benefit greatly from data predicting expected peak torque values according to age, sex, size, and body type, as well as the extent of side-to-side strength differences in normal subjects.

REFERENCES

1. Moffroid M, Whipple R, Hofkosh J, et al: A study of isokinetic exercise. Phys Ther 49:735, 1969
2. Laird C, Rozier C: Toward understanding the terminology of exercise mechanics. Phys Ther 59:287, 1979
3. Davies G: A Compendium of Isokinetics in Clinical Usage: Workshop and Clinical Notes. S & S Publishers, LaCrosse, WI, 1984
4. Cybex: Isolated Joint Testing and Exercise: A Handbook for Using Cybex II and the UBXT. Cybex, Ronkokoma, NY, 1983
5. Moffroid M, Whipple R: Specificity of speed of exercise. Phys Ther 50:1693, 1970
6. Barnes WS: The relationship of motor unit activation to isokinetic muscular contraction at different contractile velocities. Phys Ther 60:1152, 1980
7. Thorstensson A, Grimby G, Karlsson J: Force velocity relations and fiber composition in human knee extension muscles. J Appl Physiol 40:12, 1976
8. Smith M, Melton P: Isokinetic versus isotonic variable resistance training. Am J Sports Med 9:275, 1981
9. Rasch P, Burke R: Kinesiology and Applied Anatomy. 3rd Ed. Lea and Febiger, Philadelphia, 1967
10. Williams P, Warwick R: Gray's Anatomy. 36th Ed. WB Saunders Co, Philadelphia, 1980

11. Knott M, Voss D: Proprioceptive Neuromuscular Facilitation: patterns and Techniques. 2nd Ed. Harper and Row, New York, 1968
12. Gardner E, Gray D, O'Rahilly R: Anatomy: A Regional Study of Human Structure. 2nd Ed. WB Saunders Co, New York 1963
13. Johnston T: The movements of the shoulder joint. A plea for use of the "plane of the scapula" as the plane of reference for movements occurring at the humero-scapular joint. Br J Surg 25:252, 1952

4 | Posture and the Upper Quarter

Edward Ayub

The upper quarter consists of the occiput, cervical spine, and the upper extremities, including the clavicles and scapulas. Through an interdependent process, positions of the component parts are related so that a change in the position of one structure may influence the position of related structures. An immediate relationship is perceived when one realizes that the occiput is connected to the cervical spine which, through muscular attachments, is connected to the shoulder girdle.

A disturbance in upper quarter muscle balance may lead to observable deviations in structural position and become evident as a postural deviation. Muscles which become tight tend to pull body segments to which they attach, causing deviations in alignment. The antagonistic muscles may become weak and allow deviation of body parts due to their lack of support.[1] The muscle tone will change via afferent impulses from the joint structures such as capsule, synovial membrane, ligaments, and tendons.[2] These impulses reflexively influence the tone of muscles.[2] Although the function of a joint is movement, a disturbance in mobility may lead to pathology.[2] A joint may have a restriction in movement or an abnormal range of movement that results in shortening or lengthening of the muscles acting on it. These changes may result in impaired movement patterns which in turn result in pain or disability in the upper quarter. The most frequent clinically observed postural deviation of the upper quarter involves abnormal positioning of the head and cervical spine. However, the evaluation of faulty positional mechanics necessitates an understanding of normal posture in order to judge the degree of deviation.

POSTURE

By definition, good posture is that state of muscular and skeletal balance which protects the supporting structures of the body against injury or progressive deformity, irrespective of the attitudes, (erect, lying, sitting, squatting, stooping) in which the structures are working or resting.[3] Although posture is described as a matter of alignment, observable changes in body contours may translate to some degree of variation in skeletal alignment. The spinal curve must transect a plumb line to remain in balance with gravity, such that an increase in any one curve may be compensated by a proportionate increase or decrease in the other curves. Around this line, the body is hypothetically in a position of equilibrium, which implies a balanced distribution of weight as well as a stable position of each joint. Balance is efficient with less expenditure of energy if the body remains in line with the vertical axis. Body deviation from this efficient positioning may be significant in understanding how posture may influence the upper quarter.

Faulty posture may cause prolonged mechanical deformation of a tissue and cause a structural change in inherent form. This prolonged deformation may produce a pain felt distally if pressure on pain-sensitive tissue is acute, whereas loss of function is more likely to occur if pressure is prolonged and continuous.[4] Maintenance of erect upright posture and performance of voluntary movements are highly integrated coordinated functions of groups of skeletal muscles. Inhibition of select postural muscles may be reflected in abnormal upper quarter postural deviations.

Of importance in the evaluation of the upper quarter is the position of the head, which is significant in the determination of overall body posture, as well as limb control.[5] Abnormal positioning of the head on the cervical spine is increasingly significant when one considers the importance of the upper cervical spine, (occiput on atlas and atlas on axis) on the regulation of body posture. The essential afferent impulses for the static and dynamic regulation of body posture, as well as the ability to produce reflex changes in the motor unit activity of all four limb muscles, arise from the receptor systems located in the connective tissue structures and muscles within the upper vertebral synovial joints.[5] One may view the balancing of the head on the cervical column as a lever system whose fulcrum lies at the level of the occipital condyles, whereas the center of gravity of the head is near the sella turcica. The apex of the cervical lordosis is located at the posterior–inferior border of C4.[6]

Therefore, the center of gravity lies anterior to the fulcrum. It becomes apparent that motionless, erect posture is maintained by the antagonistic pull of the posterior cervical muscles against the force of gravity and the anterior neck muscles.[6]

An important group of muscles in the determination of head position are the suboccipital muscles, which have their origin as well as their insertion between occiput and atlas, occiput and axis, or between atlas and axis. These are short, deep muscles which run in oblique directions and have a high innervation ratio (three to five fibers per neuron), signifying that the number of muscle fibers per motor neuron is small.[7] Consequently, the potential rate of contraction of these muscles is similar to that of the extrinsic eye muscles. Therefore, they are well suited to their role of producing rapid movements as well as fine-tuning action capable of elimination of undesirable components of movement derived from the lower vertebral column.[6,7]

By design, the mobility of the cervical spine allows for its component parts to function unimpaired; that is, the discs are allowed to distort and recover, the ligaments have sufficient ability to permit movement, the apophyseal joints are free of bony disturbance and possess adequate capsular elasticity to permit their freedom of motion, and the soft tissues and muscles have adequate length to allow the bony structures free movement. Loss of movement of any part of the cervical spine may result in pain or disability in the upper quarter.

ABNORMAL POSTURE

Relaxed Postural Position

The relaxed postural position typifies a postural deviation reflective of inhibition of muscle activity. In this abnormal postural position, responsibility for the maintenance of upright spinal posturing is transferred from the contractile muscle unit to the noncontractile structural unit. The contractile unit consists of the muscle and muscle tendon, whereas the noncontractile unit consists of bone, ligaments, cartilage, and connective tissue. By their inherent design, the contractile units are well suited to their postural and movement roles. However, the noncontractile units, as a result of increased postural stress, tend to deform over time, which may result in dysfunction such as pain or instability.

An observable structural deviation which occurs with the relaxed postural position is an anterior displacement of the head relative to the thorax when compared with the anatomical points of reference that occur in standard posture.[3] With the head moving forward, the occipital condyles slide anteriorly on the oval-shaped articular facets of the atlas into a position of increased backward bending. Consequently, the occipital bone moves closer to atlas, resulting in the approximation of the posterior arches of atlas and axis. This position may be a factor in the mechanical production of headaches (Rocobado, course notes, Institute of Graduate Health Science, 1981). This postural position produces suboccipital muscle shortening at the atlanto-occipital joint of the rectus posterior minor and the superior oblique muscles and at the atlantoaxial joint of the rectus posterior major and the inferior oblique muscles. The position of increased backward bending of the head on the upper cervical spine will shorten the muscles forming the suboccipital triangle—the rectus posterior major and the superior and inferior obliques. This shortening may cause irritation to, or interfere with the normal physiology of, the structures passing through this triangle, namely the dorsal root of the first cervical nerve as well as the vertebral artery.[8] The decreased suboccipital mobility has far-reaching consequences because this region plays a significant role in the production of arthrokinetic reflexes. Specialized mechanoreceptors are numerous in the cervical facet joint capsules as well as in the skin overlying these joints, and contribute to the consciously perceived system subserving postural and kinesthetic sensations. A disturbance in mobility may lead to degenerative changes, possibly altering these afferent impulses and decreasing their reflexogenic efficiency.[5,7]

Abnormal Mechanics and Dysfunction

According to biomechanical principles, when a force is applied to a curved structure, the area on the convex side is stretched while that on the concave side is compressed.[9] With the increased concavity in the suboccipital region as a result of shortening of the suboccipital muscles, one would anticipate lengthening on the convex side of this curve. Because tight muscles tend to inhibit their antagonists,[1] weakness of the anterior vertebral cervical flexors may be anticipated. The increased suboccipital backward bending, coupled with the diminished stabilizing role of the anterior prevertebral cervical stabilizers, results in lengthening of the middle and lower portions of the cervical spine. As a result, the apex of the cervical lordosis moves cephalad, possibly to the posterior–inferior portion of C1. Consequently, there is a forward displacement in the active segment of the vertebral column, consisting of the intervertebral disc, the intervertebral foramen, the articular processes, the ligamentum flavum, and the interspinous ligament.[6] The passive segment of the vertebral column consists of the vertebra itself. The mobility of the active segment underlies the movement of the vertebral column.[6] Due to loss of middle and lower cervical lordosis, an increased compression force is applied to the posterior aspect of the active segment and a tilting or tension force on its anterior portion, which shortens the interspinous ligament as well as the posterior portion of the apophyseal capsules while lengthening the ligamentum flavum and the anterior portion of the apophyseal capsule. This may interfere with the role of the ligamentum flavum in the prevention of impingement of the apophyseal capsule between its two articular surfaces during movement. In addition, one would expect an increase in compression on the posterior surface of the vertebral bodies,[10] which may result in increased tension anteriorly. Posteriorly, this may lead to early degenerative changes,[10] whereas traction spurs may be seen anteriorly, particularly on the anterior–inferior portion of the superior vertebral segment and on the anterior–superior position of the inferior segment.

Changes occur in the muscles and soft tissue in response to the forward head position.[11] Shortening of the suboccipital muscles moves the occiput posteriorly–inferiorly, which results in an upward and backward displacement of the mandible in the glenoid fossa. As a result, there is shortening of the suprahyoid muscles, which are the digastric, stylohyoid, geniohyoid, and mylohyoid muscles, while lengthening occurs of the antagonistic infrahyoid mus-

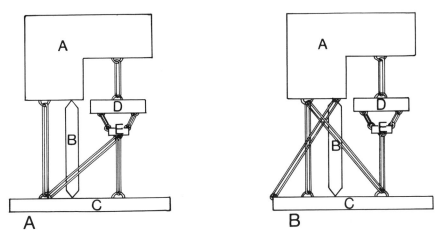

Fig. 4-1. (A) Schematic representation of the interdependent relationship of the upper quarter structures. A, occiput; B, cervical spine; C, shoulder girdle; D, mandible; E, hyoid bone. The elastics show the posterior cervical, supramandibular, suprahyoid, and infrahyoid muscles. The omohyoid muscle is displayed to demonstrate the connection between the hyoid bone and the scapula. (B) Same as (A) with the addition of the levator scapula muscle and the sternomastoid muscle. The omohyoid muscle has been omitted.

cles, consisting of the sternohyoid, sternothyroid, thyrohyoid, and the omohyoid muscles, resulting in elevation of the hyoid bone.[11] These positions would leave the mouth open if not for excessive contraction of the supramandibular muscles—the masseter and temporalis muscle.[11] Therefore, the relaxed postural position appears to disrupt the normal synergism of the mandibular elevators versus the mandibular depressors. As a result of these positional and muscular changes the patient may adopt mouth breathing instead of the more desirable nasal breathing.[11] The changes are significant when one views these muscles as links in a chain which join the cranium with the mandible by the temporalis and masseter muscles, the mandible with the hyoid bone by the suprahyoid and infrahyoid muscles, and the hyoid bone with the scapula by the omohyoid muscle[12] (Fig. 1).

With the head moving anteriorly, and the posterior aspect of occiput moving posteriorly–inferiorly, there is shortening of the upper trapezius muscle, which attaches to the superior lateral portion of the scapula, as well as of the levator scapula, which attaches to the superior medial portion of the scapula. Therefore, shortening of these muscles results in scapular elevation. Shortening of the levator scapula muscle is considered clinically significant because this muscle originates from the first four cervical transverse processes, and consequently is capable of movement in the suboccipital region, especially when the shoulder is fixed. In addition, levator scapula dysfunction may refer pain to the superior medial border of the scapula.[13]

In response to the loss of the midcervical lordosis, more weight and tension is exerted at the cervical–thoracic junction, resulting from the development of a torque force at the base of the cervical spine, which no longer acts as a weight-bearing column as when the standard posture is assumed.[14] Subsequently, there is a proportionate increase in thoracic kyphosis. The increased thoracic convexity tends to abduct the scapulae and lengthen the rhomboid and lower trapezius muscles, while shortening the serratus anterior, latissimus dorsi, subscapularis, and teres major muscles.

In addition, the increased scapular abduction shortens the pectoralis major and minor muscles, which, by their attachment to the coracoid process of the scapula, tend to pull the scapula over the head of the humerus. In an effort to maintain its resting position in the glenoid, the humerus moves into internal rotation, which shortens the glenohumeral ligament. This may result in contracture of the anterior shoulder capsule, resulting in diminished shoulder abduction, lateral rotation, and extension. Because a tight muscle inhibits its antagonists,[1] numerous muscle imbalances may result. Weakness of the lower trapezius muscle may result from shortening of the upper trapezius, levator scapula, and serratus anterior muscles, whereas inhibition of the rhomboid muscles may occur in response to the shortening of the teres major muscle. Increased glenohumeral internal rotation will shorten the humeral head medial rotators, with resulting lengthening and inhibition of the lateral rotators. These changes in normal muscle length may result in alteration in the normal scapulohumeral rhythm.

The movement of the scapula into abduction may result in increased acromioclavicular joint compression and shorten the conoid ligament while lengthening the trapezoid ligament. As a result, the sternoclavicular joint slides posteriorly, shortening the anterior portion of the sternoclavicular capsule. This altered clavicular position may diminish the actual rotation at the clavicular joint and diminish total scapular rotation. The possibility of shoulder impingement is increased by the upper quarter changes seen with the relaxed postural position. The coracoacromial arch is described as an unyielding structure consisting of the coracoid anteriorly, the coracoacromial ligament running from the coracoid to the anterior edge of the acromion, and the acromion itself. Impingement may be caused by the close relationship of the tendon of the long head of the biceps and supraspinatus muscle to the coracoacromial ligament and the anterior portion of the acromion during overhead elevation. Impingement may result in a painful arc syndrome.[15] Because of limited space beneath the coracoacromial arch, rotator cuff impingement may occur if the volume of the structures passing beneath the coracoacromial arch is increased. Due to the change in length of the rotator cuff muscles and the resulting dyskinesia, abnormal thickening of these tendons may occur, resulting in less space under the coracoacromial arch. The increased glenohumeral internal rotation stretches the rotator cuff and biceps tendon over the humeral head and may be a factor in their diminished blood supply. The vascularity of the rotator cuff is most compromised when the arm is adducted.[15] Degenerative changes of the rotator cuff are frequent because of diminished blood supply at the watershed area, which translates to the distal portion of the supraspinatus tendon, proximal to its insertion into the humeral head.[16] Although the supraspinatus tendon is most involved, the infraspinatus and teres minor are also implicated. Owing to the increased length and subsequent angulation of the tendons over the head of the humerus, ischemia may occur; therefore, small attritional tears have less capacity for repair. This may occur in such a way that, with active contraction of the supraspinatus muscle, the humeral head acts as a compressive force, occluding the vessels coursing longitudinally through the substance of the tendon.[15] The prime movement muscles are largely ineffectual without the help of the rotator cuff muscles to steer the humeral head through the complex motions of roll and glide required to produce the full range of shoulder motion.[17] Repeated microtrauma in this area results in an inflammatory response with edema and increase in volume of the tendinous structures. The inflamed tissues are aggravated by their impingement during abduction. Further impingement occurs if there is a partial tear of the supra-spinatus muscle involving its inferior surface, which allows a "buckling" of the tendon as it passes beneath the coracoacromial arch, resulting in a painful catching sensation.[15]

Impingement may also occur as a result of the formation of osteophytes on the inferior and anterior aspect of the acromion, as a result of traction by the coracoacromial ligament.[18] The shortening of the pectoral muscles pulling the scapula anteriorly, as well as inferiorly, may approximate the acromion and humerus, decreasing the suprahumeral space. Activities such as abduction and shoulder elevation may impinge into this already compromised region which may, over time, lead to the formation of osteophytes, as described by Neer.[18]

The acromioclavicular joint may degenerate in a secondary phenomena because the subacromial bursa extends under the coracoacromial ligament and may be involved as an extension of the inflammatory response.[15] The increased scapular rotation required by a patient with a painful shoulder may result in recurring stress at the acromioclavicular joint, with resultant degeneration.[15,19] Owing to the close proximity of the acromioclavicular joint to the supraspinatus tendon in abduction, degenerative osteophyte lipping of this joint may further mechanically irritate the supraspinatus muscle.[15,18]

The long head of the biceps muscle is subject to impingement because of its close proximity to the coracoacromial ligament during shoulder flexion.[15] Because the biceps tendon undergoes the same motions as do the tuberosities, rotator cuff, and the subacromial bursa, an alteration in the normal movement patterns of this muscle may result from the relaxed postural position. Because the sheath of the biceps tendon is an extension of the shoulder joint's synovial lining and the synovium is intimately related to the rotator cuff, an inflammatory process involving one of these structures may affect the other. The coracoac-romial ligament and the anterior inferior surface of the acromion are known to contribute to the irritation of these tendons.[20,21] Inflammatory processes which constitute the painful arc syndrome can originate anywhere within the arch, including the acromioclavicular joint, the acromion, the rotator cuff, and the biceps tendon.[21]

Entrapment Neuropathies and Abnormal Posture

Nerve entrapment may result from the postural changes which occur with the relaxed postural position.

Suprascapular Nerve

The suprascapular nerve is derived from the upper trunk of the brachial plexus which is formed from the roots of C5 and C6. Occasionally, the nerve may pass through the body of the scalenus medius muscle and, at the upper border of the scapula, it passes through the suprascapular notch. The notch is roofed over by the transverse scapular ligament, which thus converts it to a foramen. After it passes through the notch, the nerve reaches the posterior aspect of the scapula, in the supraspinous fossa. It supplies the supraspinatus muscle, the glenohumeral and the acromioclavicular joints, and the infraspinatus muscle. The relaxed postural position may cause traction, which in turn induces tension in the brachial plexus where the suprascapular nerve is given off.[22] Fixation of the suprascapular nerve by the foramen can cause tension in the nerve, with abnormal cervical spine–scapula relationships.[22] The relaxed postural position may move the scapula laterally, forward, and medially, in relationship to the thorax. This protracted position increases the total distance from the origin of the nerve to the suprascapular notch, thus placing stress on the suprascapular nerve.[22] This becomes increasingly important in persons whose suprascapular notch is less spacious. The relaxed postural position induces shortening of the scalenus medius muscle, which in turn may irritate the suprascapular nerve. The forward head position also increases the distance between the C5-6 cervical segment and this nerve's insertion into the acromioclavicular joint, and infraspinatus muscle. The increased scapular protraction tends to create nerve tension, which may cause pain at the lateral and posterior aspects of the shoulder, as well as at the anterior aspect of the acromioclavicular joint.[22]

Dorsal Scapular Nerve

Entrapment of the dorsal scapular nerve can occur because this nerve pierces the scalenus muscle. Conditions such as scalenus anticus syndrome, scalenus medius syndrome, and thoracic outlet may lead to irritation of this nerve. The relaxed postural position, may shorten the scalene muscles, inducing abnormal tension on the dorsal scapular nerve. The scaleni muscles are accessory respiratory muscles. Hypertrophy of these muscles may be seen with abnormal breathing patterns. The relaxed postural position may induce mouth breathing as well as upper respiratory breathing and resultant scalene hypertrophy. Abnormal tension may result as these muscles are stretched with the increased scapular protraction. In addition, hypertrophy of the scalenus medius muscle may result from inadequate stabilization of the spine. This may result from ligamentous laxity due to the increased tension on the anterior cervical spine, as observed in the forward head posture.[22] When the dorsal scapular nerve is hung up at its entrapment point in the scalenus medius muscle, the slack necessary to compensate for head and arm motion is prevented. A tense nerve moving against taut muscles, (muscle fibers) can set up the initial mechanical irritation in the nerve that results in a neuropathy.[22] A dorsal scapular nerve neuropathy can cause scapular pain. Irritation to the upper trunk will cause pain along the radial C5-6 axis. In addition, an anomalous cervical rib may induce mechanical irritation to the nerve. According to Kopel[22] the most frequent cause of upper extremity disability, based on a scalene (neurological type) mechanism, is an entrapment neuropathy of the dorsal scapular nerve.

CONCLUSION

Dysfunction of any upper quarter structure may be related to abnormal posture. However, the motor system tends to function as an entity in that a local dysfunction produces a chain of reflexes which may involve the whole motor system and vice versa. Therefore, although upper quarter dysfunctions may be apparent locally, the subsequent solution to pathology may necessitate evaluation of the motor system as a whole.

REFERENCES

1. Janda V: Muscles as a pathogenic factor in back pain. In Buswell J, Smith MD (eds): The Treatment of Patients: Proceedings of the International Federation of Orthopaedic Manipulative Therapists, 4th Conference, Christchurch, New Zealand, 1980
2. Stoddard A: Manual of Osteopathic Technique. 3rd Ed., Hutchinson and Co, 1980
3. Kendall HO, Kendall FP, Boynton DA: Posture and Pain. Robert E. Krieger Publishing Co, Huntington, New York, 1977
4. Cyriax J: Textbook of Orthopaedic Medicine. 7th Ed. Vol. 1, Bailliere Tindall, London, 1978
5. Wyke B: Conference on the aging brain. Cervical articular contributions to posture and gait; their relation to senile disequilibrium. Age Aging, 8:255, 1979
6. Kapandji IA: The Physiology of the Joints. Vol. 3, Churchill Livingstone, Edinburgh, 1974
7. Grieve GP: Common Vertebral Joint Problems. Churchill, Livingstone, Edinburgh, 1981
8. Warwick R, Williams P. (eds): Gray's Anatomy. 35th British Ed. WB Saunders Co, Philadelphia, 1973
9. Radin E, Simon SR, Rose RM, Paul IL: Practical Biomechanics for the Orthopedic Surgeon. John Wiley and Sons, New York, 1979
10. Cailliet R: Neck and Arm Pain. FA Davis Co, Philadelphia, 1975

11. Ayub E, Glasheen-Wray M, Kraus S: Head posture A case study of the effects on the rest position of the mandible. J Orthop Sports Phys Ther 5:179, 1984
12. Brodie AG: Anatomy and physiology of head and neck musculature. Am J Orthop 36:831, 1950
13. Gould JA, Davies GJ: Orthopaedic and Sports Physical Therapy. CV Mosby Co, St. Louis, 1985
14. Saunders HD: Orthopaedic Physical Therapy. Evaluation and treatment of musculoskeletal disorders, Minneapolis, 1982
15. Penny JN, Welsh MB: Shoulder impingement syndromes in athletes and their surgical management. Am J Sports Med 9:11, 1981
16. Rathburn JB, Macnab I: The microvascular pattern of the rotator cuff. J Bone Joint Surg 528:540, 1970
17. Saha AK: Dynamic stability of the glenohumeral joint. Acta Orthop Scand 42:491, 1971
18. Neer CS: Anterior acromioplasty for the chronic impingement syndrome in the shoulder. A preliminary report. J Bone Joint Surg 54:41, 1972
19. Macnab I, Hastings D: Rotator cuff tendinitis. Am Med Assoc J 99:91, 1968
20. Bateman JE: Cuff tears in athletes. Orthop Clin North Am 4:721, 1973
21. Neviaser TJ, Neviaser RJ, Neviaser JS, Neviaser JS: The four-in-one arthroplasty for the painful arc syndrome, p. 107. In Clinical Orthopedics and Related Research, No. 163: JB Lippincott Co, Philadelphia, 1982
22. Kopell HP: Peripheral Entrapment Neuropathies. 2nd Ed. Robert E. Krieger Publishing Co, New York, 1976

5 | Management of Frozen Shoulder

Helen Owens-Burkhart

Patients with a diagnosis of frozen shoulder are commonly seen in the physical therapy department. Unfortunately, frozen shoulder is often a "catch-all diagnosis"[1,2] that can imply myriad shoulder problems. In the literature, confusion abounds on the subject of frozen shoulder. First, there is no consensus on the name of this clinical entity. Some of the more common terms that are synonyms for frozen shoulder are adhesive capsulitis, periarthritis, stiff and painful shoulder, periarticular adhesions, Duplay's disease, scapulo-humeral periarthritis, tendinitis of the short rotators, adherent subacromial bursitis,[3] painful stiff shoulder, bicipital tenosynovitis, subdeltoid bursitis, humeroscapular fibrositis, shoulder portion of shoulder–hand syndrome, bursitis calcarea, supraspinatus tendinitis, periarthrosis humeroscapularis, and a host of foreign language terms.[4]

Confusion in terminology probably reflects the confusion in the definition, pathology, etiology, and treatment of this clinical entity so evident in the literature. One of the difficulties in reviewing the literature of evaluation and treatment of frozen shoulder, the main thrust of this chapter, was that few studies defined frozen shoulder in the same way. As a result, inconsistencies in patient selection based on their varied definitions made it difficult to assess the value of the treatment being examined. In addition, most studies did not discuss the evaluative procedures used to reach the diagnosis of frozen shoulder. The goals of this chapter are: (1) to present a literature review of the pathology, etiology, and clinical features of frozen shoulder; (2) to establish a working definition of frozen shoulder; and (3) to present evaluative and treatment procedures for frozen shoulder. I hope that the reader can readily apply this information to clinical practice, thereby improving patient care.

LITERATURE REVIEW

Frozen shoulder is loosely defined as a painful stiff shoulder.[1] This definition appears to be more of a description of symptoms than a diagnosis. McLaughlin states that frozen shoulder is a popular medical colloquialism and not a diagnosis.[5] In this literature review, a working definition of frozen shoulder will be established.

Pathology and Definition

Historically, Duplay[6] in 1872 was first credited with describing the painful stiff shoulder, referring to the condition as humeroscapular periarthritis (periarthritescapulohumerale) secondary to subacromial bursitis. In 1934, Codman[7] coined the term frozen shoulder, attributing the painful stiff shoulder to a short rotator tendinitis. Codman devoted only nine pages of his textbook on the shoulder to frozen shoulder, summarizing this condition as difficult to define, explain, and treat. In 1945, Neviaser[3] surgically explored 10 cases of frozen shoulder, finding absence of the glenohumeral synovial fluid and the redundant axillary fold of the capsule, as well as thickening and contraction of the capsule, which had become adherent to the humeral head; thus, he used the term adhesive capsulitis. As Neviaser rotated these shoulders, it appeared at first as if the humeral head and capsule were glued together but could be separated with one or two rotational movements, thus freeing joint movement. Microscopic examinations in all 10 cases revealed reparative inflammatory changes in the capsule. Based on this work, Neviaser suggested that "adhesive capsulitis" described the pathology of frozen shoulder.

In 1938, McLaughlin[5] reported that in surgical exploration of a number of frozen shoulders he found no histologic evidence of inflammation. He too observed a loss of the inferior redundant fold, but the adhesions between the folds were easily separated and separation did not increase shoulder motion. McLaughlin consistently found that the rotator cuff tendon was contracted and shrunken, holding the humeral head tight in the glenoid and allowing little motion at this articulation. Although unsupported by examination, McLaughlin postulated that the tissue changes in the cuff were related to collagen stiffening. This appeared reasonable since McLaughlin observed that prolonged disuse of the extremity preceded a frozen shoulder. He recognized that the reason for shoulder disuse may be in or removed from the shoulder. Although many studies cite disuse of the extremity as a contributing factor,[1,8-11] McLaughlin's study is one of a few which address collagen changes as a result of immobility in the frozen shoulder. Recent research documents that changes in periarticular connective tissue collagen result from immobilization. The effects of immobilization and its relationship to frozen shoulder will be addressed later.

Simmonds[12] in 1949, like Codman, proposed that patients with frozen shoulder exhibited inflammation in the rotator cuff, particularly in the supraspinatus tendon. Inflammation of the supraspinatus tendon is secondary to degenerative changes in the tendon caused by impaired blood supply as the tendon is repeatedly traumatized by rubbing against the acromion process and cora-coacromial ligament. Histological examination of four patients with frozen shoulder confirmed the above clinical findings, showing evidence of degeneration of the supraspinatus tendon with hyperemia, a definite inflammatory reaction.

Similarly, Macnab[13] in 1973, illustrated that degenerative changes in the supraspinatus occurred first at the zone of impaired blood supply where the tendon passes over the humeral head. This area is relatively avascular, as the humeral head pressure on the tendon "wrings out" the blood vessels. The lack of circulation in this area could cause degeneration of the supraspinatus tendon. The degeneration process produces a local irritation of the tendon. In response to tissue inflammation, the body produces antibodies affecting the adjacent rotator cuff tendons. This autoimmune reaction produces a diffuse capsulitis or frozen shoulder.

Lippmann[14] in 1943, confirmed both Schrager and Pasteur's theory that bicipital tenosynovitis preceded frozen shoulder. In examining 12 surgical cases of frozen shoulder, Lippmann consistently found tenosynovitis of the long head of the biceps tendon. The tendon sheath was typically thickened and edematous, and the tendon was roughened and adherent to the sheath. In fact, Lippmann proposed that the progression of the frozen shoulder could be determined by the extent of tendinous adhesion: the more advanced the condition, the more adherent the tendon. He attributed stiffness of the shoulder to the upward spread of the tenosynovitis into the shoulder joint, causing adherence of the intracapsular tendon to the capsule and the articular surface of the humeral head. Ultimately, the intracapsular tendon would disintegrate and gradual improvement of shoulder function would occur.

Turek[15] theorized that continual trauma of the rotator cuff and biceps tendon as they are forced against the acromial arch results in degeneration and edema. The tendons thicken as a result, creating a barrier to humeral head movement under the arch. If trauma persists, healing by granulation tissue results in fibrous adhesions of the biceps tendon, the rotator cuff, subacromial bursa, capsule, humeral head, and acromion. The result is loss of motion at the glenohumeral joint.

DePalma[16] stated that the pathologic process of frozen shoulder primarily involves the fibrous capsule. The normally flexible capsule becomes nonelastic and shrunken. The mechanism responsible for these changes is unknown. As the condition progresses, the synovial fluid, fascial covering, rotator cuff, biceps tendon, its sheath, and the subacromial bursa can all become involved. DePalma has observed involvement of these structures in various stages of frozen shoulder.[16] In the early stages, the capsule becomes contracted, with loss of the inferior capsular fold. In the later phases, increased capsular fibrosis occurs. The synovial membrane becomes thickened and hypervascular. These tissues lose their elasticity and easily tear as the humerus is rotated or abducted. The coracohumeral ligament becomes a thick, contracted cord as it spans the tuberosities to the coracoid process. The subscapularis tendon also becomes fibrotic, thereby limiting shoulder external rotation. In addition to the subscapularis, the supraspinatus and infraspinatus are also tight, resulting in restricted glenohumeral motion as the head is held high in the glenoid by these fibrotic tendons, thereby limiting downward humeral excursion. The biceps tendon was found to be adhered to the sheath and the groove. Like Lippmann,[14] DePalma[16] speculates that once the gliding mechanism of the biceps tendon is gone as the tendon becomes anchored to the humerus by adhesions, shoulder function begins to return.

Cyriax,[17] like Neviaser[3] states that the term frozen shoulder is misused and abused. Cyriax says that "frozen" describes a symptom of stiffness. According to Cyriax, frozen shoulder is "arthritis," which implies that the entire glenohumeral joint capsule is affected, limiting both active and passive movement.

For clarity's sake, I will explain a point of Cyriax's examination of the shoulder which ultimately will help to clarify the pathology and definition of frozen shoulder. Cyriax[17] has contributed to a very thorough examination process of the shoulder that is used by many physical therapists. His examination includes selective tension testing of the shoulder complex whereby different structures are stressed by active, passive, and resisted motions to determine the site of the lesion. Both contractile elements (muscle, tendon, tendoperiosteal unit, and musculoperiosteal unit) and noncontractile or inert elements (ligaments, synovial membrane, joint capsule, articular surfaces, bursa, dura, fascia, nerve root, and fat pads) are tested.

In the examination, active shoulder motion is initially tested. Although active motion may incriminate both contractile and noncontractile elements, the results, when correlated with passive and resistive testing, frequently can give additional information about the soft tissue lesion. Second, passive shoulder motion is tested to evaluate the inert tissues, since the contractile elements are totally relaxed during passive testing. Last, with resisted shoulder motion, only the contractile elements are evaluated, since the tests are performed isometrically, thus preventing joint movement. Based on this exam procedure, Cyriax has observed that patients with "arthritis" causing glenohumeral stiffness have pain and limitation of movement with active and passive testing only. Resisted testing is negative, thereby ruling out any of the contractile structures previously mentioned as the cause of frozen shoulder.

Limitation in both active and passive glenohumeral movement has been observed by others.[8,9,18–20] Cyriax[17] further clarifies that arthritis exhibits limitation of passive motion in characteristic proportions—what he calls the capsular pattern. The capsular pattern of frozen shoulder is most limited in external rotation, followed by abduction, then by internal rotation. Both Neviaser[3] and Kozin[18] noted limitations in these same motions. Others observed loss of glenohumeral movement in all directions[12,15,21,22]; in external rotation and abduction only[23]; and in abduction, external rotation, and flexion.[24]

Reeves[25] substantiated the capsular pattern in arthrograms of 17 patients with frozen shoulder. He consistently noted that more contrast dye was deposited posteriorly than in any other areas of the joint capsule and that the joint capacity was grossly reduced and the inferior capsular fold, subscapularis bursa, and biceps sheath were obliterated. Therefore, based on the arthrokinematics of shoulder motion, it follows that if the anterior capsule were more contracted than the posterior capsule, external rotation would be more limited than internal rotation. In addition, abduction would be limited by the loss of the inferior redundant fold and limited external rotation.

Scientific research and clinical observation point to capsular adhesions as the cause of the glenohumeral stiffness in frozen shoulder. Therefore, frozen shoulder will be defined as a shoulder condition in which active and passive motion is painful and restricted at the glenohumeral joint. Passive mobility is limited in a capsular pattern, with external rotation being limited most, followed by abduction, and then internal rotation. This however, does not rule out that the patient with frozen shoulder may have had a contractile structure initially involved, as pointed out by the authors previously mentioned. The frozen shoulder may indeed be the end result of such a lesion.[16] According to this working definition, however, a frozen shoulder does not exhibit objective findings of a contractile lesion unless the lesion is concurrent with a noncontractile capsular lesion.

In summary, various pathologies have been outlined as characteristic in frozen shoulder, including both inert and contractile elements of the shoulder. Based primarily on the work of Neviaser[3] and Cyriax[17], the frozen shoulder will be defined as glenohumeral stiffness resulting from capsular restrictions.

Etiology

Although much has been reported on the pathogenesis of frozen shoulder, its exact cause remains unknown. However, certain factors—pain, disuse, and a periarthritic personality—are considered to contribute to the development of frozen shoulder.

Pain in the shoulder can result from various intrinsic and extrinsic sources.[10,26–28] Whatever the source, pain usually forces the patient to protect the arm from use. Immobilization of a synovial joint has been shown to have detrimental effects on the periarticular connective tissue.[29–36]

Lundberg[37] examined the synovial membrane and fibrous layer of the anterior–inferior capsule of 14 frozen and 13 normal shoulders. He found an increased amount of hexosamine in the frozen shoulder as compared with normal shoulders. This difference was caused by an increase in the total content of glycosaminoglycans (GAG), namely an increase in heparan sulfate, chondroitin-6 sulfate, and dermatan sulfate, and a decrease in hyaluronic acid in the frozen shoulders. These changes in GAG content reflect a process of fibrosis occurring in the tissue. There was marked fibroblastic proliferation, indicating remodeling of the collagenous portion of the connective tissue. The cause for the increased collagen production is unknown. The end result of increased fibrosis is a "subsequent loss of biologic properties of the connective tissue" in the shoulder joint, namely "loss of capsular flexibility and toughness."[37]

Therefore, the clinically observed loss of shoulder motion resulting from disuse is definitely the result of underlying capsular connective tissue changes.

The third factor associated with the development of frozen shoulder is that of the periarthritic personality. Some authors[5,8,9,16] state that psychological factors, especially depression, apathy, and emotional stress contribute to frozen shoulder. Patients with periarthritic personalities have a low pain threshold[9]; therefore, any shoulder pain will probably lead to early voluntary immobilization of the extremity. These patients take no active role in any treatment such as exercise for shoulder pain[9] and therefore are more likely to develop a more severe case of frozen shoulder. Wright and Haq[38] however, tested 186 patients with frozen shoulder and found no such personality.

Clinical Features

In the literature, a few clinical features appear consistently in patients with frozen shoulder. These common observations include arthrographic and x-ray findings, age of onset, type of onset, and course of the condition.

Arthrographic findings appear to be one of the most prevalent characteristics of frozen shoulder. So that the abnormal arthrogram may be better understood, the normal shoulder arthrogram is discussed first. The joint capsule normally attaches to the humeral head just proximal to the greater tuberosity, then extends medially at the level of the anatomic neck of the humerus and inserts into the bony rim of the glenoid.[39] The redundant fold of the capsule hangs in the axilla (Fig. 5-1). In addition, the shoulder joint can accept 28 to 35 ml of solution, with 16 ml of contrast fluid allowing the best viewing of the normal joint.[39]

In frozen shoulder arthrograms, the contrast dye is injected posteriorly since the capsule is usually contracted superiorly, anteriorly, and inferiorly.[40] Abnormal findings include retraction of the joint capsule away from the greater tuberosity (Fig. 5-2),[38] a ragged and irregular outline of the capsule,[39] and absence of the axillary redundant fold (Fig. 5-2).[41-43] Frequently, there is no filling of the subscapularis bursa and bicipital sheath[41,43,44] and pain is usually experienced as the capacity is reached.

Some authors believe that arthrography is essential in diagnosing frozen shoulder.[45,46] Others find it helpful but not essential to rule out other shoulder lesions in addition to confirming frozen shoulder.[39,41] Arthrography, however, gives no clues to what initiates the capsular changes.

Plain film findings in frozen shoulder are usually negative, except that occasionally they show some osteoporosis from disuse.[22,24,39,40,47,48] Seldom is frozen shoulder encountered in a patient < 40 years of age.[4,11,16,39,40,46,47] Wright and Haq[38] and DePalma[16] speculate that this age coincides with normal degenerative changes of connective tissue, a factor which may precipitate frozen shoulder. Reeves' study[49] confirms that the strength of the anterior inferior capsule and capsular ligament decreases with age, especially in the fifth decade. Some authors associate frozen shoulder with the post-menopausal stage, when

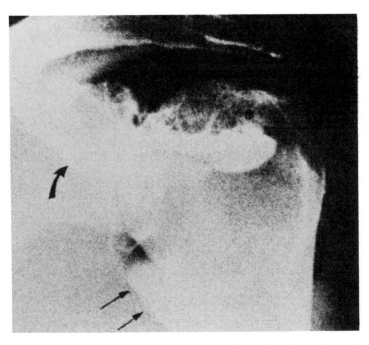

Fig. 5-1. Normal shoulder arthrogram. An external rotation view shows the insertion along the humeral neck, the axillary recess (black arrows), and the subscapularis bursa (black curved arrow). Note that the capsular insertion has a smooth contour. (Goldman A: Shoulder Arthrography. Technique, Diagnosis, and Clinical Correlation, p. 140. Little, Brown, and Co, Boston, 1982.)

hormonal changes may alter connective tissue also.[7] Most studies of frozen shoulder consider the onset to be insidious.[2,11,15,21] Trauma including minor injuries was only occasionally recalled by some patients.[40]

Although many studies describe frozen shoulder as being self-limiting,[12,19,22,50,51] there are very few documented studies of the natural course of frozen shoulder.[21,50] Reeves[21] studied 41 patients with frozen shoulder for 5 to 10 years (average 30 months), always to their greatest recovery. He defined frozen shoulder as an "idiopathic condition of the shoulder characterized by the spontaneous onset of pain with restriction of movement in every direction." He noted three consecutive stages of frozen shoulder: pain, stiffness, and recovery. The early painful period lasted from 10 to 36 weeks in this study. During this stage, arthrographic findings included decreased joint volume and obliteration of the subscapularis bursa and sometimes of the biceps sheath. The painful period gradually subsided but, at the end of this stage, the shoulder capsule was the tightest and the joint capacity was smallest. Treatment during this painful period included resting the extremity in a sling and analgesics.

The second phase was the stiff period, lasting between 4 and 12 months, during which there was no improvement in joint mobility. Treatment included encouraging the patient to use the shoulder but to rest the extremity in a sling

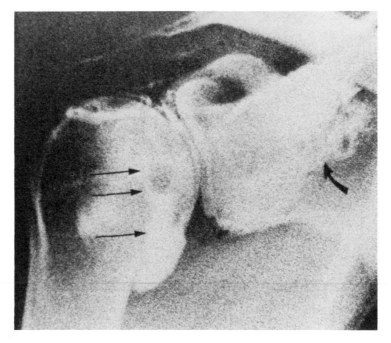

Fig. 5-2. Adhesive capsulitis. The capsule is retracted away from the tuberosities (black arrows). The axillary recess is small, and extravasation has occurred prior to exercise (curved black arrow). (Goldman A: Shoulder Arthrography. Technique, Diagnosis, and Clinical Correlation, p. 141. Little, Brown, and Co, Boston, 1982.)

as discomfort dictated. Pain was generally noted on resumption of activity in this stage.

The last stage noted was spontaneous recovery of motion lasting from 5 months to 2 years and 2 months. Initially, there was a gradual return of external rotation which coincided with the arthrographic reappearance of the subscapular bursa. Next, there was gradual return of abduction and internal rotation. Treatment during this phase was a home exercise program for external rotation and abduction. This is the same phase that DePalma[16] and Lippmann[14] associated with obliteration of the intracapsular bicipital tendon. The total time for greatest recovery was between 1 and 4 years after the onset of symptoms.

One observation gleaned from this study was that the length of the painful period corresponded to the length of the recovery period. A short painful period was associated with a short recovery period, and a long painful period was associated with a long recovery. More than half of the patients[21] were left with permanent loss of shoulder motion, as compared with the uninvolved "normal" shoulder's range of motion (ROM), but had no limitation in any functional activities. Three patients had functional limitations. Reeves' study[21] contradicts other research indicating full recovery or slight loss of motion in 18 to 24 months from the onset of symptoms.[11,15,19,47,50]

Cyriax also classified frozen shoulder into three stages.[17] The first stage exists when the pain is confined to the deltoid area or at least does not extend distal to the elbow, when the patient can lie on the involved extremity at night, when pain is present only with movement, and when the end-feel is elastic. The second stage is present if only some of the criteria in stage one are met. The third stage is characterized by severe pain extending from the shoulder into the forearm and wrist, inability to lie on the involved extremity at night, pain at rest and greatest at night, and an abrupt end-feel. Treatment varies according to the stage of the condition and will be addressed later.

In a small series of 21 patients with frozen shoulder, Simmonds[12] observed that after 3 years only 6 regained normal function, 9 had weakness and pain, and 6 had either weakness or decreased mobility. Gray[50] noted that 24 of 25 patients regained normal glenohumeral motion within 2 years from the onset of symptoms. This success was achieved with treatment of reassurance and occasional simple analgesics and hypnosis.[50] Lipmann and colleagues[47] noted that it is uncommon to outwait the natural course of frozen shoulder without intervention. Simon[22] further emphasizes that simply outwaiting the condition does not assure the patient a full painless ROM.

In addition to the previously mentioned clinical features, others are found with less consistency. Opinion varies on their relationship to the incidence of frozen shoulder. These features include sex, side involved, occupation (manual vs sedentary),[19,38] the presence of immunological factors such as HLA-B27,[45,52,53] serum IgA levels,[54] raised C-reactive protein (CRP) and immune complexes (IC) levels,[53] and association with other diseases (hemiparesis,[23,38] ischemic heart disease, thyroid disease, pulmonary tuberculosis, chronic bronchitis,[38] and diabetes[48,55,56]).

Diabetes and the incidence of frozen shoulder has been under closer scrutiny, with some interesting results. Lequesne and co-workers[48] tested 60 consecutive patients with frozen shoulder and found that 17 of these had diabetes. In a larger sample, Bridgman[55] found that > 10 percent of 800 diabetics had frozen shoulder as compared with 2 percent of 600 nondiabetic control subjects. These authors contend that the prevalence of diabetes in frozen shoulder is significant.

In summary, the onset of frozen shoulder is usually insiduous and occurs in patients > 40 years of age. The course of the condition has been documented to be as long as 10 years. During this time, the level of pain and restriction can vary greatly. Other typical features of frozen shoulder include abnormal arthrograms with marked capsular changes and normal x-rays.

EXAMINATION

A complete description of the examination of the frozen shoulder is beyond the scope of this chapter. Emphasis will be placed on the physical therapist's objective assessment and the way in which findings relate to treatment of frozen shoulder.

Subjective Findings

In my clinical experience, most patients with frozen shoulder have had the condition for several weeks to several months before seeking treatment. When referred to physical therapy, the patient probably has taken or is currently taking a course of anti-inflammatory medication and has used self-treatment with a heating pad, warm showers, aspirin, and rest of the extremity. Pain motivates the patient to seek medical attention,[9,16] as does decreased function of the extremity.[57] Subjectively, the patient complains of a vague, dull pain over the deltoid which increases with motion[2,40,47] and disturbs sleep.[21,23,24,40,47,58] Functionally, the patient will be unable to sleep on the affected side,[2,6,17] hook a brassiere in the back, comb the hair, or reach for a wallet in a back pocket. The patient usually cannot recall an injury and frequently is unable to determine when the pain and/or loss of function began. If the condition is more advanced, the patient may complain of pain spreading from the shoulder down the forearm[12,17] up to the cervical spine and into the ipsilateral scapula, and pain at rest.[17]

These complaints correspond well to Cyriax's stages of capsular lesions. Although Reeves'[21] study documents arthrographic changes in the first and last stages of frozen shoulder, from a practical standpoint Cyriax's division is more clinically applicable. In the patient population that I saw, very few patients were examined arthrographically. It appears that arthrography was reserved for those patients who did not respond to a long-term conservative program of physical therapy and medication. Even if arthrography is performed, Cyriax's stages can also be clinically helpful in treatment planning.

During the interview, it is also important to ask questions concerning the patient's general health in order to assess any other disease process that may be referring pain to the shoulder. The same applies to pertinent questioning concerning the shoulder complex, the cervical spine, and brachial plexus structures, although these areas will be examined.

Objective Findings

Initial observation of the patient frequently reveals a stooped posture with rounded shoulders; the involved extremity is adducted and internally rotated, resting in the patient's lap.[59]

In gait, the arm swing is usually limited or absent on the affected side. A therapist observing the patient disrobe, notices that the patient's shirt is usually removed as though the arm were in a cast. The uninvolved extremity is removed first, with very little movement of the opposite side. The reverse occurs when the patient dresses. The patient usually wears shirts that button down the front and require no overhead action to remove.

The levels of the shoulders are frequently uneven, with the involved side usually elevated in a protective manner. As a result of maintaining this posture, there may be tenderness and trigger points along the ipsilateral upper trapezius, with perceived pain along its course to the suboccipital area. The scapula on the involved side is usually elevated, laterally rotated, and abducted as a result of excessive scapular motion to compensate for the impaired glenohumeral motion. The abnormal scapula position can cause stretch weakness of the rhomboids[59] and levator scapulae tightness, giving rise to local pain. If the condition is longstanding and there has been a long period of disuse, muscle atrophy around the involved shoulder and scapula may be evident.

Because cervical spine dysfunction can refer pain to the shoulder, this area must be assessed.[10,26,27] It is not the objective of this chapter to outline a complete cervical examination, but a few important tests are mentioned. If active cervical ROM is normal, overpressure should be applied at the end of each range.[60] This involves a gentle passive movement at the end of the available range. There should be a slight pain-free increase in the ROM. If active ROM and active ROM with overpressure are negative for provocation of symptoms, the cervical quadrant test can be performed. This involves guiding the head into extension toward one side and then adding cervical rotation to the same side.[60] Gross passive ROM can be performed to rule out any muscular influence in cervical mobility.

Individual cervical segmental mobility should then be tested to ascertain any joint dysfunction. Physical therapists trained in these methods have a variety of testing techniques that can be performed to check segmental mobility in all directions of motion. Cervical compression and traction tests complete the passive cervical spine examination. Additional information concerning the cervical influence on the shoulder pain may be obtained by having the patient elevate the involved shoulder while traction is being applied to the cervical spine and noting if there is any improvement in shoulder pain or ROM.[26] Finally, resistive testing of cervical ROM will provide information concerning the contractile structures of the neck.

The integrity of the brachial plexus must be evaluated in cases of shoulder pain.[26] The standard Addson, hyperabduction, and costoclavicular tests may not be valid with limited shoulder motion. Wells[26] reports a brachial plexus tension test developed by Elvey, an Australian physical therapist, which can adequately be performed in spite of restricted shoulder motion. The reader is encouraged to refer to this text for the details.

Acromioclavicular, sternoclavicular, and scapulothoracic dysfunction and first rib syndrome can also give rise to shoulder pain.[26,61] Acromioclavicular joint pain is usually very localized and can easily be pinpointed by the patient.[17] This local pain differs from the diffuse dull pain common with frozen shoulder. Scapulothoracic dysfunction usually results from excessive scapular compensatory motion and sternoclavicular dysfunction usually results from abnormal shoulder mechanics. First rib dysfunction can result from a variety of problems. The mobility of the sternoclavicular, scapulothoracic,[26,61] acromioclavicular, and first rib[26] should be tested to rule out their involvement in shoulder pain. In summary, careful examination of the cervical spine, brachial plexus, acromioclavicular, sternoclavicular, scapulothoracic joints, and first rib is essential in a complete assessment of shoulder pain.

Much of the remaining objective assessment of the shoulder is based on Cyriax's[17] examination principles. The entire exam is presented because the negative findings are as important as the positive findings in assessing frozen shoulder. All examination procedures mentioned should be performed bilaterally, using the uninvolved extremity as "normal" for the individual who is being assessed.

Twelve movements are included in the examination, and the order of their performance is important. Active motion assesses both contractile and noncontractile elements, passive motion assesses inert structures, and resisted motion assesses contractile structures.

1. Active elevation—Elevation is movement away from the side in the coronal plane, with 180° possible. During active elevation, the patient's willingness to move, the muscular power, and the ROM can be assessed.

2. Passive elevation—The ROM, the location in the range where pain is produced, and the end-feel should be noted. End-feel is the sensation detected by the examiner at the extreme of the passive ROM.[17,62] The normal end-feel of the shoulder is capsular, which is similar to the sensation encountered when "two pieces of tough rubber are squeezed together." There is a firm arrest to movement but some "give" is noted.[17] Both the end-feel and the point in the range where pain is provoked are important in deciding treatment. This will be further discussed in the section stretching as treatment.

3. Painful arc—This can only be tested when 90° of abduction is present actively or passively. Abduction is defined as the amount of movement between the scapula and humerus, with 90° being normal. The patient actively elevates the extremity and notes if there is a painful point in the range bordered on either side by nonpainful motion. The same arc of pain can be felt as the arm is brought down from the elevated position or if elevation is performed passively. A positive finding indicates that a structure is being pinched during the movement.

4. Passive scapulohumeral abduction—The scapula is stabilized at its inferior angle as the therapist passively elevates the extremity, noting when the inferior angle begins to move; 90° is the normal range before the scapula moves.

5. Passive lateral rotation.
6. Passive medial rotation.

> As with passive elevation, ROM, the point in the range at which pain is provoked, and the end-feel should be noted.

7. Resisted adduction.
8. Resisted abduction.
9. Resisted lateral rotation.
10. Resisted medial rotation.
11. Resisted elbow extension.
12. Resisted elbow flexion.

> All resisted tests are performed isometrically. Both pain and muscle weakness are noted.

As previously mentioned confusion occurs when more than one lesion exists. With this concise examination, both contractile and inert structures can be assessed.

In summary, because frozen shoulder is a capsular lesion, active elevation and all passive testing is limited and painful. In addition, limitation of passive movement is in a capsular proportion, with most limitation in external rotation, followed by abduction, then internal rotation.

Further information in determining which areas of the capsule are involved in frozen shoulder can be obtained by assessing motions of glenohumeral joint play. Mennel[61] coined the term and defines joint play as small, involuntary movement essential for normal joint motion. He based this definition on joint mechanics, in which rotations, glides and long axis extension (traction) are normal joint plane motions. Joint play motion is often not more than $\frac{1}{8}$-in movement in any plane. When joint play is lost, joint dysfunction exists. Mennel proposes that manipulation is the preferred treatment to restore joint play.

According to Mennel, there are seven joint play motions at the glenohumeral joint. He recognizes that normal glenohumeral movement depends on normal acromioclavicular, sternoclavicular, and scapulothoracic joint movement. The reader is referred to chapter 1 on mechanics of the shoulder joint for review of this necessary harmony. All of the joint play motions are actually rolls and glides of the humeral head within the glenoid. In the shoulder, where the convex humeral head is moving on the stationary glenoid, roll and glide occur in opposite directions.[62] Any discrepancies in joint play assessment will direct the therapist with a knowledge of normal joint mechanics to the involved area of the capsule. Furthermore, treatment can be directed to these specific areas.

The normal joint play motions of the glenohumeral joint are anterior glide; posterior glide; lateral glide; inferior and posterior glide, lateral and posterior glide, and external rotation of the humeral head within the glenoid fossa; and posterior glide of the humeral head within the glenoid fossa with the shoulder flexed to 90°.[61] Although the above joint play motions are assessment techniques, they are also treatment techniques which can be used to restore normal shoulder mechanics by stretching the involved portions of the capsule. This will be discussed in the treatment section.

All joint play motions can be quantified using a 0-6 scale.[63] Although the assessment of joint play is subjective, grading the movement allows easy documentation of the motion. Again, the uninvolved extremity should be tested to assess ''normal'' for the patient. Zero grade indicates no joint movement as in an ankylosed joint; a grade of 1-a indicates marked loss of motion; 2, a slight limitation in motion; 3, normal mobility; 4, a slight increase in mobility; 5, a marked increase in motion; and 6, joint instability. In frozen shoulder with capsular restrictions, grade 1 and 2 will be encountered most frequently.

A final examination tool is palpation. Cyriax[17] cautions that palpation gives very little information and is often irritable to the involved structures. For these reasons, palpation is reserved until the very end of the exam. In frozen shoulder, palpatory findings are generally negative. There may be tenderness over the acromioclavicular joint as a result of improper shoulder mechanics. In addition, any secondary muscular involvement resulting from posture or abnormal scapular motion may exhibit painful trigger points. In a contractile lesion coexisting with frozen shoulder, there will probably be tenderness over the lesioned structure.

Although this evaluation is lengthy, it is imperative that an accurate assessment of the shoulder lesion be made. Proper treatment is based on an accurate assessment.[24,61,64]

TREATMENT

Prevention is the best treatment of frozen shoulder.[19,40] Although there is little agreement on its treatment when it occurs, there is agreement on the treatment goals: pain relief and restoration of normal shoulder movement.[51,65] Unfortunately, few controlled studies in the literature examine treatment of frozen shoulder. One of the problems in studies of frozen shoulder is the variable patient selection due to the variable definitions of what frozen shoulder constitutes. Another problem, so frequently encountered in any human subject study, is the ethics of the necessity of an untreated control group.

Hazleman[51] studied 130 cases of frozen shoulder retrospectively and found no difference in treatment of local corticosteroid injections, physical therapy consisting of pendulum and pulley exercises with shortwave diathermy, or manipulation under anesthesia. Binder and colleagues[66] followed 42 patients with frozen shoulder for 8 months and found no long-term difference in treatment by intraarticular steroids, Maitland-type passive mobilization, ice, or no treatment. Hamer and Kirk[67] documented no significant advantage in ice or ultrasound treatments, but both were beneficial in decreasing the painful stage and hastening recovery. Lee and co-workers[68] found no difference in patients who received local hydrocortisone and exercises or infrared irradiation and exercises. However, both groups receiving exercises did significantly better than patients receiving analgesics alone.

Biswas and colleagues[57] found that patients receiving intraarticular hydrocortisone, shortwave diathermy, and aspirin as well as active and passive mobilization exercises all benefited. Furthermore, these authors concluded that exercise is the most important treatment in frozen shoulder. Liang and Lien[69] found no difference in active exercises when combined with intraarticular injection and heat (shortwave diathermy, ultrasound, or moist heat), with heat alone, or injection alone. Similarly, they concluded that exercises were probably the only useful treatment for frozen shoulder. Risk[70] and colleagues found that transcutaneous electrical nerve stimulation (TENS) with prolonged pulley traction was superior to a variety of heat modalities and exercises. Pothmann and others[71] found that one acupuncture treatment of point ST-38 cured acute frozen shoulder.

Fig. 5-3. TENS electrode placement for frozen shoulder. (1A) In depression bordered by the acromion laterally, spine of scapula posteriorly, and clavicle anteriorly; acupuncture point LI 16. (1B) Insertion of deltoid at lateral aspect of arm; acupuncture point LI 14, (channel 1). (2A) In depression below acromion anteriorly; acupuncture point LI 15. (2B) In depression below acromion posteriorly; acupuncture point TW 14, (channel 2). (Modified from Mannheimer J, Lampe G: Clinical TENS. p. 477. F.A. Davis Co, Philadelphia, 1948.)

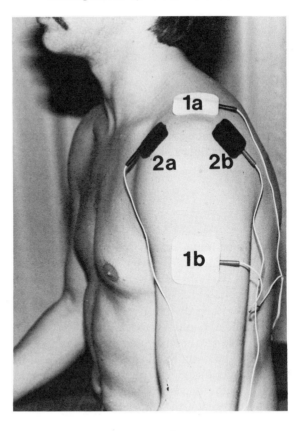

Transcutaneous Electrical Nerve Stimulation

Various treatments can be used to achieve the goals of pain relief and restoration of mobility, but documentation of their effectiveness in frozen shoulder is lacking. TENS can be used to decrease the symptoms of pain in both the early and later stages of frozen shoulder. Figure 5-3 illustrates an effective TENS application for frozen shoulder.[72] The analgesia provided by TENS allows other therapeutic procedures such as exercises to be performed more comfortably. For maximal effectiveness, the TENS should be applied before and/or during the exercises.[72] Decreasing the pain during stretching of the frozen shoulder will gain the confidence of the patient as well as facilitate joint relaxation, which is essential for passive joint manipulation.

TENS is significantly more effective in reducing the acute pain.[72] Therefore, TENS is an excellent treatment choice when the patient is in too acute a stage for active treatment. Such is the case in stage three of frozen shoulder as defined by Cyriax.[17] If TENS can reduce the discomfort, the patient will use the extremity more and probably avoid the stiffening results of disuse.

Other useful acupuncture points which can be used as electrode sites for TENS include a combination of ST 38 and UB 57 or a combination of LI 15, SI 10, GB 34, and LI 11.[73] (See ref. 73 for exact point location.)

Heat

Heat application is a very common treatment used to decrease pain and increase soft tissue extensibility. A variety of modalities including shortwave and microwave diathermy, ultrasound, moist packs, paraffin baths, whirlpools, and infrared irradiation create hyperthermia in the tissue.[72] The result of hyperthermia is increased circulation and vasodilation to the tissues.[72] Other authors recommend heating the joint capsule prior to stretching, since the increased circulation acts as an analgesic.[17] The analgesic effect, however, tends to be temporary.[72]

Ultrasound

Ultrasound research in frozen shoulder began in the 1950s when ultrasound was a new form of therapy. Mueller and colleagues[74] found that ultrasound at 2 W/cm^2 was of no value in treating subacute frozen shoulder. Quin[75] found no difference in groups receiving ultrasound at 0.5 W/cm^2 and exercises and those receiving diathermy and exercises.

Clinically, ultrasound is used for its thermal and mechanical effects on tissue.[75] In frozen shoulder, it is often used prior to stretching of the capsule. Because the sound waves are so focal, the therapist must be very specific as to the target tissue.[76] With the inferior capsule so frequently involved in frozen shoulder, the extremity may need to be positioned in abduction and external rotation to reach the inferior portion effectively. Similarly, any portion of the capsule can be treated specifically with proper positioning of the joint. The therapist may also put the target capsule on stretch as ultrasound is applied.

A home program of heat prior to exercises can be helpful, especially when the patients can exercise with less discomfort. Warm showers and warm moist compresses are easily applied. Heating pads, especially those with a moist heat feature, are useful as long as the patient does not apply a pad for long periods.[64] Patients frequently abuse heating pads by falling asleep with them. Even with the pad on the lowest setting, the patient should be strictly instructed to apply it only for short intervals. Most of us have seen the mottled skin of a patient who has abused the heating pad.

Cryotherapy

Cryotherapy, like heat application, produces increased circulation and vasodilation to the area. There is however, an intial vasoconstriction with cold application.[72] Ice packs, ice massage, ice whirlpools, and vapocoolant sprays are all effective cold treatments.

Ice packs can easily be constructed at home with a plastic bag. A proportional amount of rubbing alcohol added to ice keeps it from refreezing solidly. Convincing a patient to use ice at home—especially one who thrives on warm showers and a heating pad—is often difficult. Ice, like heat, prior to exercises will help the patient perform with less pain. Pain after exercises for > 1 to 2 hours[17] is abnormal. Ice can prove beneficial in reducing any post-exercise soreness.

In the acute phase, when the extremity is generally rested, ice for its analgesic effect is very useful. In addition, if there is a concurrent lesion such as a rotator cuff tendinitis or bicipital tenosynovitis, ice can combat the inflammation and edema, thereby decreasing pain. With lessened pain, the patient will be more willing to use the extremity and prevent subsequent stiffness.

Exercise

Exercise is the most useful treatment in frozen shoulder.[57,69] In the acute stage or stage three as defined by Cyriax,[17] all active treatment is contraindicated. Treatment in this stage should be directed at pain relief. As mentioned, rest, ice, and TENS are helpful at this time. In the subacute stage or stage two, exercises both active and passive may be cautiously initiated, but the patient's reaction must be constantly monitored. Increased pain or pain lasting > 2 hours after exercises is abnormal.[17] In stage one, active and passive exercises can usually safely and vigorously be performed. A good physical therapist must be able to judge when to initiate exercise, the amount and vigor of exercises, and when the patient is aggravated by exercise. Experience helps in this decision making, but each patient is different and must be individually evaluated.

Other guidelines to determine when and to what degree of exercise should be used can be based on the end-feel and the pain and resistance sequence.[17] An end-feel other than the capsular resistance is abnormal at the shoulder. With the limited range of frozen shoulder, the end-feel is still capsular only in that it will occur at the end of the reduced ROM.

During passive motion testing, both the location of pain in the range and the end-feel where noted.[17] Combining these two factors will indicate the severity of the condition, thereby guiding treatment. If during passive movement the patient perceives pain before the therapist reaches the end of range, the joint is probably acute and active exercises are contraindicated. During this situation, the therapist will obviously not have a chance to evaluate the end-feel, but this can be done in subsequent visits as the pain subsides. If pain is experienced as the end of range is reached, the patient is less acute and exercises may be cautiously attempted. If exercises exacerbate the pain, they should be delayed. Last, if the end of the limited range is reached and no pain is provoked, exercises will probably be tolerated without problems.[17]

In summary, certain factors can help the therapist determine when and what exercises are indicated for the patient with frozen shoulder. The three stages as outlined by Cyriax, the end-feel, and the pain/resistance sequence are three such guides.[17] A good therapist will pace the patient through a graded active and passive exercise program and constantly reassess the effect of the program on pain and stiffness.

Manipulation

Manipulation, or mobilization as it is frequently called, is a form of passive exercise designed to restore joint play motions of roll, glide, and joint separation.[61] Very few controlled studies involve joint manipulation in the treatment of frozen shoulder. Bulgen and co-workers[77] found no superiority of Maitland-type manipulative techniques in patients with frozen shoulder for > 1 month over treatment with ice, intraarticular steroid injections, or no treatment. In fact, after 6 weeks of treatment, the group receiving manipulation had greater loss of motion than did the other groups. Bulgen and co-workers explain that the detrimental effect of physical therapy occurred when manipulation was performed during the active stage, an error that must be avoided.[77]

For normal shoulder function, all areas of the capsule must be extensible to allow joint play motion. Capsular extensibility depends on friction-free sliding of the collagen fibers within the capsule.[29] Hyaluronic acid with water is the lubricant between the collagen fibers[29,78,79] that allows this free gliding to occur.

Lundberg's study of the capsular changes in frozen shoulder revealed a marked increase in fibroblastic formation of collagen, a loss of hyaluronic acid, and an increase in sulfated GAGs.[37] The newly formed collagen in the capsule depends on motion for proper alignment and deposition. Without movement, the new collagen is laid down in a haphazard manner. Abnormal collagen deposition occurs between the newly synthesized fibril and preexisting collagen fibers[29] resulting in a mechanical block to collagen movement. Multiple adhesions between collagen fibrils and fibers is manifested as joint stiffness. In addition, with the decrease in hyaluronic acid, the lubricant between the fibers is lost, contributing to further impairment of free collagen movement.

Based on these considerations, it seems reasonable to assume that movement of the joint will prevent or limit adhesive formation. Although this is not documented, movement to prevent adhesions is a clinical goal of exercise. In the event that capsular adhesions have formed, manipulation can be used to break the adhesions and restore joint play. Further research is obviously needed in this area.

It is beyond the scope of this chapter to outline every manipulative technique for frozen shoulder. Demonstrations can be found in the texts of Maitland,[60] Mennel,[61] and Kaltenborn.[63] Techniques for each area of the shoulder capsule, acromioclavicular, sternoclavicular, and scapulothoracic joints are illustrated here. The physical therapist benefits by becoming as familiar with as many techniques as possible to afford better treatment to their patients. Any of the techniques illustrated can be adapted as oscillatory or static stretching techniques and can be performed in any part of the range. The goal of treatment, whether for pain relief or increasing ROM, will influence the choice of treatment technique. The mobilization techniques are illustrated in Chapter 12.

Cervical as well as shoulder pain may be present. This may result from overuse of the upper trapezius and levator scapula with excessive scapular elevation to compensaate for the loss of glenohumeral motion.[59] The upper

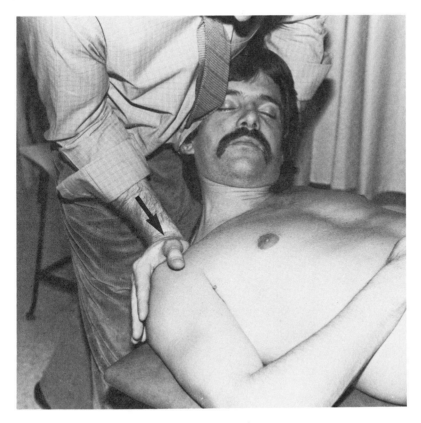

Fig. 5-4. Upper trapezius stretch.

trapezius and levator scapula are usually shortened and will need treatment to decrease pain and restore normal physiological length. Any of the physical modalities are useful to decrease pain. Massage is relaxing as well as beneficial in moving any excessive fluid accumulation. It also can assist in mobilizing the soft tissue. Stretching of the upper trapezius can be done in a number of ways. Figure 5-4 illustrates a passive upper trapezius stretch.

Patient position: Supine with the head off the edge of the table.

Therapist position: Left hand under the occiput with the head on the forearm stabilizing the head and neck in the desired amount of flexion and sidebending left and rotation right. Right palm over the clavicle and scapula medial to the acromioclavicular joint.

Technique: Left hand maintains head and neck position. Right hand pushes the clavicle and scapula inferiorly.

In a good home exercise for stretching the upper trapezius, the patient simply reaches behind the back and grasps the involved distal humerus. The patient should sidebend and rotate away from the involved side and flex the neck to a comfortable position. Once positioned, the stretch is imparted by pulling downward on the involved humerus.

Frequently, pain may be provoked while the shoulder is being manipulated. Although such pain is not desirable, it is often difficult to manipulate a frozen shoulder without some discomfort to the patient. "Shaking" the extremity and momentary pauses will help decrease pain and maintain patient relaxation.[59] Simple gentle shaking of the extremity while in any position will stimulate the joint mechanoreceptors and decrease nociceptive input.[80]

Both Maitland[60] and Kaltenborn[63] offer guidelines to the amount of manipulation to perform in one session. Reassessment is important before and during each treatment session. Treatment can continue as long as pain is decreased and motion is improved.[63] Overtreating can cause increased pain and inflammatory reactions[59] and may push the patient into an acute stage. The therapist should progress slowly until familiar with the patient's response to treatment. It is well documented that the course of frozen shoulder is slow[21,50]; therefore, the therapist should not expect too much improvement too quickly. A patient who is informed that improvement will be slow will be less frustrated.

Liebolt[81] has recommended four passive stretches which, performed over a period of time, will increase shoulder ROM in frozen shoulder. The four exercises are glenohumeral abduction, external rotation, flexion with external rotation, and flexion performed at the end of the available ROM. These exercises, however, do not deal with the loss of joint play. I have found that these exercises in the cardinal planes often provoke pain and do little to increase ROM.

Mechanical exercises with shoulder wheels, pulleys, and wands are often standard exercises in treating frozen shoulder. Unfortunately, like the stretching in the cardinal plane, these do not address the loss of joint play. Murray[59] outlines three disadvantages of the overhead pulley system: (1) there is no stabilization of the scapula to avoid excessive abduction and upward rotation, (2) there is no force to depress the humeral head, and (3) there is a tendency for the patient to extend the spine to decrease glenohumeral motion. These same three points are applicable to the shoulder wheel, finger ladder, and wand exercises. To improve the use of these apparatuses, stabilization of the scapula can be improved by placing a strap around the scapula and the chair. The therapist or a reliable family member who has been taught the exercises can depress the humeral head while using the apparatus. Last, the patient can be instructed to keep his spine flat against the chair while performing these exercises. Despite these efforts to improve the exercises, Murray[59] contends that these apparatuses should be used only when normal gliding is present.

Active exercises allow more patient control than do mechanical exercises. Active exercises are essential in maintaining the capsular extensibility obtained through manipulation. They are best performed in a pain-free range to prevent any inflammatory reaction by forcing joint movement. The same principles of mechanical exercises apply to forced active exercises; that is, the active range will not be available if normal joint play is lacking.

Codman or pendulum[7] exercises performed with gravity are usually pain-free. With the patient bent at the waist and the extremity dangling, the weight of the extremity produces joint separation and eliminates a fulcrum at the glenoid or acromion with movement.[7] With traction at the joint, the patient will usually find the exercises more comfortable. For additional traction, the patient can grasp a light weight, such as an iron. The exercises include forward and backward, medial to lateral, and circular motions made with the entire extremity. The object is have the patient increase the arc of movement within a painful ROM.

Cardinal plane or diagonal active motion can be performed as a home program if the necessary joint play movements are available. Home exercise programs should be kept simple and to a minimum, requiring no special equipment, so the patient will comply with the program, which in frozen shoulder is usually a long course. The number of repetitions as well as the vigor will have to be determined for each patient. As mentioned, for their analgesic effects, preparatory heat or ice may be used prior to performance of exercises.

Last, muscle reeducation and strengthening may be needed to restore normal physiological balance to the entire shoulder complex and cervical spine. "Muscles cannot be restored to normal if the joints which they move are not free to move."[61] Because there is often excessive scapular motion, stabilization exercises to the scapular area can be performed before full glenohumeral motion is restored. Otherwise, I do not advise strengthening exercises until near normal ROM is achieved. This will avoid strengthening a muscle in a shortened range that may impede the restoration of motion.

Isometric, isotonic, both concentric and eccentric, isokinetic, free-weights, and PNF are all useful in restoring muscle strength. Various exercise equipment such as Cybex, Universal, and Nautilus are frequently commonplace in many health clubs, and individual programs should be developed for the patients. After pain abates and ROM is restored, most patients will not continue physical therapy for a strengthening program. Therefore, intermittent follow-up visits should be made to review and alter the exercise program as needed and to assess the patient's progress.

CONCLUSION

In summary, a physical therapy treatment course for a frozen shoulder may include preparatory modalities to decrease pain, passive manipulation, muscle reeducation and strengthening, and a home exercise program. The course is long and often tedious to both the patient and therapist since progress is very slow. The goal of treatment is the restoration of normal pain-free shoulder function.

Cortisone injections and manipulation under anesthesia are two other common treatments for frozen shoulder. The literature is filled with arguments for and against manipulations under anesthesia.[82–88] The same varied opinions are documented for treatment by cortisone injection.[65,89–91]

Various manipulative procedures are described in the literature. A common caution, however, is to use short lever arms with very gentle force to avoid injury, such as a fractured humerus. Arthrographic studies following manipulation under anesthesia show that the adherent inferior fold of the capsule is torn, allowing the dye to escape into the axillary space and along the medial humerus.[41,42] Some authors reported rotator cuff tears following manipulation under anesthesia,[43] whereas others did not find any tears of the cuff.[42]

Clinically, if a patient has been treated with manipulation, it is helpful to know the ROM obtained and the complications, if any, that were encountered during the procedure. It is very common for a patient to have less motion following manipulation even if therapy is initiated immediately. This may be owing to an acute inflammatory reaction and muscle splinting due to pain. Pain is frequently increased for several days following manipulation. TENS and ice are very helpful in this stage. Exercises are essential following manipulation under anesthesia. The therapist frequently sees the patient four times a day in the hospital beginning the day of the procedure. Reassurance and encouragement are needed to motivate the patient to exercise in the presence of pain.

The physical therapist should be aware of the location, number, and frequency of cortisone injections administered to the patient. Because of reports of spontaneous tendon ruptures following multiple injection, care should be exercised with these patients.

Other treatments in the literature include a combination of manipulation under anesthesia and cortisone and arthrographic joint distention to rupture capsular adhesions. Knowledge of any procedure performed on the patient enhances treatment decisions.

In summary, this chapter has presented the varied theories on pathogenesis, definition, etiology, clinical features, and treatment of the frozen shoulder. Physical therapy management, including physical modalities and passive and active exercises, have been presented. Further research in all of the above areas is needed to prevent and better treat the common musculoskeletal complain of frozen shoulder.

ACKNOWLEDGMENT

I wish to thank Rita K. Owens, B.S., P.T., for assistance in the preparation of the manuscript, and William Boissonnault, M.S., P.T., and Steve Janos, M.S., P.T., for their assistance with the photographs.

REFERENCES

1. Bateman J: The Shoulder and Neck. WB Saunders Co, Philadelphia, 1978
2. Neviaser JS: Adhesive capsulitis and the stiff and painful shoulder. Orthop Clin North Am 11:327, 1980

3. Neviaser JS: Adhesive capsulitis of the shoulder: study of pathological findings in periarthritis of the shoulder. J Bone Joint Surg 27:211, 1945

4. Meulengracht E, Schwartz M: The course and prognosis of periarthrosis humeroscapularis with special regard to cases with general symptoms. Acta Med Scand 143:350, 1952

5. McLaughlin HL: The "frozen shoulder." Clin Orthop 20:126, 1961

6. Rizk TE, Pinals RS: Frozen shoulder. Semin Arthritis Rheum 11:440, 1982

7. Codman EA: The Shoulder. Robert E Kreiger Publishing Co, Malabar, FL, 1934

8. Coventry MB: The problem of the painful shoulder. J Am Med Assoc 151:177, 1953

9. Cailliet R: Shoulder Pain. 2nd Ed. FA Davis Co, Philadelphia, 1981

10. Neviaser RJ: Painful conditions affecting the shoulder. Clin Orthop 173:63, 1983

11. Thompson M: The frozen shoulder and shoulder-hand syndromes. Practioner 189:380, 1962

12. Simmonds FA: Shoulder Pain with particular reference to the "frozen" shoulder. J Bone Joint Surg 31B:426, 1949

13. Macnab I: Rotator cuff tendinitis. Ann R Coll Surg Engl 53:271, 1973

14. Lippmann RK: Frozen shoulder; periarthritis; bicipital tenosynovitis. Arch Surg 47:283, 1943

15. Turek S: Orthopaedics. Principles and their Application. JB Lippincott Co, Philadelphia, 1977

16. DePalma AF: Surgery of the Shoulder. JB Lippincott Co, Philadelphia, 1983

17. Cyriax J: Textbook of Orthopaedic Medicine. 7th Ed. Vol 1. Bailliere Tindall, London, 1978

18. Kozin F: Two unique shoulder disorders. Adhesive capsulitis and reflex sympathetic dystrophy syndrome. Postgrad Med 73:207, 1983

19. Jayson MV: Frozen Shoulder: adhesive capsulitis. Br Med J 283:1003, 1981

20. Morgensen E: Painful shoulder. Aetiological and pathogenetic problems. Acta Med Scand 155:195, 1956

21. Reeves B: The natural history of the frozen shoulder syndrome. Scand J Rheumatol 4:193, 1975

22. Simon WH: Soft tissue disorders of the shoulder. Frozen shoulder, calcific tendinitis, and bicipital tendinitis. Orthop Clin North Am 6:521, 1975

23. Bruckner FE, Nye CJS: A prospective study of adhesive capsulitis of the shoulder ('frozen shoulder') in a high risk population. Quart J Med 198:191, 1981

24. Flicker PL: The painful shoulder. Primary Care 7:271, 1980

25. Reeves B: Arthrographic changes in frozen shoulder and post-traumatic stiff shoulders. Proc Soc Med 59:827, 1966

26. Wells P: Cervical dysfunction and shoulder problems. Physiotherapy 68:66, 1982

27. Leach RE, Schepsis AA: Shoulder pain. Clin Sports Med 2:123, 1983

28. Neviaser JS: Musculoskeletal disorders of the shoulder region causing cervicobrachial pain. Differential diagnosis and treatment. Surg Clin North Am 43:1703, 1963

29. Akeson WH, Amiel D, LaViolette D: The connective tissue response to immobility: a study of the chondroitin 4- and 6-sulphate and dermatan sulphate changes in periarticular connective tissue of control and immobilized knees of dogs. Clin Orthop 51:183, 1967

30. Akeson WH, Amiel D, LaViolette D, et al: The connective tissue response to immobility: an accelerated aging response. Exp Gerontol 3:289, 1968

31. Akeson WH, Amiel D, Mechanic GL, et al: Collagen crosslinking alterations in joint contractures: changes in reducible crosslinks in periarticular connective tissue collagen after nine weeks of immobilization. Connect Tissue Res 5:5, 1977

32. Akeson WH, Amiel D, Woo S: Immobility effects of synovial joints: the patho-mechanics of joint contracture. Biorheology 17:95, 1980
33. Enneking W, Horowitz M: The intra-articular effects of immobilization on the human knee. J Bone Joint Surg 54A:973, 1972
34. Evans E, Eggers G, Butler J, et al: Immobilization and remobilization of rats' knee joints. J Bone Joint Surg 42A:737, 1960
35. LaVigne A, Watkins R: Preliminary results on immobilization: induced stiffness of monkey knee joints and posterior capsule. Perspectives in Biomedical Engineering. Proceedings of a symposium of Biological Engineering Society, University of Strathclyde, Glasgow, June 1972. University Park Press, Baltimore, 1973
36. Woo S, Matthews JV, Akeson WH, et al: Connective tissue response to immobility: correlative study of biomechanical and biochemical measurements of normal and immobilized rabbit knees. Arthritis Rheum 18:257, 1975
37. Lundberg BJ: Glycosaminoglycans of the normal and frozen shoulder—joint cap-sule. Clin Orthop 69:279, 1970
38. Wright V, Haq AMMM: Periarthritis of the shoulder. Aetiological considerations with particular reference to personality factors. Ann Rheum Dis 35:213, 1976
39. Goldman A: Shoulder Arthrography. Technique, Diagnosis, and Clinical Correla-tion. Little, Brown, and Co, Boston, 1982
40. Neviaser JS: Adhesive capsulitis of the shoulder (frozen shoulder). Med Times 90:783, 1962
41. Neviaser JS: Arthrography of the Shoulder. The Diagnosis and Management of the Lesions Visualized. Charles C Thomas, Springfield, Ill, 1975
42. Lundberg BJ: Arthrography and manipulation in rigidity of the shoulder joint. Acta Orthop Scand 36:35, 1965
43. Samilson RL, Raphael L, Post L, et al: Arthrography of the shoulder joint. Clin Orthop 20:21, 1961
44. Neviaser JS: Arthrography of the shoulder joint. Study of the findings in adhesive capsulitis of the shoulder. J Bone Joint Surg 44A:1321, 1962
45. Rizk TE, Christopher RP, Pinals RS, et al: Arthrographic studies in painful hem-iplegic shoulder. Arch Phys Med Rehabil 65:254, 1984
46. Loyd JA, Loyd HM: Adhesive capsulitis of the shoulder: arthrographic diagnosis and treatment. South Med J 76:879, 1983
47. Lipmann K, Bayley I, Young A: The upper limb. The frozen shoulder. Br J Hosp Med 25:334, 1981
48. Lequesne M, Dang N, Bensasson M, et al: Increased association of diabetes mellitus with capsulitis of the shoulder and shoulder-hand syndrome. Scand J Rheumatol 6:53, 1977
49. Reeves B: Experiments on the tensile strength of the anterior capsular structures of the shoulder in man. J Bone Joint Surg 50B:858, 1968
50. Gray RG: The natural history of "idiopathic" frozen shoulder. J Bone Joint Surg 60B:564, 1978
51. Hazleman BL: The painful stiff shoulder. Rheumatol Phys Med 11:413, 1972
52. Bulgen DY, Hazleman BL, Voak D: HLA-B27 and frozen shoulder. Lancet 1:1042, 1976
53. Bulgen DY, Binder A, Hazleman BL, et al: Immunological studies in frozen shoul-der. J Rheumatol 9:893, 1982
54. Bulgen DY, Hazleman B, Ward M, et al. Immunological studies in frozen shoulder. Ann Rheum Dis 37:135, 1978
55. Bridgman JF: Periarthritis of the shoulder and diabetes mellitus. Ann Rheum Dis 31:69, 1972

56. Erhard R: Diabetic capsulitis of the shoulder. Proceedings of the International Federation of Orthopaedic Manipulative Therapists. Christchurch, New Zealand, 1980
57. Biswas AK, Sur BN, Gupta CR: Treatment of periathritis shoulder. J Indian Med Assoc 72:276, 1979
58. Olsson O: Degenerative changes of the shoulder joint and their connection with shoulder pain. Acta Chir Scand, suppl., 181:104–107, 1935
59. Murray W: The chronic frozen shoulder. Phys Ther Rev 40:866, 1960
60. Maitland GD: Peripheral Manipulation. 2nd Ed. Butterworths, Boston, 1977
61. Mennel J: Joint Pain. Diagnosis, Treatment using Manipulative Techniques. Little, Brown, and Co, Boston, 1964
62. Warwick R, Williams PL: Gray's Anatomy. 35th Brit. Ed. WB Saunders Co, Philadelphia, 1973
63. Kaltenborn FM: Mobilization of the Extremity Joints. Examination and Basic Treatment Techniques. Olaf Bokhandel, Oslo, 1980
64. Nelson PA: Physical treatment of the painful arm and shoulder. J Am Med Assoc 169:814, 1959
65. Valtonen E: Subacromial betamethasone therapy. The effect of subacromial injection of betamethasone in cases of painful shoulder resistant to physical therapy. Ann Chir Gynaecol Fenn 63: suppl. 188, 5–8, 1974
66. Binder AI, Bulgen DY, Hazleman BL, et al: Frozen shoulder: a long-term prospective study. Ann Rheum Dis 43:361, 1984
67. Hamer J, Kirk JA: Physiotherapy and the frozen shoulder: a comparative trial of ice and ultrasonic therapy. NZ Med J 83:191, 1976
68. Lee M, Haq AMMM, Wright V, et al: Periarthritis of the shoulder: a controlled trial of physiotherapy. Physiotherapy 59:312, 1972
69. Liang H, Lien I: Comparative study in the management of frozen shoulder. J Formosan Med Assoc 72:243, 1973
70. Rizk TE, Christopher RP, Pinals RS, et al: Adhesive capsulitis (frozen shoulder): a new approach to its management. Arch Phys Med Rehabil 64:29, 1983
71. Pothmann R, Weigel A, Stux G: Frozen shoulder: differential acupuncture therapy with point ST-38. Am J Acupuncture 8:65, 1980
72. Mannheimer J, Lampe G: Clinical Transcutaneous Electrical Nerve Stimulation. F.A. Davis, Philadelphia, 1984
73. The Academy of Traditional Chinese Medicine: An Outline of Chinese Acupuncture. Foreign Languages Press, Peking, 1975
74. Mueller EE, Mead S, Schulz B, et al: A placebo-controlled study of ultrasound treatment for periarthritis. Am J Phys Med 33:31, 1954
75. Quin CE: Humeroscapular periarthritis. Observations on the effects of x-ray therapy and ultrasonic therapy in cases of "frozen shoulder". Ann Phys Med 10:64, 1967
76. Hayes KW: Manual for Physical Agents. 3rd Ed. Northwestern University Press, Chicago, 1984
77. Bulgen DY, Binder AI, Hazleman BL, et al: Frozen shoulder: prospective clinical study with an evaluation of three treatment regimens. Ann Rheum Dis 43:353, 1984
78. Ham A, Cormack D: Histology. 8th Ed. JB Lippincott Co, Philadelphia, 1979
79. Swann D, Radin E, Nazimiec M: Role of hyaluronic acid in joint lubrication. Ann Rheum Dis 33:318, 1974
80. Wyke BW: Articular neurology—a review. Physiotherapy 58:94, 1972
81. Liebolt FL: Frozen shoulder. Passive exercises for treatment. NY State J Med 70:2085, 1970

82. Haggart GE, Dignam RJ, Sullivan TS: Management of the "frozen" shoulder. J Am Med Assoc 161:1219, 1956
83. Srivastava KP, Bhan BL, Bhatia IL: Scapulohumeral periarthritis. A clinical study and evaluation of end results of its treatment. J Indian Med Assoc 59:275, 1972
84. Quigley TB: Indications for manipulation and corticosteroids in the treatment of stiff shoulders. Surg Clin North Am 43:1715, 1963
85. Helbig B, Wagner P, Dohler R: Mobilization of frozen shoulder under general anaesthesia. Acta Orthop Belg 49:267, 1983
86. Coombes WN: Frozen shoulder. J Roy Soc Med 76:711, 1983
87. Quigley TB: Treatment of checkrein shoulder by use of manipulation and cortisone. J Am Med Assoc 161:850, 1956
88. Weiser HI: Painful primary frozen shoulder mobilization under local anesthesia. Arch Phys Med Rehabil 58:406, 1977
89. Steinbocker O, Argyros TG: Frozen shoulder: treatment by local injections of depot corticosteroids. Arch Phys Med Rehabil 55:209, 1974
90. Murnaghem GF, McIntosh D: Hydrocortisone in painful shoulder. Lancet 1:798, 1955
91. Roy S, Oldham R: Management of painful shoulder. Lancet 1:1322, 1976
92. Cyriax J, Trosier O: Hydrocortisone and soft tissue lesions. Br Med J 2:966, 1953
93. Crisp EJ, Kendall PH: Treatment of periarthritis of the shoulder with hydrocortisone. Br Med J 1:1500, 1955

6 | The Shoulder in Hemiplegia

Susan Ryerson
Kathryn Levit

Hemiplegia, a paralysis of one side of the body, occurs with strokes or cerebrovascular accidents (CVAs) involving the cerebral hemisphere or brainstem. Although hemiplegia is the classic and most obvious sign of neurovascular disease of the brain, it can also occur as a result of cerebral tumor or trauma.[1]

One of the most worrisome physical problems for clients with hemiplegia is the shoulder.[2] Shoulder pain, subluxation, loss of muscular activity, and loss of functional use are the most common complaints. These problems can be avoided with proper assessment and treatment and can be ameliorated if they already exist. This chapter reviews biomechanical and motor control impairments and presents a framework for the clinical management of these shoulder problems in hemiplegia.

NORMAL SHOULDER GIRDLE MECHANICS

Before beginning a study of the shoulder girdle in hemiplegia, it is important to review the normal mechanics of the shoulder (see Ch. 1). Three areas of normal shoulder mechanics should be emphasized: (1) the mobility of the scapula on the thorax,[3] (2) scapulohumeral rhythm and the factors influencing both humeral mobility and humeral stability in the glenoid fossa,[4,5] and (3) the muscular attachments of the shoulder–girdle complex.[3,6] Because muscles that move the scapula and humerus have attachments to the cervical, thoracic, and lumbar spine and rib cage, a loss of motor control and alignment will have multiple effects on the shoulder girdle.

ABNORMAL BIOMECHANICS

The loss of motor control of the shoulder in patients with a hemiplegia affects the operation of normal biomechanical principles. In hemiplegia, three factors prevent normal shoulder biomechanical patterns from occurring: (1) loss of muscular control; (2) the development of abnormal movement patterns and spasticity; and (3) secondary soft tissue changes that block motion.

Loss of Muscular Control

Following the onset of a cerebrovascular accident with hemiplegia, a low tone or flaccid state is present. The length of the lower tone state varies from a short period of hours or days to a period of weeks or months. This state is characterized by a decrease in active postural tone and a loss of motor control in the musculature of the head, neck, trunk, and extremities. As recovery progresses, three predictable patterns (I, II, III) of movement occur.

Pattern I

With a severe insult to the central nervous system, head and trunk control are virtually absent. Initially, the scapula assumes a downwardly rotated position (the superolateral angle moves inferiorly), and the inferior angle becomes

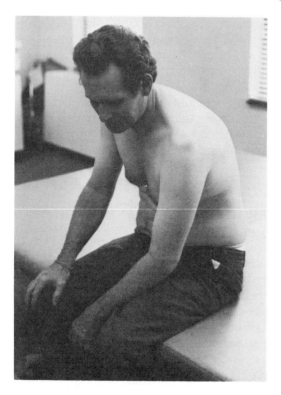

Fig. 6-1. Pattern I, left hemiplegia: Forward flexion of trunk with scapula riding high on thorax.

adducted. With scapular downward rotation, the glenoid fossa orients downward, and the passive locking mechanism of the shoulder joint, as described by Basmajian, is lost.[6] The loss of this mechanism, the loss of postural tone, and the loss of tension of the shoulder capsule result in a humeral subluxation of the hemiplegic shoulder.

When placed in an upright position, the body falls into gravity. If the upper trunk assumes a forward, flexed position, the scapula will ride "higher" up on the thorax (Fig. 6-1). Conversely, if the upper trunk assumes a laterally flexed position, the scapula will be depressed or "lower" down on the thorax (Fig. 6-2A). In either case, the humerus will hang by the side in internal rotation, the elbow will extend passively, the forearm will pronate and, eventually, the carpals will pronate on the radius (Fig. 6-2B). With carpal pronation, the hand will lose its arches and have a "claw-like" appearance.

Upper extremity problems resulting from this pattern (I) include:

1. Downward rotation of the scapula
2. Inferior angle and/or vertebral border winging of the scapula

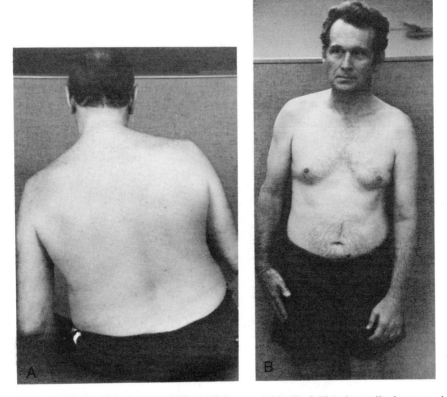

Fig. 6-2. (A) Pattern I, left hemiplegia: left side of body falling laterally into gravity; scapula lower on thorax. (B) Pattern I, left hemiplegia: humerus hangs by the side in internal rotation, elbow extension, and forearm pronation.

3. Severe humeral subluxation inferiorly
4. Humeral internal rotation tightness
5. Collapse of palmar arches and finger "clawing".

Pattern II

A second pattern appears with a less severe insult. This pattern develops as the trunk gains more extension control than flexion control. An increase in cervical and lumbar extension is evident. The head and neck assume a position of ipsilateral flexion and contralateral rotation (Fig. 6-3). At the thoracic level, this imbalance results in a unilateral loss of control of the abdominals. Therefore, the rib cage loses its abdominal "anchor" and will flare laterally and/or rotate backward (Fig. 6-4A and B). The scapula and humerus are strongly influenced mechanically by this rib cage deviation. The downwardly rotated scapula begins to move superiorly on the thorax, and the humerus hyperextends with internal rotation. This combination of rib cage rotation and humeral hyperextension allows the elbow to flex and the forearm to pronate (Fig. 6-5). As the scapula continues to elevate on the thorax, and the subluxed, internally rotated humerus moves into stronger hyperextension, the humeral head protrudes forward against the proximal end of the biceps tendon. This forward pressure of the humerus against the already shortened biceps tendon will mechanically move the forearm into a supinated position (Fig. 6-6). The wrist will appear to be less flexed as the carpals move dorsolaterally.

Upper extremity problems resulting from this pattern (II) include: (1) downward rotation and elevation of the scapula, and vertebral border winging;

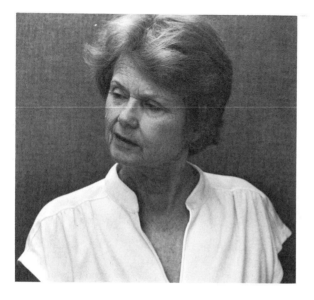

Fig. 6-3. Pattern II, left hemiplegia: head and neck are in ipsilateral flexion and contralateral rotation.

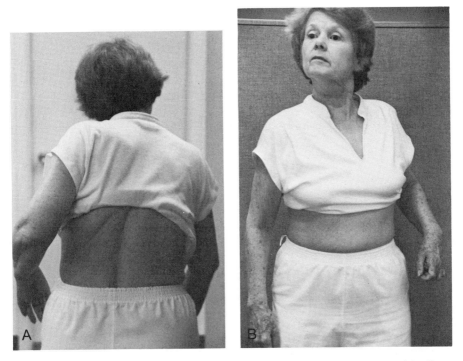

Fig. 6-4.   (A and B) Pattern II, left hemiplegia: loss of rib cage anchor with rib cage rotated backward and humeral hyperextension with internal rotation.

(2) humeral subluxation anteriorly on the abnormally aligned scapula; and (3) humeral adductor tightness.

Pattern III

The third movement pattern is characterized by abnormal coactivation of the limb muscles. This gives an appearance of "mass" flexion in the hemiplegic upper extremity. The neck and trunk control in clients with this upper extremity pattern contain elements of both flexion and extension. The control patterns are not sufficiently integrated to allow selective combinations of movement, and the sequential flow of motor activity is interrupted. The scapula is usually elevated and abducted on the thorax. The head of the humerus is held tightly beneath the acromial process. Although the deltoid and biceps attempt to initiate humeral motion, no disassociation occurs between the humerus and scapula. The upper extremity pattern that is available as a result of the position of the scapula and humerus is shoulder elevation with slight humeral abduction, severe internal rotation, and elbow flexion (Fig. 6-7). Activity in the long thumb flexors synergistically accompanies the shoulder motion. The wrist and fingers assume a flexed and radially deviated position. This moves the forearm me-

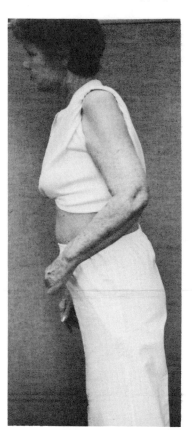

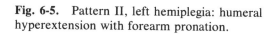

Fig. 6-5. Pattern II, left hemiplegia: humeral hyperextension with forearm pronation.

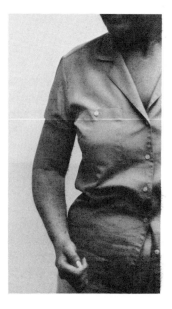

Fig. 6-6. Pattern II, right hemiplegia: humeral hyperextension with forearm supination.

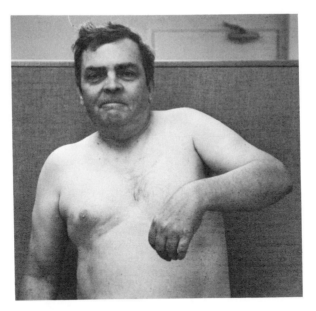

Fig. 6-7. Pattern III, left hemiplegia: active motion available in shoulder elevation, humeral abduction, internal rotation, and elbow flexion.

chanically from pronation in the direction of more supination. Problems resulting from this movement pattern (III) include:

1. Scapula elevation and abduction with vertebral border winging
2. Humeral impingement under the acromial process
3. Humeral internal rotation
4. Lack of disassociation between the scapula and humerus
5. Strong wrist flexion with radial deviation.

The development of these three upper extremity patterns affects the hemiplegic patient's ability to move the arm functionally in three ways. First, the loss of antigravity postural tone and the subsequent patterns of motor return will change the relationship of the scapula to the trunk and the relationship of the distal arm to the scapula. This change in position will alter the anatomical relationship of the joints. Second, the changes in bony alignment will change the resting length and direction of pull of the major muscle groups of the shoulder and arm. Biomechanically, this will lead to muscle imbalance and problems of motor control. Third, changes in muscle excitation and recruitment patterns may occur in these muscles whose resting lengths have been altered. Patterns of spasticity or abnormal coactivation of muscles may result in problems in any or all of these areas and will contribute to the abnormal and inefficient motor patterns associated with hemiplegia. Clinically, it is necessary to analyze the patient's motor patterns to identify the segments of abnormal motion. This will facilitate more effective treatment.

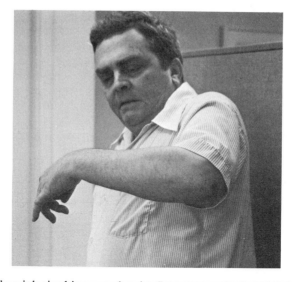

Fig. 6-8. Left hemiplegia: biceps and wrist flexors recruited to help move shoulder.

Development of Abnormal Movement and Spasticity

Early patterns of motor return pull the scapula and arm into abnormal postures. When the scapula and humerus are pulled severely out of alignment, certain muscle groups are positioned in shortened ranges. This results in lengthening or mechanical disadvantage in opposing muscle groups. Because the shortened muscles are available to the patient to use actively, muscle activity in these shortened groups is reinforced cortically with the attempt to move the arm. Muscle firing in these groups may also be reinforced by associated movements.[7] Thus, "functional spasticity" can develop when muscles of the upper extremity are maintained in an almost constant state of excitation.

In other patients, this abnormal motor recruitment sequence can develop slightly differently. Distal muscle groups can be recruited abnormally in what appears to be an attempt to substitute for proximal weakness. As an example, the biceps and wrist flexors may be recruited to help lift the weight of the arm during shoulder flexion while no contraction of the deltoid can be palpated (Fig. 6-8). Over time, a more constant state of excitation develops in the biceps and wrist flexor muscles, leading to muscle shortening. The constant muscle firing in these shortened groups can quickly pull the carpal bones out of alignment, leading to deformities in the forearm, wrist, and hand. The emergence of spasticity will perpetuate abnormal alignment. However, inhibition of spasticity alone will not produce a functional arm. Motor reeducation must be directed toward both the recruitment or strengthening of absent or weak muscle groups and the retraining of spastic muscles to fire appropriately. Thus, treatment must address the abnormal tonal state, the abnormal movement components, and the abnormal joint alignment to restore normal movement. To restore the normal mechanical relationships of the bones, soft tissue stretching and mobilization may be necessary.

Soft Tissue Blocks to Motion

Soft tissue blocks to motion can be categorized as loss of scapular mobility, loss of glenohumeral mobility, and loss of the ability to disassociate the scapula and humerus. The loss of scapular stability on the thorax occurs in all but the most minor strokes and is influenced initially by such factors as the pull of the arm into gravity, the development of postural asymmetry, and the influence of patterns of motor return and treatment. As the scapula assumes a position that combines elements of elevation, downward rotation, and abduction, the position of the scapula prevents forward flexion of the arm past 60 to 80°. Because upward rotation is not available for the scapula, glenohumeral movement > 60° is not possible.

Without treatment, the scapula loses its mobility on the thorax and becomes fixed, thus eliminating the scapular component of scapulohumeral

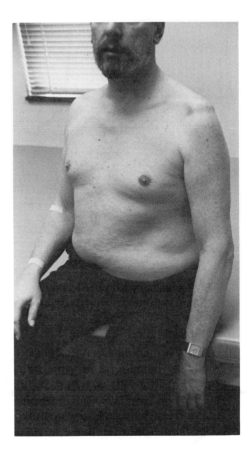

Fig. 6-9. Left hemiplegia: inferior subluxation.

rhythm. The loss of this scapular component results in the substitution of scapula elevation, consisting of scapular protraction and upward rotation. The loss of scapula upward rotation and protraction is important functionally because it is necessary for reach and pain-free elevation of the arm. However, loss of scapular adduction and depression has equal functional importance for resistive tasks such as lifting, pushing, carrying, and upper extremity weight-bearing. The goal in treatment is to restore the normal resting position of the scapula on the thorax and to regain mobility and motor control in all planes of motion.

Changes in scapula position will alter the orientation of the glenoid fossa and affect the resting position of the humerus. In cases of chronic hemiplegia, the humerus always postures in some degree of internal rotation, but its position relative to the glenoid fossa will depend on the position of the scapula. With a downwardly rotated and depressed scapula, inferior subluxation and internal rotation result (Fig. 6-9). In patients with an elevated, abducted scapula and a hyperextended humerus, the humeral head will be positioned anteriorly in the fossa. In patients with an elevated, abducted scapula and a humerus that postures in abduction and internal rotation, the humeral greater tuberosity will impinge under the acromion (Fig. 6-10).

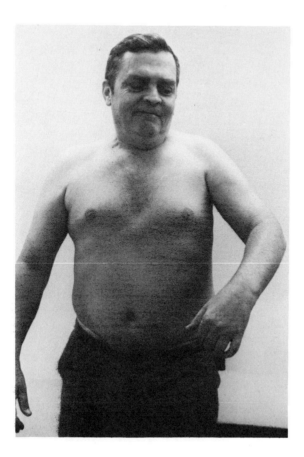

Fig. 6-10. Left hemiplegia: impingement of humeral greater tuberosity beneath acromion.

Loss of disassociation of the humerus from the scapula is the third block to normal movement. In this case, the scapula has mobility on the thorax and the humerus retains mobility in the glenoid fossa, but any movement of the humerus into flexion or abduction results in simultaneous scapular abduction.

MUSCULOSKELETAL CONSIDERATIONS

Shoulder Subluxation

Shoulder subluxation occurs in hemiplegia when any of the biomechanical factors contributing to glenohumeral stability are disturbed. The most important factor is the position of the scapula on the thorax. The scapula is normally held on the thorax at an angle of 30° from the frontal plane.[3] When the slope of the glenoid fossa becomes less oblique and no longer faces upward, the humerus "slides down" the slope of the fossa and inferior subluxation occurs.[4,6]

As subluxation occurs, the shoulder capsule is vulnerable to stretch, especially when the humerus is hanging by the side of the body. In this position, the superior portion of the capsule is taut.[4] The weight of the dependent humerus will place an immediate stretch on the taut capsule. Over time, the superior portion of the capsule will become lax and remain that way.[8]

In the flaccid or low-tone stage of hemiplegia, three situations lead to subluxation. First, the loss of scapular muscle activity allows the scapula to lose its normal orientation on the thorax and rotate downward (the superolateral angle moves inferiorly). Second, loss of trunk control results in increased lateral trunk flexion. The scapula, moving on this laterally flexed trunk, becomes relatively downwardly rotated, and the glenoid fossa faces inferiorly.[3,4] Third, the weight of the arm, if not supported, will pull the weakened scapula downward and place the humerus in relative abduction. With humeral abduction, the shoulder capsule is lax superiorly, and the head of the humerus can slide down the glenoid fossa.[4]

As recovery progresses, two other forms of subluxation exist. In patients with type II movement patterns, anterior humeral subluxation can occur. The scapula in these patients is superior and abducted on the thorax, lying more in a sagittal plane. The glenoid fossa faces directly anteriorly.[3] The humerus, which postures in hyperextension and internal rotation, moves forward out of the fossa (Fig. 6-5).

In patients with type III movement pattern, the humerus can become lodged under the acromial process (superior subluxation). This occurs as a result of humeral abduction activity without appropriate scapular rotation. The scapula in these patients is elevated, downwardly rotated, and abducted on the thorax. Although the glenoid fossa is oriented anteriorly, the strong abduction, internal rotation pattern of the humerus allows the humeral greater tuberosity to become displaced under the acromial process. Passive motion of the humerus is severely limited and, if attempted, may be painful.

Subluxation is not painful as long as the scapula is mobile.[7] However, the subluxed shoulder should not be allowed to progress into a painful shoulder with loss of passive range of motion (ROM).

Shoulder Pain

Shoulder pain is one of the major problem areas in hemiplegia.[2] Pain occurs in the hemiplegic shoulder as a result of muscle imbalance with loss of joint range, impingement of the shoulder capsule during improper ROM, improper muscle stretching, tendinitis, hyper- or hyposensitivity; pain also is caused by sympathetic changes.

To plan a treatment program, the nature of the pain, the precise anatomical location of the pain, the duration of the pain, and the body position during the movement that causes the pain must be assessed. Four categories of shoulder pain can be identified: joint pain, muscle pain, pain from altered sensitivity, and shoulder–hand pain syndrome.

Joint Pain

Joint pain in hemiplegia occurs whenever a joint is placed in a biomechanically compromised position as a result of either shoulder muscle imbalance or improper movement patterns. When the joint is improperly aligned, passive or active motion either with or without weight-bearing will result in joint pain. This pain is sharp and stabbing in nature. It is relieved immediately when joint alignment is corrected. At the shoulder, joint pain occurs when glenohumeral alignment and rhythm is not maintained. The most frequent reasons for poor alignment occurring are (1) lack of appropriate humeral rotation during forward flexion, and (2) improper placement of the humeral head in the glenoid fossa.

Treatment for this type of pain begins with immediate cessation of the movement pattern. Forced motion with pain must *never* be allowed. The movement should STOP; the limb should be lowered and the bones must be correctly realigned before treatment begins again. If soft tissue or joint tightness exists, realignment may not be possible unless soft tissue or joint mobility is improved or increased.

Muscle Pain

Muscle pain occurs as a shortened or spastic muscle is lengthened too fast or lengthened beyond the range to which the shortened muscle is "accustomed." Often, this type of pain occurs when the upper extremity is in a weight-bearing position and the patient is asked to move the body on the limb (Fig. 6-11). Muscle pain is perceived as a "pulling" sensation and is localized to the region of the muscle belly that is being stretched. The pain is immediately

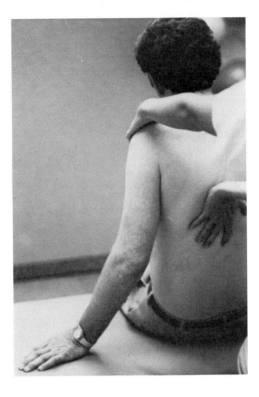

Fig. 6-11. Left hemiplegia: body moving on weight-bearing upper extremity.

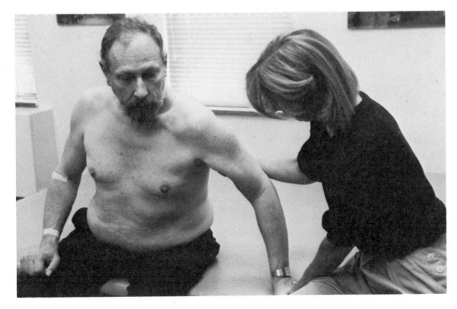

Fig. 6-12. Left hemiplegia: weight-bearing with improper alignment.

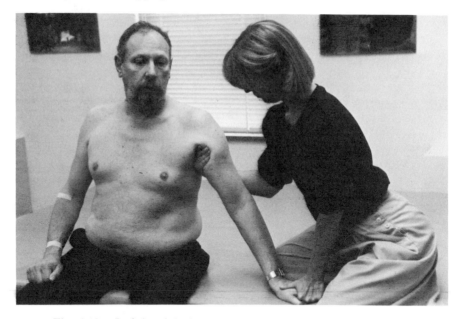

Fig. 6-13. Left hemiplegia: weight-bearing with proper alignment.

relieved if the amount of severe stretch is decreased a few degrees. Because lengthening shortened muscles is a goal of treatment, the muscle is not allowed to move back to the shortened range, but is allowed to shorten until the pain is relieved. Treatment can proceed with careful attention given to speed and progression of movement.

The pain which accompanies tendinitis is related to muscle pain, for it is caused by the same mechanism. Overstretching of a limb muscle followed by overaggressive weight-bearing with poor joint alignment results in tendinitis. The pain is described as aching or sharp, remains after the weight-bearing is stopped, and is referred to other locations. In the hemiplegic upper extremity, the two most common types are bicipital groove tendinitis with pain referred down into the muscle belly, and bicipital tendinitis across the elbow with pain referred down the volar aspect of the forearm.

The inappropriate weight-bearing pattern that leads to tendinitis in these cases is severe humeral internal rotation with forced elbow extension, along with an inactive trunk and "leaning" on a weak scapula (Fig. 6-12).

The weight-bearing extended arm activity should be stopped until the pain subsides. When weight-bearing treatment is resumed, particular care should be given to proper joint alignment, and active trunk scapular pattern (Fig. 6-13).

Altered Sensitivity

The pain that occurs because of altered sensitivity of the central nervous system (CNS) to sensory input is found at the acute stage of recovery following an insult.

This pain occurs in the upper extremity and is described as both diffuse and aching and localized to the shoulder and sharp. It typically occurs during the middle of a treatment session that has included tactile, sensory, kinesthetic, and proprioceptive stimuli. One explanation for its occurrence is that the levels of "tolerance" of the impaired CNS have been reached. The treatment should stop for that session, and the duration of treatment and the nature of the treatment should be noted. Subsequent treatment should be graded to allow movement to continue but not to exceed the patient's sensory tolerance. If treatment is stopped completely, these patients may proceed to a shoulder–hand syndrome.

Shoulder–hand syndrome begins with diffuse "aching pain" in the shoulder and entire arm. Because this pain interferes with the desire to move the arm, the hand soon becomes swollen and tender. If passive motion is forced on a swollen wrist and hand, the joints will become sharply painful.

The second stage is characterized by decreased ROM of the shoulder girdle, hand, and fingers. Skin changes are also present because of the lack of motion and loss of tactile input.

The syndrome culminates with presence of atrophied bone and severe soft tissue deformity and joint contractures. Shoulder–hand syndrome can be prevented by a program that

1. grades the motor program in stages with increasing sensitivity to movement.
2. gradually but consistently uses weight-bearing activities for the entire shoulder girdle and upper extremity.
3. reeducates open-ended activities (nonweight bearing) with appropriate scapulohumeral rhythm.
4. prevents edema.
5. teaches patients how to care for their arms.

TREATMENT PLANNING

The treatment of the deficits in motor control in the patient with hemiplegia focuses on the improvement of function and the prevention of further disability from secondary complications. In this section, treatment objectives for the hemiplegic shoulder will be presented in three major categories. The first category of objectives is designed to help the patient relearn basic postural control. The second set of objectives focuses on the neuromuscular deficits of hemiplegia: loss of extremity motor control and function. In the third category, the objectives for the secondary complications of hemiplegia—subluxation, pain, loss of motion and spasticity—will be discussed.

Reestablishment of Postural Control

The objectives for establishing postural control include:

1. the facilitation of righting reactions, equilibrium reactions, and protective reactions.

2. the provision of normal tactile, proprioceptive, and kinesthetic input.

Before specific retraining of the shoulder in patients with hemiplegia can begin, postural control of the head, neck, and trunk must be present. This postural trunk control provides the body with the ability to shift weight. The ability of the body to shift and bear weight to one side frees the opposite extremity for the functions of reaching, grasping, and releasing. Along with sensory feedback (tactile, proprioceptive, kinesthetic, visual, and vestibular) movement requires a base of stability or base of support, a point of mobility, and a weight shift. Weight shift, either anterior, posterior, lateral, or diagonal, is followed by one or more of the following: righting reactions, equilibrium reactions, protective reactions, or falling. The establishment of head and neck control allows the shoulder girdle to disassociate or move freely from the thorax and the humerus to disassociate from the scapula. To establish good motor control, the body (trunk) must be able to adjust posture automatically so that an upper extremity movement may achieve its purpose.

Neuromuscular Deficits

Objectives for reestablishing motor control and function of the hemiplegic arm include

1. establishment of normal weight-bearing patterns in the upper extremity.
2. initiation and "holding" of proximal patterns.
3. reeducation of distal or "open-ended" (nonweight bearing) movement for functional skills.

Establishing Weight-Bearing

The ability to accept and bear weight on the affected arm following a stroke is one of the most important goals of a therapeutic program. Active weight-bearing on either a partially flexed or extended upper extremity is used as a means of increasing mobility; increasing postural control of the trunk; improving motor control of the affected arm; introducing and grading tactile, proprioceptive, and kinesthetic stimulation; and preventing edema and pain. Positions that provide weight-bearing for a hemiplegia shoulder and arm include: (1) rolling onto the affected side in preparation for getting out of bed (Fig. 6-14A and B); (2) supporting the forearm on a pillow placed in the lap or on a lap board or on a table when sitting (Fig. 6-14C), and (3) extending the weight-bearing arm down onto a countertop while standing (Fig. 6-14D).

An active weight-bearing program for the paretic arm stresses "active" patterns in the trunk and does not allow the patient to lean or "hang" on the

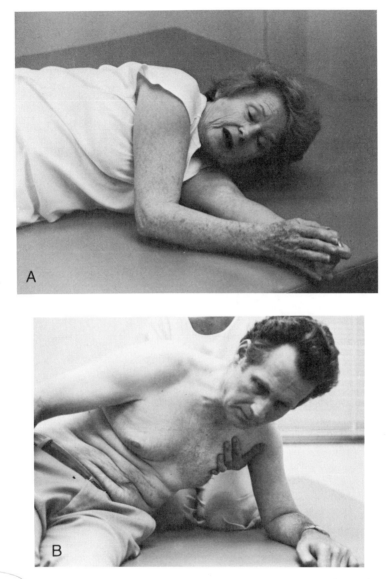

Fig. 6-14. Weight-bearing positions for the upper extremity. (A) Left hemiplegia: rolling onto affected side. (B) Left hemiplegia: moving onto affected forearm. (*Figure Continues.*)

ligaments of the affected extremity (Fig. 6-15). This active participation of the trunk is accomplished by placing the upper extremity in an aligned weight-bearing position and asking the trunk or "body" to move on the stable arm in anterior/posterior, lateral, and rotational directions.

In the acute stage of hemiplegia when very little postural control is present, upper extremity weight-bearing is used to facilitate proximal motor control.

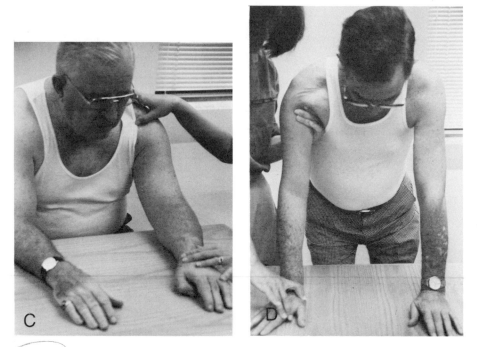

Fig. 6-14 (*Continued*). (C) Left hemiplegia: supporting forearm on table, (D) Right hemiplegia: extended arm weight-bearing.

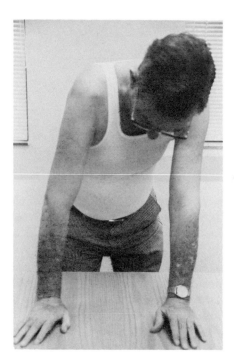

Fig. 6-15. Right hemiplegia: improper weight-bearing on extended arm—"hanging" on shoulder and mechanically locking elbow.

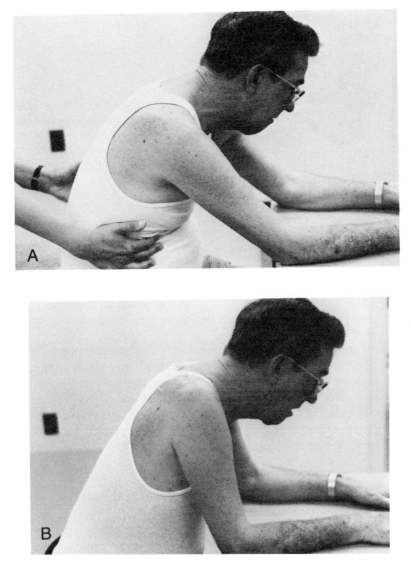

Fig. 6-16. (A) Right hemiplegia: moving body away from weight-bearing arm. (B) Moving body toward weight-bearing arm.

When the upper extremities are "fixed" onto the supporting surface through forearm weight-bearing activities, the arm becomes a point of stability for movements of the trunk and pelvis. As the body moves away from the arm, scapular protraction and upward rotation, humeral flexion, and upper trunk flexion are encouraged (Fig. 6-16A). As the body moves toward the arm, scapular adduction and trunk extension are encouraged as the humerus moves into more extension (Fig. 6-16B). When the pelvis and trunk move laterally, the scapulae move in opposite directions, one into more abduction and one

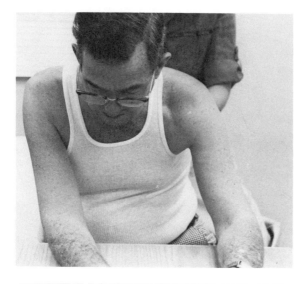

Fig. 6-17. Right hemiplegia: weight shifting to right moves right humerus into more external rotation while left humerus begins to move into the direction of internal rotation.

into more adduction. The humerus on the side of the lateral weight shift becomes more externally rotated, while the other humerus becomes more internally rotated (Fig. 6-17).

For patients with available but synergistic movement patterns, upper extremity weight-bearing can be used to lengthen or inhibit tight or spastic muscles while simultaneously facilitating muscles that are not active. When the person sits with hands down and open, a rotational movement of the body toward the affected upper extremity will lengthen tight shoulder depressors and downward rotators, tight humeral internal rotators, and elbow flexors while simultaneously activating the opposing groups (Fig. 6-18A and B).

Initiation and "Holding" of Proximal Patterns

When the hand or arm is placed in a position of weight-bearing, the motions of the shoulder girdle occur as a reaction to the body's movement over the fixed extremity. When the arm is taken out of weight-bearing and is asked to move in space, the demands on the shoulder girdle are different from weight-bearing demands. The motor demands on the shoulder for nonweight-bearing (open-ended) activities can be divided into (1) the ability to hold the weight of the limb against gravity; (2) the ability to initiate anti-gravity movement patterns; including the ability to switch from glenohumeral movement to scapulohumeral as needed; and (3) the ability to reciprocate and coordinate the combinations of mobility and stability needed for reaching, grasping, carrying, and releasing.

Motor reeducation aimed at training the hemiplegic arm to move against gravity will vary according to the patterns of return present and variables such as pain, spasticity, or malalignment. Techniques for managing pain and spas-

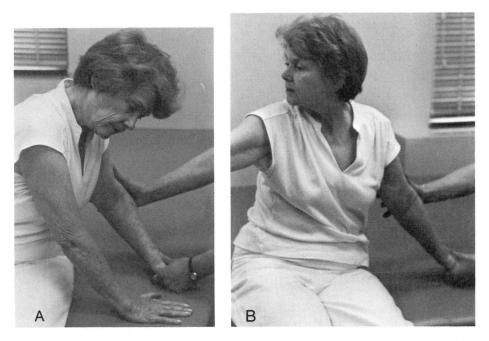

Fig. 6-18.   (A and B) Left hemiplegia: rotational body movements over a weight-bearing upper extremity.

ticity are discussed separately (see Treatment of Secondary Complications) and should be used before treatment of motor control proceeds. Orthopedic changes, particularly those that are long-standing, represent a particular treatment challenge because although orthopedic malignment at the shoulder will necessitate compensation or abnormal movement, it is frequently impossible within a treatment session to reposition the scapula or humerus in normal alignment before proceeding with movement reeducation. In these cases, the goal is to gain some increase in mobility in the direction of normal alignment, followed immediately by a movement pattern that uses this new mobility. Over successive treatments, as soft tissue mobility is increased and passive resting positions become closer to normal alignment, the types and combinations of movement can be increased.

When pain, spasticity, and malalignment of the shoulder joints are not problems, treatment can be directed immediately to improving motor control. In the acute stage, in which muscle tone is low and little motion is present, teaching the patient to manage the weight of the arm against gravity is the first stage of motor control to be introduced. This is done by teaching the patient to "hold" the scapula and humerus in an anti-gravity position (Fig. 6-19).[7,9]

"Place and hold" activities are practiced in supine and, later, in sitting positions until the patient develops control of the arm in various combinations of scapula and humeral patterns. The patient is then taught to move actively

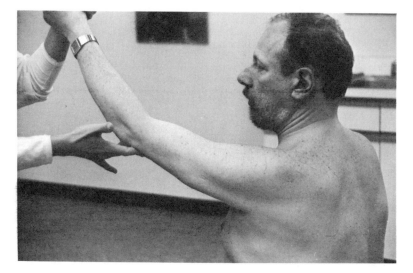

Fig. 6-19. Left hemiplegia: Place and hold position.

within his range of control. When the concept of holding has been achieved, the patient is asked to initiate patterns at the shoulder. This is done by moving the hemiplegic arm in many functional patterns combined with strong sensory stimulation during each treatment session.

Moving the hand on a table or wall seems most effective initially in introducing the sensation of normal movement into the nervous system.

When the patient has movement available, but efforts to move the arm produce abnormal patterns, treatment is directed toward establishing more normal coordination. This may involve both inhibiting the abnormal way in which muscles are recruited and retraining in the correct pattern of motor recruitment. Problems in motor recruitment can best be addressed by teaching the patient to identify and quiet muscles which are firing inappropriately whether through techniques of inhibition or biofeedback. The patient is then taught to allow passive motion of the arm without firing muscles inappropriately or allowing muscle tone in the arm to increase. The patient is then encouraged to try to "follow" the movement and finally to perform it actively with less assistance from the therapist. Place and hold exercises are useful in helping the patient use the correct muscles at the shoulder girdle without inappropriately firing distal muscle groups. While new recruitment patterns are being established, the patient is also taught appropriate control of the previously "over-used" muscles. Thus, the patient learns to inhibit biceps activity when reaching, but to use the biceps appropriately to bring the hand to the mouth.

Patients who have less spasticity or more complete motor return have fewer problems with abnormal recruitment but more problems with motor control. This category of patients has missing components of motor activity. Compensatory motions resembling an abnormal pattern result. For example, lack of active external rotation of the humerus will lead to a substitution pattern of

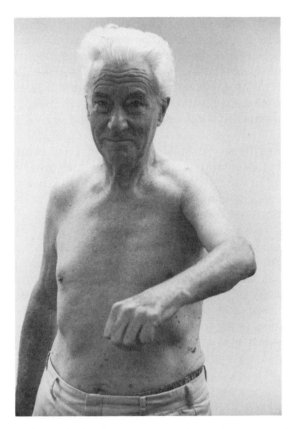

Fig. 6-20. Left hemiplegia: lack of active external rotation results in compensation pattern of humeral abduction and internal rotation.

abduction, internal rotation of the humerus, and scapula elevation (Fig. 6-20). If this motor pattern is being used because the client cannot actively externally rotate the humerus, the goal of treatment must be to make external rotation available during active shoulder movement and to establish the ability to hold the humerus in external rotation while moving distally. Similarly, other patients may have difficulties with protraction and upward rotation of the scapula. In this case, the therapist must control the motion of the scapula proximally to facilitate the correct motion of the scapula while the patient works on upper extremity placing or movement sequences.

Reeducate Distal Movements

Distal motor control, to be accurate, must be based on normal patterns of mobility and stability in the scapula and glenohumeral joint. Once the patient can initiate normal motion at the glenohumeral and scapulothoracic joints and can maintain the shoulder in positions against gravity, the patient must learn to add combinations of elbow position and forearm rotation to the control established at the shoulder. In order to use the hand functionally for grasping, carrying, and releasing, the hemiplegic patient must be able to position the hand appropriately for grasp by selecting appropriate forearm and wrist positions, hold the hand in position while the fingers move, and sustain grasp while moving proximally. Problems in any of the above may interfere with adaptive grasp.

As shoulder girdle control builds, the positions and movements of the distal segments must be added in treatment so that various distal positions are available to the patient to use functionally. As new combinations of motor behavior are learned, the patient should be taught a functional task using this pattern to insure carry-over from exercise into everyday life.

Different grasp patterns require varying wrist and forearm positions. In addition, the transition from grasp to manipulation involves the addition of complex fine motor patterns that are often task-specific. Improving the level of hand function is thus a separate treatment process that requires good motor control of the shoulder, elbow, forearm, and wrist as a precursor of success.

When the hemiplegic client has biomechanical shoulder girdle problems accurate positioning of the hand for function is difficult as they attempt to hold the shoulder against gravity and initiate appropriate antigravity movement patterns.[10]

Treatment of Secondary Complications

The objectives for each of the secondary complications—subluxation, pain, loss of motion, and spasticity—are discussed separately.

Subluxation

Acutely, if subluxation is not present, treatment follows the objectives listed under Treatment Planning. If subluxation has occurred, treatment must be preceded by careful assessment.

Proper assessment of subluxation includes determination of

1. the exact position of the humeral head, scapula, ribcage, and spine.
2. mobility or passive range of motion.
3. tone.
4. amount and location of motor control.

The assessment will reveal the cause of the subluxation (i.e., loss of motor control of scapula and/or humerus, soft tissue tightness, and hypotonus or hypertonus). Appropriate treatment can then begin.

Treatment of subluxation includes the following goals:

1.   manual alignment and support of scapula of the thorax and humerus in the glenoid fossa.

2.   increase in motor control in shoulder girdle muscle groups.

3.   inhibition of spasticity or stretching of soft tissue tightness.

4.   maintenance of pain-free ROM with proper glenohumeral rhythm.

5.   prevention of stretching of shoulder capsule through proper positioning.

This can be achieved through the use of lapboards, tables, armrests, or pillows when sitting; self-assisted motion during functional activities; weight-bearing on the forearm or hand. Although slings are often used to support the shoulder and protect the shoulder capsule from stretch, they do not correct the cause of the subluxation.[2] The ideal shoulder sling is one that maintains the normal angular alignment of the glenoid fossa and decreases the tendency of the humerus to rotate internally, yet allows movement in the shoulder and upper extremity. Smith and Okamoto offer a review of shoulder slings for hemiplegic clients.[11] Slings should not be expected to cure a subluxation, inhibit spastic muscles, or facilitate movement patterns. At best, they relieve some of the downward pull of gravity on the arm.

Pain

The causes of shoulder pain have been described in detail. Treatment of the painful shoulder and arm should include

1.   immediate cessation of any movement or activity that causes or increases the pain.

2.   removal of edema, if present.

3.   realignment of the shoulder girdle/trunk complex either by the therapist manually (passively) or by the client actively: this includes lengthening or inhibition of the shortened or spastic muscle groups and realignment of malaligned joints.

4.   reeducation of the inactive muscle groups through functional activities.

5.   a graded program of weight-bearing through the shoulder, forearm, and hand.

Loss of range

Loss of ROM at the shoulder can lead to decreased arm function and impaired balance in patients with hemiplegia. Although classic stretching procedures (nonweight-bearing) are often used for loss of shoulder motion in hemiplegia, slow maintained stretching or elongation through weight-bearing (i.e., functional stretching in conjunction with retraining motor control) is more effective.

Spasticity

The importance of spasticity in the treatment of hemiplegia is a controversial subject.[7,12,13] Spasticity is one of the positive symptoms of hemiplegia, along with clonus and disinhibition of primitive reflexes. Although spasticity must be dealt with during the treatment of the hemiplegic shoulder, the negative symptoms, paresis, loss of force production, delayed initiation of movement, and pathological co-contraction of muscles, must also be addressed.[14] Inhibition of spasticity alone will not result in a functional upper extremity.

Campbell hypothesizes that by preventing the development of abnormal compensatory motor patterns through activation of normal motor control, therapists may decrease or even prevent the development of spasticity.[12] From a movement point of view, existing spasticity in the upper extremity can be inhibited by (1) maintained elongation or lengthening in the pattern of shortened muscle groups; or (2) activation of the trunk musculature through upper extremity weight-bearing.

CONCLUSION

The importance of identifying the exact location and nature of shoulder girdle dysfunction in hemiplegia has been stressed in this chapter. Because the abnormal motor patterns of hemiplegia can arise from a combination of abnormal alignment, unbalanced motor return, and abnormal patterns of muscle excitation and recruitment, treatment strategies must be based on a thorough understanding of the interrelationships between orthopedic and neurologic factors. The presence of subluxation and pain are additional problems that must be addressed before neuromuscular reeducation can begin. The positive results of any treatment regimen will ultimately depend on the clinician's systematic evaluation and skill in implementing appropriate treatment of the shoulder girdle complex.

REFERENCES

1. Adams RD, Victor M: Principles of Neurology. McGraw-Hill, New York, 1981
2. Davis PM: Steps to Follow. Springer-Verlag, Berlin, 1985
3. Kapandji IA: The Physiology of the Joints: Upper Limb. Churchill Livingstone, Edinburgh, 1970
4. Cailliet R: The Shoulder in Hemiplegia. FA Davis Co, Philadelphia, 1980
5. Codman EA: The Shoulder. Thomas Todd Co, Boston, 1934
6. Basmajian JV: Muscles Alive. Williams & Wilkins, Baltimore, 1979
7. Bobath B: Adult Hemiplegia: Evaluation and Treatment, 2nd Ed. William Heinneman Medical Books, London, 1979
8. Jensen M: The Hemiplegic Shoulder, Scand J Rehabil Med (Suppl) 7:113, 1980
9. Carr JH, Shepherd R: A Motor Relearning Programme for Stroke. Aspen Systems, London, 1983

10. Tubiana R: Examination of the Hand and Upper Limb. WB Saunders Co, Philadelphia, 1984

11. Smith RO, Okamoto GA: Checklist for the prescriptions of slings for the hemiplegic patient. Am J Occup Ther 35:91, 1981

12. Campbell S: Pediatric Neurologic Physical Therapy. Churchill Livingstone, New York, 1984

13. Sahrmann S, Norton BJ: The relationship of voluntary movement to spasticity in the upper motor neuron syndrome. Ann Neurol 2:460, 1977

14. Lance JW: The control of muscle tone, reflexes and movement: Robert Wartenberg lecture. Neurology 30:1303, 1980

7 | Evaluation and Management of Thoracic Outlet Syndrome

Julianne Wright Howell

Thoracic outlet syndrome (TOS) represents a multitude of syndromes involving the upper quarter and hand that are believed to be caused by proximal compression of the subclavian artery, vein, and/or brachial plexus.[1-5] Most authors agree that at least one of these structures must be compressed at some point between the superior opening of the thorax and the axilla to qualify as TOS.

This chapter focuses on this diagnosis; however, I have elected not to perpetuate the use of the term thoracic outlet syndrome, because the term thoracic outlet is anatomically incorrect when used to describe the superior opening of the thoracic cavity. According to the classic anatomists, the superior opening of the thorax is the thoracic inlet, and it is simply an anatomical misnomer to refer to the superior opening as the outlet.[6,7] Therefore, for the sake of anatomical correctness, the area bordered anteriorly by the clavicle and first thoracic rib and posteriorly by the first thoracic vertebra is the inlet, not the outlet, of the thorax. I recognize that most of the literature refers to this area as the outlet; however, the reader should take note of the change in nomenclature from TOS to thoracic inlet syndrome (TIS) in this chapter.

The amount of literature on TIS available to the clinician is overwhelming and relates primarily to its etiology, its differential diagnosis, and the surgical management of the TIS patient. Because of the vast number of reports on TIS, the reader may be totally unaware that many authors question the frequency of its occurrence and that some even doubt the existence of the syndrome![8-10] To support their claim, those who question the existence of TIS cite as evidence: (1) the lack of "proof positive," i.e., a single diagnostic test or battery of tests that is a valid indicator(s) of neurovascular compression in the proximity of the inlet; (2) the failure of surgical intervention to relieve the patient's symptoms consistently, as well as the high percentage of patients whose symptoms reoccur postsurgically; and (3) the fact that 50 to 90 percent of these patients respond to conservative management, i.e., physical therapy, despite the claims that excision of a muscle and/or rib is necessary to decompress the neurovascular structures of the inlet adequately.

In addition to the above factors, the risk of surgical complications, such as brachial plexus palsy, pneumothorax, and recurrence of symptoms have convinced even the staunch endorser of TIS to take a more conservative approach in their management of these patients.[5] As a result of this change in philosophy, physical therapy is often the first line of treatment prescribed for these patients. Unfortunately, for the physical therapist who desires more information on this topic, documentation of physical therapy evaluation, treatment, and results of therapeutic intervention is scarce and, at best, sorely lacking in scientific organization.

Therefore, it is the purpose of this chapter to provide the reader with background information relative to special testing for TIS, a review of the existing literature on physical therapy management of TIS, and suggestions that I have found helpful in the evaluation and treatment of these patients. Last, it is hoped that this chapter will provide food for thought to persuade the reader that only by careful documentation of their clinical findings and results of treatment will the understanding of this syndrome improve.

CLINICAL PRESENTATION

Characteristically, the persons who develop TIS are usually women (outnumbering men three to one) and middle-aged. The onset of symptoms is generally insidious, but has been reported by some authors to follow trauma involving the shoulder girdle.[11-13] Patient complaints include inability to raise or maintain the arm in a static posture for short periods of time without the onset of their symptoms. Typical examples of activities which evoke symptoms include: styling hair, driving, needlework, lifting, overhead use of the arm, carrying a briefcase, and typing. The patient may describe the sensation of heaviness and fatigue in the upper extremity, swelling, blotchy skin discoloration, and pain throughout the neck and arm, frequently extending into the hand.

The symptoms of TIS are assumed to be of neurovascular origin, involving compression of the subclavian artery, vein, and brachial plexus. Generally, these structures are compressed in combination, but cases of single structure compression have been reported.[14,15] Symptoms related to compression of the brachial plexus have been documented in 90 percent of all TIS cases.[13,16,17]

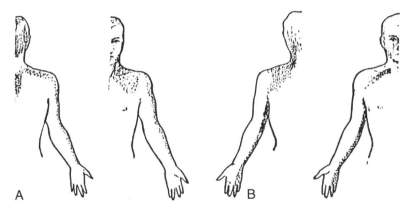

Fig. 7-1. TIS symptom patterns for (A) upper plexus involvement, and (B) lower plexus involvement.

Those symptoms, as reported in frequency of occurrence, include: pain, paresthesia, and paresis of the neck, upper extremity and hand. Roos, in a retrospective analysis of 3,630 TIS patients, identified two distinct neurological symptom patterns in these patients.[16] One pattern involves the upper roots of the plexus (C5–C7), and the other involves the lower roots of the plexus (C8 and T1). Some patients within the sample were found to have atypical symptoms which involved both upper and lower plexus compression[16] (Fig. 7-1).

Symptoms of vascular origin occur in 5 to 10 percent of all cases and are rarely the only complaint.[18] The most widely reported complaints which suggest vascular involvement include: edema, heaviness or weakness of the upper extremity, and the triad of cyanosis, blanching, and erythema mimicking Raynaud's phenomenon.[4,19]

ETIOLOGY

The list of probable etiologies for compression of these neurovascular structures is endless (Table 7-1). Those causes most commonly implicated and surgically removed include: an anomalous cervical rib,[20] the first thoracic rib,[21] the scalene anticus,[22] and anomalous fibromuscular bands.[23] I have found the classification scheme of primary and secondary TIS useful to simplify this confusing list of etiologic mechanisms.[24] According to Jaeger et al, the primary form of TIS is caused by compression from a bony or soft tissue abnormality. These structures may include, but are not limited to, a cervical rib, a malunion of the clavicle, anomalous fibromuscular bands of the scalenei, or a Pancoast's tumor of the apex of the lung. Secondary TIS, on the other hand, occurs in the absence of any anatomic variation, and is the direct result of trauma to the upper extremity or cervical spine. As a result of this trauma cervicothoracic posture is altered and, in turn, produces intermittent compression of the plexus and subclavian vessels.[24] Although this classification scheme has helped me

Table 7-1. Suggested Etiologies of Neurovascular Compression Against First Thoracic Rib

Primary TIS		Secondary TIS
Soft Tissue	Bony	
Anterior scalene	Cervical rib	Trauma
Middle scalene	Clavicle malunion	Occupational stresses
Pectoralis minor	Transverse processes	Shoulder girdle descent
Subclavius		Overweight conditions
Costocoracoid fascia		Pendulous breasts
Fibromuscular bands		
Pancoast's tumor		

TIS, thoracic inlet syndrome. Primary TIS has an anatomical basis and secondary TIS is situational.

to simplify the list of etiologies, I have not found that patients with either form of TIS initially have any different clinical presentation or that this scheme has much predictive value in selecting the most successful management plan for these patients.

SPECIAL TESTS FOR THORACIC INLET SYNDROME

The difficulty in making the diagnosis of TIS is well documented.[5,8] Subsequently, a barrage of tests is used to localize the cause of the patient's symptoms. Among the most familiar are the provocative maneuver tests, which include the scalene anticus, costoclavicular, hyperabduction, and 3-minute elevated arm exercise tests. Although there are many other tests and methods of testing, this chapter will be limited to reviewing the related literature and testing methods performed by the physical therapist.

Provocative Maneuver Tests

The scalene anticus or Adson's test is used to evaluate the muscle's role in the compression of the subclavian artery as it passes between the anterior and middle scalenei enroute to the axilla.[22] To compress the artery, the anterior scalene must be stretched from its origins on the anterior tubercles of the transverse processes of C4, C5, C6, and C7 to its insertion on the scalene tubercle of the first thoracic rib. To stretch the anterior scalene, Adson stipulated that the patient must hyperextend and rotate the head toward the affected side and take a deep breath. Meanwhile, the examiner must monitor the radial pulse of the affected upper extremity as it is held in a relaxed position at the patient's side (Fig. 7-2). A positive test for the anterior scalene is indicated by an obliteration or a decrease in the pulse rate.[22]

The space between the first rib and the clavicle has also been implicated in the compression of these neurovascular structures. Falconer and Weddell described the costoclavicular or exaggerated military position which is designed to narrow the space between the first rib and the clavicle, thus compressing

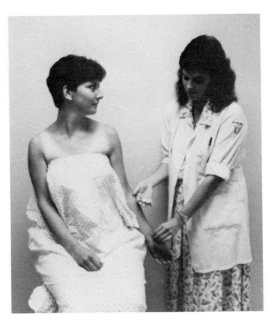

Fig. 7-2. Left scalene anticus test.

the subclavian vessels and/or the brachial plexus.[21] To perform the test, the subject is seated with arms held comfortably at the sides to approximate the anterior surface of the rib to the posterior surface of the clavicle; the subject then retracts and depresses the shoulder girdle. Simultaneously, the examiner monitors for a change in the radial pulse. A positive costoclavicular test is

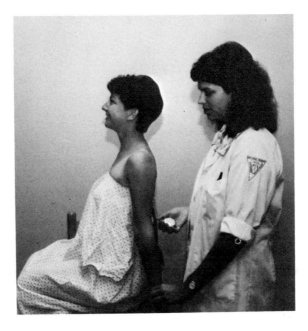

Fig. 7-3. Costoclavicular provocative maneuver.

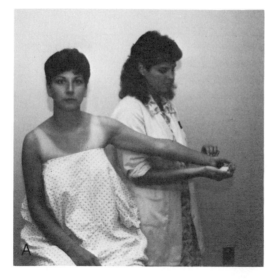

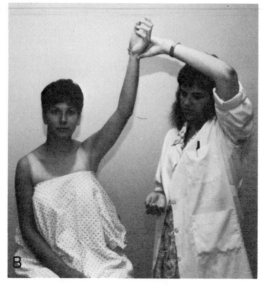

Fig. 7-4. Hyperabduction maneuver at (A) midway position and (B) on completion.

indicated by obliteration or decrease in pulse rate and/or the onset of symptoms[21] (Fig. 7-3).

The hyperabduction maneuver as described by Wright involves passive circumduction of the affected upper extremity overhead while the examiner monitors the radial pulse.[25] It is important that the examiner monitor the pulse while the arm is slowly moved into the overhead position to localize the point in the arc of motion where the pulse changes (Fig. 7-4A and B). Hypothetically, there are two potential sites of torsion for the neurovascular bundle during this maneuver. The first site is between 0° and 90° of shoulder abduction when the

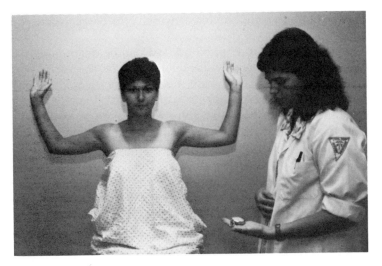

Fig. 7-5.   Three-minute elevated arm exercise test.

subclavian vessels and the plexus are stretched around the coracoid process and the other is at the costoclavicular space as it narrows, with shoulder abduction beyond 90°. The hyperabduction test is considered positive if the pulse rate changes and/or symptoms are elicited.[25]

The 3-minute elevated arm exercise test has gained in popularity since it was described by Roos.[26] This test is performed with the patient sitting, arms abducted 90° from the thorax and the elbow flexed 90° with the shoulders braced slightly. The patient is then asked to open and close his fist slowly and steadily for a full 3 minutes (Fig. 7-5). The examiner watches for dropping of the elevated arms and decreased rate of fisting on the onset of the patient's symptoms. According to Roos, a person can normally perform this test without symptoms other than mild fatigue; however, a patient with suspected TIS who is asked to perform the test will complain of the usual symptoms. Furthermore, Roos states that this test will evaluate involvement of all three of the neurovascular structures since the test position places the structures in the position for greatest compression. A positive elevated arm exercise test is indicated by the patient's inability to complete the full 3 minutes and the onset of the patient's symptoms.[3]

The four provocative maneuvers discussed above are the most commonly used tests for obliteration of the pulse and reproduction of symptoms when TIS is suspected. However, the reader should realize that there are vascular testing instruments such as the photoplethysmograph (PPG) and the Doppler ultrasound (Doppler) which are often used to monitor blood flow in place of examiner palpation of the radial pulse during the provocative maneuver. I believe that monitoring vascular flow with instrumentation rather than palpation offers several advantages that are worth consideration.

1.   Both instruments are noninvasive monitors, therefore the patient is not at risk, as would be the case with an arteriogram or venogram.

2. Instruments may offer better sensitivity to detect subtle changes in blood flow.

3. A change in the volume of blood flow can be quantitated with instruments, whereas only a change in pulse quality can be detected by palpation.

4. If the examiner is unsure which subclavian vessel is involved, the Doppler can be used to differentiate venous from arterial flow.

5. A permanent record of the pulse tracing can be produced by both instruments and can then be used as an objective finding in the patient's medical record.

6. For patients whose symptoms are produced by overhead or repetitive motion, the PPG monitor can be secured, and the subject can move the extremity while being simultaneously monitored, a task not easily performed with palpation.

7. The Doppler probe flow detector can be placed externally over the vessel along its entire course through the neck and upper extremity to localize the site of compression.

A few physical therapists are fortunate enough to be trained in vascular testing; for those who are not, there may be a vascular testing center located in the therapist's facility or community with which the therapist can consult. In addition, if the therapist is treating several such patients, chances are that many of them will have undergone vascular testing; therefore, the therapist may want to be able to interpret or compare the results of their tests with clinical findings. Similarly, the TIS literature is filled with references to the PPG and Doppler as a mechanism to diagnose and evaluate the effectiveness of treatment. To critique these results, the therapist needs some basic background knowledge.

If at this point the reader understands that provocative maneuver tests are used for exactly what their name implies—to provoke a change in blood flow and/or to evoke symptoms in a patient suspected of TIS—all is well and good! However, I caution the reader not to assume, without the benefit of additional information, that a positive response to any of these special tests implies that a patient has TIS. Interesting documentation shows that these special maneuvers produce changes in blood flow and evoke symptoms not only in TIS patients, but also in a large percentage of normal asymptomatic individuals. Geroudis and Barnes studied the prevalence of vascular compression during provocative maneuver testing in 130 asymptomatic normal individuals.[19] The PPG was used to monitor digital blood flow during these maneuvers, and the response was categorized by these authors based on the change in the amplitude of the digital pulse. A response was classified as normal if <76 percent reduction in pulse amplitude was noted and as abnormal if > 75 percent of the pulse amplitude was reduced or if there was complete absence of the digital pulse. Based on this classification scheme, abnormal responses were noted in 60 percent of the subjects for at least one of the provocative maneuvers; 55 percent of these were abnormal bilaterally. In addition, abnormal flow patterns were recorded in 27 percent of the subjects for two of the three maneuvers.

Specific results for each individual test revealed that Adson's test reduced the pulse amplitude in more than half of the sample, and the hyperabduction test occluded the blood flow in 10 percent of the sample.[19] This prevalence of false-positive results for provocative maneuver testing of 160 normal individuals was also reported by Pisko-Dubienski and Hollingsworth.[18] These authors used a Doppler to document alterations in blood flow and the onset of symptoms during performance of the costoclavicular and hyperabduction tests, Adson's maneuver, and a position of 90° of shoulder abduction.[19]

Occlusion of the subclavian artery with hyperabduction of the arm overhead was shown to be a frequent phenomenon, occurring in varying degree in a sample of 150 normal subjects.[25] Wright found that for positions from neutral to directly overhead, the radial pulse obliterated bilaterally 80 percent of the time in 125 of these normal subjects. These results were obtained provided the head was held in midline or the cervical spine was flexed; however, if the head was rotated or hyperextended to stretch the anterior scalene, the frequency of obliteration was increased. Furthermore, when the provoking position was held for at least an additional 2 minutes, neurological symptoms were elicited.[25]

Because the validity of these maneuvers is questionable, it behooves the reader to use these tests with this in mind. After provocative maneuver testing of more than 160 asymptomatic undergraduate physical therapy students, I found that it is not unusual to tally ~50 percent of the students as responding positively to at least one of the provocative maneuvers! The test which has consistently produced the most false-positive results in these students is the hyperabduction maneuver, followed closely by Adson's test.

The previous information illustrates the frequency of false-positives in a population of normal subjects. The reader may ask whether a patient with established TIS responds positively to these maneuvers if normal subjects can be symptomatic and falsely positive. If so, what happens in provocative maneuver tests after surgical removal of the offending structure, i.e., do the tests then become normal? Is there a relationship between the patient's pre- and postoperative clinical status and their pre- and postoperative provocative maneuver test results? The reports by several authors who have documented pre- and postoperative information for both the patient's clinical status and response to provocative maneuvers findings may help to answer these questions. Of 29 TIS patients, Sanders found that all were symptomatic but that only 13 had abnormal preoperative PPG tracings.[26] Following surgery, eight of these 13 patients were reexamined and half of these, despite the fact that they reported relief of symptoms, continued to demonstrate abnormal PPG tracings.[26] In another report, a high percentage of 47 preoperative TIS patients had changes in blood flow as shown by Doppler monitoring for the costoclavicular, hyperabduction, Adson's maneuver, and 90° of shoulder abduction. Postoperatively, none of the patients had residual symptoms despite the fact that five patients still demonstrated minor flow disturbances.[18] Although the results from both of these authors might lead one to conclude that there is no relationship between clinical status and provocative maneuver testing, perhaps the following should be taken into consideration. In these reports, all patients had relief of their symptoms postsurgically. Ninety percent of all TIS patients have neurological complaints and only 10 percent are known to have vascular symptoms. Because both Sanders and colleagues[27] and Pisko-Dubienski and Hollingsworth[18] noted that the patients' symptoms were relieved, perhaps (1) their complaint was primarily neurologic and was adequately relieved with surgery, since neither group noted the onset of symptoms with postsurgical maneuver testing; and (2) the positive vascular response may have occurred because a large number of individuals normally respond with false positives to these tests.

On the other hand, 45 TIS patients were studied with Doppler by Stanton and co-workers, who found that 44 of 45 had positive results prior to surgery.[27] After surgical intervention, only two of the patients' tests remained abnormal, although eight patients still complained of residual and recurrent symptoms.[27] Based on this information, I believe that there is not enough evidence to conclude anything concerning the relationship between clinical status and results of provocative maneuver testing.

Motor Nerve Conduction Velocity Studies

Most TIS patients present with neurological complaints as opposed to the few with strictly vascular symptoms. Many of the symptoms of TIS are also associated with other compression neuropathies of the upper extremity; therefore, motor nerve conduction velocities (MNCVs) are often used to localize the site of compression.[11] The conduction velocity of the ulnar nerve (UNCV) is reported most frequently by these authors who use this test extensively with the TIS patient. This is in keeping with the neurological symptom pattern outlined by Roos for compression of the lower roots of the brachial plexus.[16] Although many authors obtain MNCVs in these patients, the information from the test result is often used in very different ways. For instance, Urschel uses the velocity of conduction as criteria to operate or not. This decision was based on a comparison of the clinical status of 79 patients to the patient's pre- and postoperative UNCVs. Urschel found that the patients who had total relief following surgery also had presurgical UNCV of <60 m/sec as compared with those patients who continued to complain of residual or no change in their symptoms who had initial UNCV of >60 m/sec.[17] Although a normal UNCV from Erb's point is considered by Urschel to be 70 m/sec, patients with an initial UNCV of >60 m/sec are now referred to physical therapy instead of being advised to have surgery.[17] On the other hand, the results of MNCV studies are used by others as just one of the many pieces of the diagnostic puzzle. Caldwell and co-workers suggest that to allow MNCV results to dictate the course of management for these patients is a mistake. They recommend that additional evidence be obtained (such as positive EMG studies, documentation of sensory loss, and positive provocative maneuvers) before the course of management is decided.[12]

One possible source that may create this apparent disagreement concerning the exact usefulness of conduction velocity studies with TIS is the variability

Table 7-2. Comparison of Normal Ulnar Nerve Conduction
Velocities for Erb's Segment and Measurement
Technique

Reference	Measurement Technique	Velocity
London[28]	Calipers	58.9 ± 4.2
Cherington[51]	?[a]	59.0
Daube[52]	?	60.0 ± 5.4
Jebsen[29]	Calipers	61.3 ± 5.4
London[28]	Steel tape	70.2 ± 5.02
McGough[13]	?	70.0
Urschel and Razzuk[17]	?	70.0
Caldwell et al.[12]	Steel tape	72.0

[a] Unknown.
Velocity measured in meters per second.

in normal UNCV for Erb's point. Urschel considers 70 m/sec a normal value for this segment. Table 7-2 shows that there is no universal agreement as to what normal value is. The range of UNCV for Erb's point varies from 58.9 m/sec[28] to 72.2 m/sec.[12]

Numerous explanations have been given for the variation in this conduction value, and these include: (1) different tools such as steel tape are used rather than calipers to measure the distance between the point of supramaximal stimulation and the area under investigation[28]; (2) failure to maintain the ambient temperature constant can produce a difference of 2.4 m/sec for each degree Centigrade[29]; and (3) each individual's own MNCVs are known to vary on a day-to-day basis.[30] Because of these inconsistencies, many use standard MNCVs as a guide and establish the normal value for the segment under study for their particular center. London suggested that the subject's contralateral MNCV could be used as the "control" for normal to compare velocities on an individual basis.[28]

Obviously, the diagnosis of TIS is not made any easier by the use of electrophysiological studies. Jaeger et al have pointed out that some of the seemingly contradictory results of UNCV may be explained by the fact that Erb's point is the most proximal point of the lower trunk being stimulated.[24] These authors suggest that the portion of the lower trunk not currently studied is the point where the nerve crosses over the first rib. To assess the entire length of the lower trunk thoroughly, the technique of C8 root stimulation has been described.[24] The importance of reproducing the patient's chief complaint has also been addressed by these authors with this technique. Instead of placing the patient in the standard position with the affected upper extremity slightly abducted from the body, various positions are used to provoke the patient's symptoms.[24]

Most of these patients have sensory symptoms, i.e., pain and paresthesia, not motor dysfunction. Evoked somatosensory potential testing has recently been used by several groups for evaluation of the sensory fibers in the hope that this method will bring us one step closer to simplifying the diagnosis of TIS.[31] It is still too early to determine whether evoked somatosensory testing is worthwhile, since data are still being collected. Although not every therapist has such sophisticated equipment, sensory and sympathetic testing is readily available and is worth including in the evaluation of the TIS patient. I have found that while most of these patients show very little motor involvement, abnormalities appear on sensory and sympathetic tests.

Summary of Special Tests

This section has only scratched the surface of tests available to the physical therapist in evaluation of TIS; I hope, however, that I have made it very clear why there is no universally agreed-on diagnostic protocol for this syndrome. A fundamental evaluation scheme for the physical therapist which may be of assistance in establishing which of these tests are useful is presented later in this chapter.

The provocative maneuvers are commonly used to diagnose TIS; however, when using them, the therapist must remember that specific positions were originally described for each maneuver and any modification may change the test's intended purpose. Second, Adson's, Wright's, and the hyperabduction tests were all designed to evaluate the effect of position change of the upper extremity on the blood flow to the limb; however, only 5 to 10 percent of all TIS cases have vascular involvement. Third, although many TIS patients respond positively to the maneuvers, many asymptomatic normal persons also respond positively. Therefore, a positive test does not necessarily indicate TIS; other factors should be taken into consideration. Fourth, the relationship between the patient's clinical status and the response to provocative maneuver testing is still uncertain. Last, instruments such as Doppler ultrasound and photoplethysmography are often used in place of palpation during provocative maneuver testing with some advantages. However, there is no evidence to support the use of instrumentation over palpation.

Because 90 percent of all TI patients have neurologic complaints, many authorities believe that the site of compression can be better localized with nerve conduction studies. The information obtained from MNCVs was used in various ways by different authors. Urschel and Razzuk establish the diagnosis and select the course of treatment based on conduction velocity.[17] Others authors use the information as a mechanism of differential diagnosis.[2,5,12,32]

In addition, what is considered a normal conduction velocity for the segment from Erb's point distally is widely variable, and multiple factors have been cited for the discrepancy. As in provocative maneuver testing, no relationship has been confirmed between the patient's clinical status and the conduction velocity of the nerve.

CONSERVATIVE MANAGEMENT OF TIS

Historical Perspective: The Role of the Physical Therapist

In the literature and perhaps in personal experience, the physical therapist will encounter varied opinions regarding the role of physical therapy (PT) in the treatment of TIS. The therapist's role as described in one well-known protocol has been that of instructing the patient in a standardized set of exercises. The exercises were carried out for a 2- or 3-week period, unless the patient's symptoms worsened.[2,32] All patients were instructed by the therapist in shoulder girdle elevation and stabilization exercises, flexibility exercises for the chest and cervical musculature, and controlled breathing routines. If no symptomatic relief was obtained by the end of the trial exercise period, 1 to 3 weeks of cervical traction was ordered to rule out cervical disc or nerve root involvement.[2,32]

The therapist may also encounter those who believe that specific structures are responsible for the patient's symptoms, and that surgery—not therapy— is preferred as the ultimate treatment. According to Roos, the results of formal PT in the management of TIS are often disappointing except for patients with mild to moderate symptoms.[3] Those who experience severe neurological symptoms, Roos believes, have anomalous fibromuscular bands or irregularities of the anterior scalene which irritate the plexus, and if these patients are to feel better, those structures must be surgically removed. Furthermore, it has been Roos' experience that exercise, transcutaneous electrical nerve stimulation (TENS), and biofeedback only aggravate the symptoms and make the patient worse. PT involvement in the treatment of this physician's patients is then limited to the use of heat and massage to lessen the severity of symptoms for the patient in the advance stage of this syndrome awaiting surgery, or to postural exercises for patients with mild to moderate symptoms.[3,16,33]

Until recently, the role of the physical therapist has been either one of instituting a prescribed exercise protocol or of providing comfort for the patient awaiting surgery. However, over the last decade many physicians have elected to postpone surgical intervention in favor of a more exhaustive trial of conservative management.[5,13] McGough et al extended medical management for as long as 2 years before surgical intervention. As a result, 90 percent of their 1,200 patients were successfully relieved without surgery. In addition, these authors also reported a higher success rate for those patients who ultimately required surgery.[13]

The decision to exhaust conservative treatment affords the physical therapist the opportunity to redefine the role of PT in the management of the TIS patient. The door is open for the therapist to use specialized upper quarter musculoskeletal evaluation skills to localize the patient's problem. The therapist can then consult with the physician on these findings and together they can develop treatment tailored to the patient's needs instead of using treatment dictated by standard protocol. Perhaps in time, the results of treatment tailored to a patient's requirements will be reflected in a consistently high percentage of successful outcomes rather than the 50 to 90 percent success now anticipated from PT management.

Philosophy of PT Management

Unlike the surgical literature which is flooded with possible etiologies for this syndrome, those who manage TIS patients conservatively contend that faulty posture of the cervicothoracic spine and shoulder girdle is responsible for the symptoms. According to many authors, this altered posture places the brachial plexus and subclavian vessels in a position which makes them more vulnerable to being stretched, compressed, and rubbed by surrounding structures.[34-40] Although it is unknown whether faulty posture is the cause or the effect, the observation has been made that the symptoms of TIS correspond to a loss of muscular support and/or increased muscular tautness in the cervicothoracic and shoulder girdle region.[1,13,34-40]

Those who argue in favor of this hypothesis question whether a bony structure, such as a cervical or thoracic rib, should be held solely responsible for the symptoms associated with TIS, especially considering the fact that most of the general population are asymptomatic, even though they have a first thoracic rib; others have some type of bony abnormality but never manifest any of the TIS symptoms. For example, cervical ribs occur in ~0.5 percent of the population; of those, only 5 to 10 percent ever become symptomatic.[22] Admittedly, when a cervical rib is identified in a symptomatic person, it has become common practice to implicate it as the cause and for excision of the structure to ensue. However, several authors have reported that postural correction has relieved the symptoms of some of these patients even though they have cervical ribs. Peet et al included both patients with positive and patients with negative cervical radiographs in their treatment regime directed at postural correction. After an intensive program of strengthening and flexibility exercises, these authors concluded that all of the patients, regardless of x-ray findings, had the same 70 percent chance to achieve relief from their symptoms.[1] Similarly, Haggart reported successful treatment results for a single case study involving a patient with a cervical rib who had followed a program of strengthening for the muscles of the shoulder girdle.[37]

Perhaps, for some patients, it is imperative that a muscle be excised and/ or the first thoracic rib removed before they experience symptomatic relief. However, patients have undergone surgery and have had recurrence of their symptoms within a short time. Sanders et al reported recurrence of symptoms in 17 percent of the 239 scalenectomy patients and in 16 percent of the 214 patients who had excision of the first rib.[26] Recurrence of the patient's symptoms following removal of anatomical structures seems puzzling unless something other than the structure created the original symptoms.

The best argument in favor of the hypothesis of faulty posture is the fact that treatment programs for correction of upper quarter posture have successfully relieved the symptoms in 50 to 90 percent of all TIS patients. Therefore, the remainder of this chapter addresses PT evaluation and treatment of the TIS patient.

PHYSICAL THERAPY EVALUATION OF THE TIS PATIENT

According to Roos, "Thoracic outlet syndrome is a clinical diagnosis that depends on a careful history and physical examination."[16]

Patient History

Generally, the patient with TIS may initially have what appears to be an overwhelming problem. However, if time is set aside initially for a well-organized interview, the acquired information will be an invaluable guide for structuring the treatment plan. The interview will not tell you whether the patient has TIS or not, but the list of probable diagnoses will be narrowed and the physical examination will be expedited. The first rule of thumb when working with these patients is not to underestimate the importance of the patient interview!

Any interview format for questioning patients with upper quarter dysfunction may be used; however, it is best to choose one with which you are comfortable. I have found that a few key questions are useful when working with TIS patients. The interviewer should not be disconcerted if patients cannot recall an incident or accident that may be responsible for their current condition. Insidious onset of the symptoms of TIS is well documented. I have also found that some persons have conditions generally not considered trauma per se, such as a recent gain in weight and pregnancy. After careful questioning, the weight gain and pregnancy has proved to correspond to the onset of symptoms. Very often, not the pregnancy itself but the effect of carrying an infant or toddler was identified with the onset of symptoms. Similarly, a change in job or increased workload may also justify further investigation, since eventually this may provoke conditions that will need to be addressed and corrected.

Ninety percent of all TIS patients complain of pain, paresthesia, and paresis. More often than not the patient will have pain or paresthesia as the primary complaint. If so, the patient should be asked to sketch on a body diagram the exact location of the pain/numbness and to highlight the areas which are the worst (Fig. 7-6). Roos found that patients with nerve involvement of the upper plexus, i.e., C5–C7, report pain on the side of the neck which may radiate to the face, cranium, and anterior chest, over the scapulae, and along the lateral aspect of the forearm into the hand (Fig. 7-1). Headaches and numbness of these areas are also commonly associated with upper plexus problem.[16] According to Roos, patients with nerve involvement of the lower plexus, i.e., C8 and T1, report that the distribution of pain and numbness includes the suprascapular region, posterior neck and shoulder, and medial aspect of the arm and forearm and ulnar digits of the hand. In addition, these patients complain that the upper extremity and hand feel weak, tired, heavy, and cold[16] (Fig. 7-1).

Last, the therapist should find out if the patient's symptoms are predictable, that is, what aggravates the symptoms and what relieves or lessens them. Usually, I have found that most patients, if guided, can relate a change in their symptoms to an activity or particular posture. Upper plexus involvement may be indicated if the patient states that certain movements of the head or lifting produces their symptoms.[16] Involvement of the lower nerves of the plexus should be considered if the patient lists activities which depress the shoulder girdle, such as lifting, elevating the arm to drive, or styling the hair.[16] I have

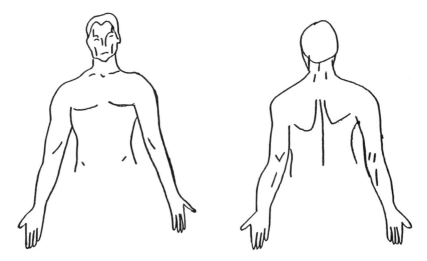

Fig. 7-6. Patient sketches location of symptoms on body diagram.

found that information pertaining to activities that produce the symptoms (i.e., upper versus lower plexus) coupled with the body diagram of the symptom pattern is sufficient to localize the area of the upper quarter to be initially examined.

Any additional questions related to past medical history such as previous cervical, thoracic, shoulder, or hand problems that display similar symptoms should be explored. Carpal tunnel syndrome and cervical disc and nerve root involvement can have the same pattern of involvement as TIS.

Physical Examination

Because multiple systems may be involved in TIS, the therapist must establish a systematic plan for evaluation. I have found it effective to organize the physical examination into two sections. The first section, a general upper quarter screen, should be done to rule out cervical disc and nerve root compression, shoulder dysfunction, and peripheral neuropathies. If this information is negative, the following six part format should be used to localize the patient's problem (Fig. 7-7). First, upper quarter posture and respiratory pattern are noted. Second, active and passive range of the head and shoulder are determined to locate soft tissue restrictions, particularly those which reproduce the patient's symptoms. Based on these findings, individual muscles are checked for tautness that might compress the neurovascular structures or refer pain. Third, the amount of bony restriction is assessed by accessory motion testing of the shoulder girdle and thoracic rib articulations. Fourth, the patient's response to the classic provocative maneuvers is recorded according to the recommendations already described. Fifth, if the patient complains of pain and paresthesia, the amount of sensory and sympathetic involvement of the upper

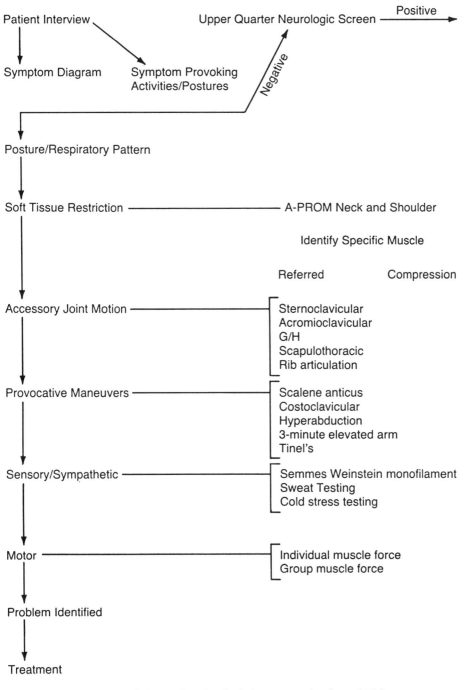

Fig. 7-7. Scheme for physical therapy evaluation of TIS.

extremity and hand is documented. Last, if the condition of a patient who complains of muscle weakness allows, the amount of force that individual muscles or groups of muscles can produce is measured by manual muscle testing or dynamometer analysis.

Postural Examination

If posture is truly at fault in producing these patients' symptoms, confirmation should begin with an upper quarter postural examination. The patient should be observed from all views, and any postural deviations should be noted. However, it is not uncommon to find insignificant postural deviations coexisting with those that are pertinent to the patient's problem. To determine which postural observations are worthy of further attention, the examiner should compare the postural information with the patient's list of symptom-provoking posture/activities and the symptom pattern sketched on the body diagram. For example, if the patient listed activities/postures that require movement of the head or lifting and the symptom diagram resembled an upper plexus symptom pattern (Fig. 7-1), I would focus on those postural faults found in the cervical region. There is much documentation to show that many of the symptoms reported by these patients are a result of a taut anterior scalene which compresses the neurovascular bundle.[14,22,37,39] Often the first clue to indicate a unilaterally shortened anterior scalene can be found by postural examination. From the anterior view, involvement of this muscle is evidenced by position of lateral flexion of the head toward the affected side and rotation toward the contralateral side, from the lateral perspective it is evidenced by an increase in the amount of cervical lordosis.

Depending on the severity of the patient's symptoms, the ipsilateral sternocleidomastoid and upper trapezius may also contribute to the postural deviations. Generally involvement of these muscles is in response to the scalene dysfunction. Spasm of the sternocleidomastoid is most notable and readily seen from the anterior view of the patient. If the upper trapezius is involved the slope of the affected shoulder and scapular height will be elevated. These patients may also breathe utilizing the accessory muscle versus diaphragmatic respiration.

On the other hand, if the patient's body diagram resembles the pattern for lower plexus involvement (Fig. 7-1) and activities that involve elevation of the arm are listed, postural deviations involving the shoulder, chest and scapulothoracic regions should be taken into consideration. Narrowing of the costoclavicular space and tautness of the pectoralis minor have frequently been implicated in compression of the plexus and subclavian vessels in cases of TIS.[25,39] Postural deviations to look for are forwardly placed and abducted shoulders and/or accentuation of the thoracic curvature, indicating shortened pectoral and medial shoulder rotator muscles.[42] The affected shoulder may also be depressed, increasing the slope of the shoulder as observed from an anterior or posterior view of the patient.

If the patient's body diagram sketch doesn't match Roos' upper and lower symptoms pattern and/or the activities that aggravate the symptoms don't correspond, perhaps the patient has components of both upper and lower plexus involvement.[16] Total involvement of both cervical and anterior chest and scapulothoracic musculature is not atypical in severely involved cases. Under these circumstances, the examiner should evaluate all of the observed postural deviations. (See Chapter 4 for further discussion of posture and the shoulder.)

Evaluation of Soft Tissue Restrictions

The next step of examination is to locate the muscle(s) that are responsible for producing the patient's symptoms, a task made easier because the list of contributing postural deviations has already been narrowed. For example, if the postural examination yields evidence of shortening of the scalene anticus and medius, the next step is to assess the amount of cervical motion these muscles will permit and to note whether further stretching of the muscle aggravates the patient's symptoms. If the patient's symptoms are reproduced by stretching the scalenes, goniometric records should be kept for future assessment of treatment. Because these muscles affect three planes of cervical motion, goniometric measures should be taken of cervical extension, lateral flexion of the head toward the contralateral side, and rotation of the head toward the affected side.

The postural examination may also produce evidence suggesting involvement of the pectoralis minor. In such cases, even though range of motion (ROM) is not measurably affected by a taut pectoralis minor, the muscle's length can be assessed by having the patient lie supine on a firm surface. If the muscle is of normal length, the posterior aspect of the shoulder will lie in contact with the surface of the table. However, if the muscle is shortened, the shoulder will be held forward, since the coracoid process of the scapula is being depressed forward and downward.[40] Once again, an assumption should not be made that this soft tissue restriction is responsible for the patient's symptoms unless the symptoms are reproduced. Stretching of the pectoralis minor can be done passively by pushing the posterior aspect of the shoulder against the surface of the table.

The previous examples are only illustrations of this concept and are certainly not the only muscles which may be found to restrict motion in these patients. Whenever possible, active and passive ROM measurements should be obtained for later assessment of treatment effectiveness.

The importance of evaluating for soft tissue restriction is twofold: first, to locate restricted motion which, when exceeded, reproduces the patient's symptoms; and second, to identify the individual muscle responsible either for compressing the neurovascular structures or referring pain. The first concept of reproducing symptoms by direct compression of the brachial plexus and subclavian vessels by a taut muscle is well established and has been traditionally classified as TIS. However, similar upper extremity symptoms have also been

Table 7-3. Muscles Which Refer Myofascial Pain to Mimic TIS Upper and Lower Plexus
Symptom Patterns

Upper Plexus	Lower Plexus
Scalene anticus	Pectoralis minor
Subclavius	Sternal fibers pectoralis major
Levator scapulae	Upper trapezius
Clavicular section pectoralis major	Triceps medial head
Sternocleidomastoid	Subscapularis
Infraspinatus	Pectoralis minor[a]
Multifidus	
Scalene anticus[a]	
Scalene medius[a]	
Subclavius[a]	

[a] Muscles classically implicated in compression of the brachial plexus and subclavian vessels which result in upper and lower plexus symptom patterns.

documented in taut skeletal muscle or its fascia containing myofascial trigger points. This phenomenon has been called referred pain or myofascial dysfunction.[41-43] These authors have found that the pain that results from compression of myofascial trigger points located in the upper quarter is referred to the thorax, upper extremity, and hand in predictable patterns. Although several authors have reported points of muscle tenderness or irritability in TIS and cervicobrachial syndrome patients,[8,16] the theory of myofascial pain has not been adequately explored in these patients. It has been my experience that many symptoms of TIS patients are not the result of direct compression on the plexus and subclavian vessels by taut muscles. Instead careful examination of the taut muscle reveals irritable points within it and, if the points are compressed by fingertip pressure, forceful contraction, or by stretching, the patient experiences the "symptoms of TIS." I have found the muscles which regularly contain myofascial trigger points in some patients with upper plexus symptom patterns to be the scalenes, the levator scapula, the subclavius, and the clavicular portion of the pectoralis major. Other muscles found with less frequency include the sternocleidomastoid, the infraspinatus, and the multifidus (Table 7-3). In some patients with typical lower plexus symptom patterns, I have found myofascial trigger points frequently in the pectoralis minor and the intermediate portion of the pectoralis major. Muscles which refer with symptoms of lower plexus compression but which I have found less frequently include the upper trapezius, medial head of the triceps and subcapularis (Table 7-3).

Reproduction of the patient's pain by muscular compression of the neurovascular structures may only require that the patient actively stretch the muscle from its origin to insertion. However, often the patient will be limited by pain and therefore will not be able to stretch the involved muscle adequately or maintain the stretch long enough to reproduce the symptoms. For this reason, the examiner may need to stretch and maintain the passively muscle, i.e., to exceed the patient's available active ROM in order to elicit the patient's complaints (Table 7-3). If this does not produce the symptoms, the muscle should then be checked for myofascial trigger points. First, the examiner should palpate over the muscle to localize a hyperirritable area within the muscle or its fascia. Generally, all that the examiner need do to reproduce the symptoms (if this is a myofascial trigger point) is apply and maintain a compressive force by fingertip pressure over the hyperirritable point. If palpation is not successful, an alternative method of trigger point localization is for the patient to forcefully contract the muscle, i.e., shorten it, and maintain it until the symptoms are elicited.[41] Further discussion of trigger point evaluation may be found in Chapter 12.

Because I have seen TIS patients whose symptoms were secondary to neurovascular compression by a taut muscle as well as by referred pain from myofascial trigger points, the reader may want to become familiar with both methods.

Muscles to Examine for Tautness and Myofascial Trigger Points in TIS Patients with Upper Plexus Involvement (Table 7-3)

Anterior Scalene

Tautness of the scalene musculature can (1) entrap the brachial plexus and subclavian vessel, (2) refer pain from trigger points within the muscle itself and, (3) depending on the severity of muscle involvement, both situations can occur.[41] Referred pain from a trigger point within the scalene will be experienced on the anterior and posterior aspects of the shoulder, lateral arm, and forearm, and distally into the radial side of the hand (Fig. 7-8). Pain resulting from nerve entrapment has been reported to follow a medial distribution or the C8–T1 dermatomal pattern as well as a lateral distribution or C5–C6 dermatomal distribution.[41] To determine whether the pain is a result of active trigger points within the muscle, Travell and Simons suggest using the scalene cramp test. For this test, the subject rotates the head toward the side of pain and actively pulls the chin down toward the clavicle by flexion of the head. The trigger points will be aggravated by forced contraction of the muscle, and the pain will be referred.[41] If the subject is experiencing too much pain to perceive a change in pain with this test, these authors suggest using the scalene-relief test to relieve the pressure of the clavicle against the muscle. To perform this test, the patient places the forearm against the forehead while raising and pulling the shoulder forward. If this position is held for several minutes, relief from the pain should occur.[41] The method for compression of the plexus and subclavian vessels by the anterior scalene has been previously described in this chapter under Adson's test.

Subclavius

I have found that the subclavius muscle is a frequent offender in this syndrome. This muscle can be stretched to compress the neurovascular structures when the examiner passively lifts the affected shoulder girdle cephalad while

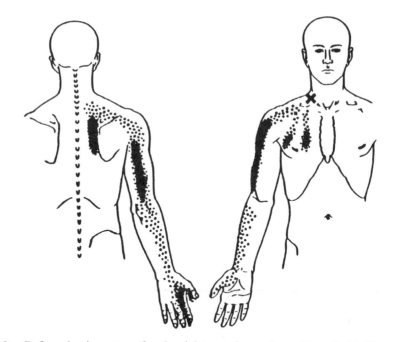

Fig. 7-8. Referred pain pattern for the right anterior scalene. (Travell JG, Simons DG: Myofascial Pain and Dysfunction. © 1983, The Williams & Wilkins Co., Baltimore.)

the subject forcefully exhales to lower the first rib.[44] The pattern of referred pain for the subclavius muscle includes the anterolateral aspect of the shoulder, arm, and forearm, both the dorsal and volar aspects of the thumb, index, and middle fingers[41] (Fig. 7-9). Myofascial trigger points within this muscle can be found by palpation of the muscle between its origin and insertion.

Levator Scapula

The levator scapula is not situated in such a way that it can compress the neurovascular structures of the thoracic inlet, but I have found that it is likely to refer pain similar to a partial upper plexus pattern in TIS. The pattern of referral includes the posterior neck, shoulder, and the area between the scapulae (Fig. 7-10). This muscle, when taut, will restrict rotation toward the affected side, neck flexion, and full abduction of the scapula.[41] Travell and Simons suggest that two trigger points may be found in this muscle by palpation along the lateral edge of the upper trapezius and the superior angle of the scapula.[41]

I have found that the clavicular portion of the pectoralis major, sterno-cleidomastoid, infraspinatus, and multifidus refer pain in a manner similar to upper plexus compression patterns. The reader may wish to consult reference 41, on myofascial pain.

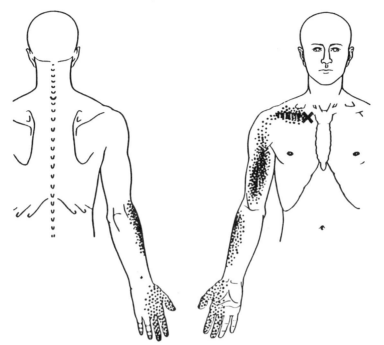

Fig. 7-9. Referred pain pattern for the (R) subclavius. (Travell JG, Simons DG: Myofascial Pain and Dysfunction. © 1983, The Williams & Wilkins Co., Baltimore.)

Fig. 7-10. Referred pain pattern for the (R) levator scapulae. (Travell JG, Simons DG: Myofascial Pain and Dysfunction. © 1983, The Williams & Wilkins Co., Baltimore.)

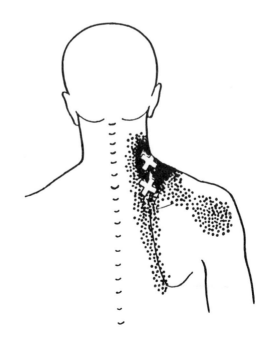

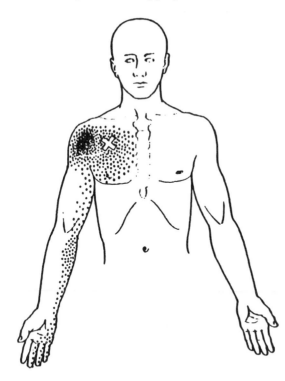

Fig. 7-11. Referred pain pattern for pectoralis minor muscle. (Travell JG, Simons DG: Myofascial Pain and Dysfunction. © 1983, The Williams & Wilkins Co., Baltimore.)

Muscles to Examine for Tautness and Myofascial Trigger Points in TIS Patients with Lower Plexus Involvement (Table 7-3)

Pectoralis Minor

Stretching of the pectoralis minor to evaluate its role in compression of the neurovascular structures can be done in the following manner. The patient should be positioned supine with the affected arm supported and with the shoulder in adduction and medial rotation. The examiner should await the onset of symptoms while simultaneously flexing the adducted and medially rotated shoulder (to rotate the coracoid process upwardly) and while the subject forcefully exhales (to lower the ribs).

To locate myofascial trigger points within this muscle, the opposite procedure is described by Travell and Simons for compression of the pectoralis minor. The supine subject forcefully raises the affected shoulder off the table, keeping the arm relaxed and inhales. During this procedure, the examiner should palpate for irritable points within the now-exposed muscle. The pattern of referral from this muscle includes the anterior chest, medial aspect of the arm and forearm, and volar aspects of the ulnar three digits[41] (Fig. 7-11). These authors believe that it is not uncommon to find associated trigger points in the pectoralis major, and I acknowledge this finding in TIS patients. The intermediate sternal fibers of this muscle refer pain in the pattern which includes the anterior chest wall and typical C8–T1 dermatomal distribution noted by Roos.[16] To locate the trigger points, Travell and Simons suggest a pinching type of palpation of the muscle with the arm abducted to 90°.[41]

Additional muscles which may refer pain mimicking a lower plexus compression pattern in part include the upper trapezius, the medial head of the triceps, and the subscapularis.

Motion Testing for TIS

I refer the reader to a manual therapy treatment protocol described by Smith explicitly for management of the TIS patient.[45] Smith describes a seven-step protocol for increasing the mobility of the shoulder girdle and the first and second thoracic ribs by joint mobilization of the sternoclavicular and acromioclavicular joints, scapula, and thoracic ribs, and by soft tissue stretching. The results of treatment are reported and support the effectiveness of this method of management. I have used some of Smith's treatment suggestions and have found that some TIS patients do not require mobilization since they have only soft tissue restrictions; other patients are initially in such pain that mobilization is not tolerated until the final stages of treatment. The fact that not all patients respond similarly emphasizes the point that a single standard treatment protocol for all patients is not always successful, and that treatment should be based on the findings of the physical examination.

Provocative Maneuver Examination

Review of the procedures and purposes of the scalene anticus, costoclavicular, and hyperabduction tests can be found in the first sections of this chapter. Although the validity of these maneuvers is still unknown, these tests are still frequently used to diagnose TIS. I propose that provocative maneuvers remain a part of the physical therapist's examination scheme, not for the purpose of diagnosis, but for research purposes. As a cursory step toward establishing the predictive validity of these tests, I suggest the following protocol.

1. Each maneuver is performed bilaterally in accordance with the classic description.
2. The patient's pulse is monitored under the criteria that a change (i.e., reduced quality of pulse or cessation of pulse) constitutes a negative response to the test and that no change is a negative response.
3. If symptoms are elicited, notation is made of the length of time it took to reproduce the symptoms with the maneuver.
4. The above information is gathered on initial evaluation, periodically during the course of therapy, and again prior to discharge of the patient. With this systematic approach, the examiner may be able to establish whether there

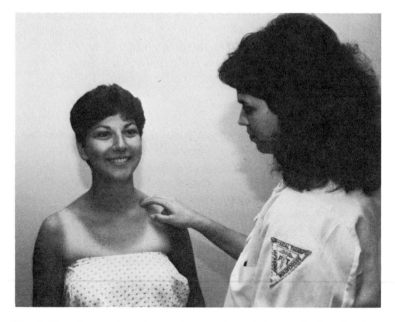

Fig. 7-12.   Percussion at superior opening of thorax for Tinel's sign.

is a relationship between the patient's clinical status and the patient's response to provocative maneuver testing.

Another provocative test described by several authors is percussion or tapping along the pathway of the plexus from the superior thoracic outlet toward the axilla (Fig. 7-12). These authors have found that percussion reveals areas of local tenderness in TIS patients.[13]

According to Kaplan's translation of the classic Tinel's sign, local pain produced by pressure applied to a nerve is a sign of nerve irritation. However, pressure on the nerve resulting in a tingling felt in the distribution of the nerve is a sign of axon regeneration.[46] In several TIS patients, I have noted that percussion of the nerve initially produces localized pain; however, as the patient's clinical status improves, the local pain response changes to the "radiating tingling" of nerve regeneration. The therapist may want to take note of the response to nerve percussion during the course of treatment in order to document whether a relationship between the nerve sign and the patient's clinical status exists.

Sensory and Sympathetic Evaluation

The TIS patient will often complain of pain and paresthesia. These symptoms suggest sensory involvement, which should be documented so that the extent of involvement is known and so that later this information can be used

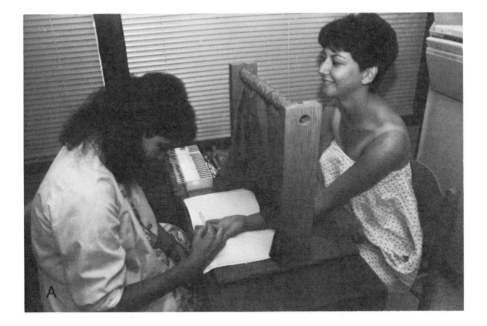

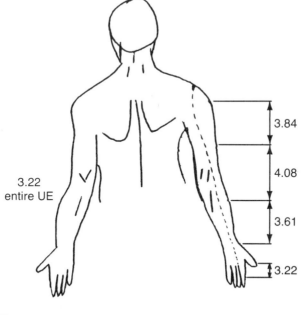

Fig. 7-13. (A) Evaluation of cutaneous sensibility with Semmes Weinstein monofilaments. (B) Monofilament mapping of upper extremity paraesthesia. (R) UE, patient's affected side; (L) UE uninvolved side.

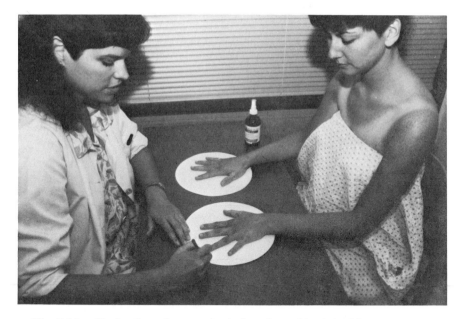

Fig. 7-14. Evaluation of sympathetic function with ninhydrin sweat test.

to evaluate effectiveness of treatment. The therapist can evaluate cutaneous sensibility of the upper extremity by using pressure-sensitive monofilaments, also known as Semmes Weinstein monofilaments (Fig. 7-13A and B). These nylon filaments are calibrated so that when a specific amount of pressure is applied to the tip, it will bend, indicating that the filament's threshold has been reached. Twenty filaments ranging from .0045 g to 447 g can be used to map out sensory localization capability.[47] Although a scale of interpretation for this test has been extensively developed for the palm of the hand, it is possible to map out sensory localization for the entire upper extremity. Because it is documented that 90 percent of all TIS patients complain of paresthesia of the upper extremity, I have recently started to use the monofilaments for TIS patients; the cutaneous sensibility mapping is done of the extremity based on the area sketched in by the patient on the body diagram. The uninvolved extremity of these patients is used as their norm (Fig. 7-12). Because these patients' complaints are more often sensory than motor in nature, this easily administered, noninvasive test may reveal more information than do tests for motor nerve involvement. Another bonus of this test is that the patient may be tested in a position that provokes the symptoms.

If sympathetic involvement is suspected, ninhydrin or sweat testing of both hands can be done (Fig. 7-14) and cold recovery times can be secured (Fig. 7-15A and B).[48,49]

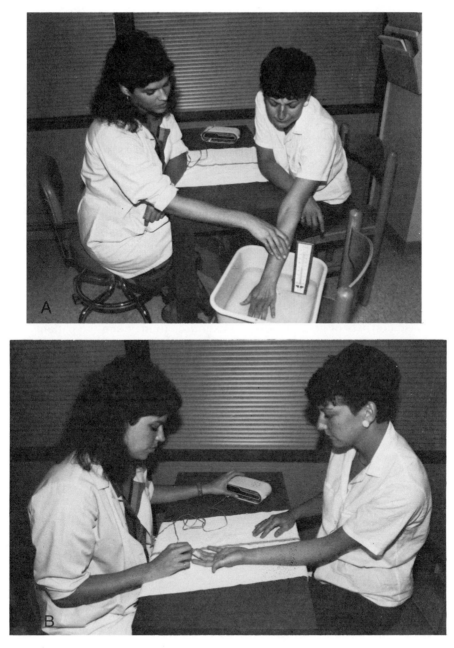

Fig. 7-15. Evaluation of cold recovery after (A) submerging hand in cold water bath, and (B) monitoring of hand temperature before and after submersion with temperature thermistor.

PHYSICAL THERAPY TREATMENT OF THE TIS PATIENT

Treatment of the TIS patient is based solely on the information collected from the patient interview and physical examination. The purpose of this section is not to describe a "cookbook protocol" for the therapist to follow, but to illustrate how very different the PT management of these patients can be. The traditional philosophy of conservative management of the TIS patient has been to correct the faulty posture. This philosophy appears to hold true whether the patient's pain is secondary to neurovascular compression or myofascial dysfunction.

To achieve postural correction, I have found that the TIS patient must pass through three phases of treatment (Fig. 7-16). In the first phase, both the therapist and the patient must be able to control the amount of pain, i.e., increase or decrease the pain. Once the patient realizes that the pain is controllable, treatment can be advanced to the next phase. In the second phase, treatment is directed at exercises to alter the symptom-producing musculoskeletal faults. Once the pain is controlled and postural corrections are attained, the final phase of treatment consists of a postural maintenance program. This final phase consists of general postural exercises to maintain the patient in the asymptomatic status, which is extremely difficult considering the frequence of recurrence in this patient population. There are no distinct dividing lines between the three phases of treatment. It is not at all uncommon for a patient in the second or third phase of treatment to report back with the original symptoms. In most cases, symptom recurrence is only temporary; however, it does

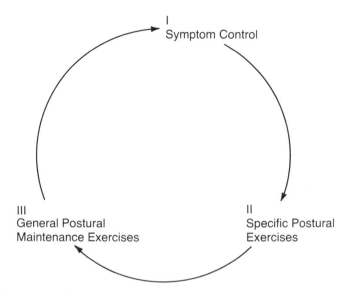

I
Symptom Control

III
General Postural
Maintenance Exercises

II
Specific Postural
Exercises

Fig. 7-16.   The three phases of physical therapy treatment for TIS.

require a return to the initial phase of treatment to bring the symptoms under control.

Throughout the remainder of this section, two clinical case studies will be used to illustrate key points of treatment. These cases are used only as examples and are by no means used to suggest that this is the only method of management. The first case illustrates myofascial dysfunction, and the second case describes neurovascular compression.

Case Study 1

J.K., a 39-year-old office manager/keypunch operator complained of pain between the scapulae radiating to the shoulder and down the lateral aspect of the arm, hypersensitivity along the lateral border of the forearm, and cold and numbness of the thumb and index finger (Fig. 7-17). She said that the forearm and hand symptoms were always present but that the arm and scapular symptoms were dull aches in the morning which intensified to constant pain by the end of a full day of typing and desk work. Her self-rating of pain on examination was three on a scale of 10, but would reach as high as a seven on bad days.

Pertinent clinical findings included reproduction of J.K.'s symptoms when fingertip pressure was applied to the (R) levator scapula, as well as with passive flexion of the head, stretching the levator scapulae. Reduction in the symptoms was achieved by the combination of passive extension and (R) rotation of the head. Semmes Weinstein monofilament testing along the lateral aspect of the upper extremity and hand demonstrated significant loss of sensation as compared with the contralateral extremity. Increased sympathetic function in the (R) hand in comparison to the (L) hand was also noted on sweat testing.

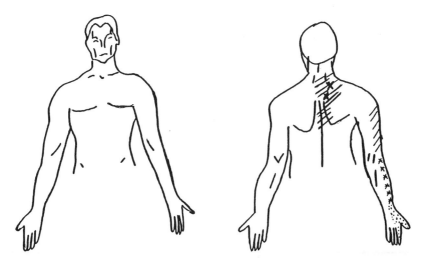

Fig. 7-17. Symptom pattern as described by J. K. in case study 1 ($\times$ = trigger point; /// = pain; ** hypersensitive; and :::, cold).

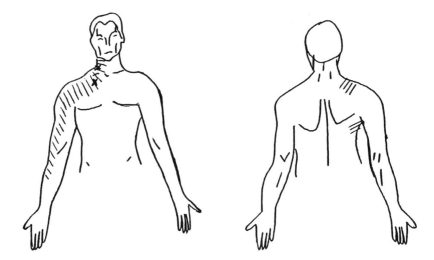

Fig. 7-18.   Symptom pattern as described by L. M. in case study 2 (///, pain).

J.K. reported a pain rating of zero and normalization of sensation after 10 treatments over a period of 20 days.

Case Study 2

L.M., a 28-year-old laborer, claimed that his symptoms were the result of operating a jackhammer 1½ years previously. His complaints included pain and swelling of the (R) anterior chest and right-sided neck pain which radiated across the shoulder and the lateral aspect of the arm and proximal third of the forearm (Fig. 7-18). At rest, L.M. rated his pain as one on a scale of 10; however, any use of the upper extremity or hand would elevate the pain to a rating of seven. This patient related that his symptoms were not any better following bilateral carpal tunnel releases, bilateral first thoracic rib resection, resection of the proximal one-third of the right (R) clavicle and a dozen (R) stellate ganglion blocks.

Pertinent physical findings included palpation tenderness of the (R) scalenes, sternocleidomastoid, upper trapezius, medial end of the clavicle, and clavectomy scars. Forced or deep inspiration was painful and lying supine was impossible. Cervical motion was restricted to 15° to 20° of left (L) lateral flexion, rotation, and extension. All plans of (R) shoulder active motion were restricted by two-thirds of the arc of full motion. Postural examination revealed abnormal forward flexion, (R) lateral flexion and (R) rotation of the head, and elevated and abducted (R) shoulder.

Initial Phase of Treatment

Modalities have traditionally been used to provide pain relief and reduce muscle spasm during the initial phase of treatment of TIS. As early as 1919, Stopford and Telford described the successful use of faradic stimulation and massage to relieve the symptoms caused by spasm of the upper trapezius.[34] To manage pain in this patient population, other therapists have included moist heat, infrared, ice, and massage as their first line of treatment.[1,13,35,48] I prefer the analgesia obtained after application of ice over an area of muscle tenderness. For example, the use of ice in myofascial dysfunction as in case 1 anesthetized the levator scapula. This was crucial to the success of the first phase of treatment, because J.K. then felt that the pain was controllable. Once in control of the pain, she permitted the treatment which was necessary to begin deactivation of the myofascial trigger point.

In severely involved cases, such as that of L.M. in case study 2, the immediate treatment goal may be only to show the patient that the amount of pain he or she is experiencing can be temporarily reduced. The patient must have the feeling of being able to control the amount of pain experienced; adding passive stretch or vigorous massage may interfere with this objective.

During the initial phase when pain control is the priority, most authors suggest that the patient avoid any activity or posture which will aggravate the symptoms.[1,13,24] The examiner should be well aware of these postures/activities, having obtained this information from the patient's initial interview and from reproduction of the patient's pain during physical examination. Because the objective of this phase of treatment is to control pain, part of the control will come from understanding what postures/activities elicit the pain. Therefore, to complete this phase, it is imperative that the therapist guide the patient so that he or she understands what postures/activities evoke symptoms in order to avoid them. Unfortunately, many patients find the job-related activities produce their symptoms. In most cases, avoidance of work is not an acceptable solution; however, task modification is a feasible option. For example, in case study 1, typing from copy placed on the right side of the typewriter aggravated this patient's symptoms by compression of an active trigger point in the (R) levator scapula. Instead of avoiding all typing, the position of the copy was changed to one directly at eye level and in front of the patient. This position eliminated the need for the constant contraction of the (R) levator scapula which contributed to this patient's symptoms.

For L.M., case study 2, merely the unsupported weight of the upper extremity depressed the shoulder girdle. Depression was then the stimulus for the (R) scalenes, sternocleidomastoid, and upper trapezius to contract continuously to elevate the shoulder girdle. To avoid continuous contraction of these muscle, which in turn compressed the upper plexus, L.M. made a conscious effort 24 hours a day to support the extremity passively. When seated, he placed the arm on a tabletop, chair armrest, or pillow. When standing, he found that the (R) arm could be cradled either by the (L) arm or by placing his hand in his pocket. Spurling and Grantham describe a position in which the hand was passively placed behind the head to relax the anterior scalene. According to these authors, 300 of the 400 patients who avoided tension on the scalene were successfully managed.[36] Hansson used other passive methods of support such as a sling, a figure-8 wrap around the shoulders similar to a clavicular sling, or an airplane splint to support the weight of the upper extremity.[48] For women

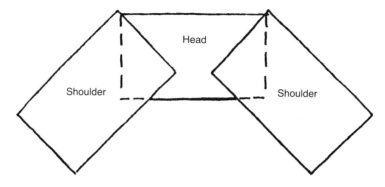

Fig. 7-19. Supine pillow arrangement for flexion for cervical spine, abduction of scapulae and support of shoulders to relieve scalene anticus spasm. (Reichert FL: Compression of the brachial plexus: the scalene anticus syndrome. JAMA 137:508, Copyright, 1942 The American Medical Association.)

with pendulous breasts, extra padding to increase the surface area of the shoulder straps or an underwire support brassiere to distribute the weight against the trunk rather than across the shoulders have been described.[13,24] Reichert suggested that these patients also required a change in their sleep habits, as positions assumed during sleep would continue to aggravate the anterior scalene. To prevent this, the author recommended strategic placement of three pillows, one pillow to support and slightly flex the cervical spine and the other to abduct the scapulae and provide support for each shoulder (Fig. 7-19). The combination of this resting posture and shoulder-shrugging exercises resulted in successful treatment in 60 out of 74 patients.[36]

In the initial phase, the patient should learn that pain can be controlled by a therapeutic modality and by avoidance of postures and activities that provoke the symptoms. Without this understanding and a conscious effort to control the symptoms, success in the final phases of treatment will be less than optimal.

Second Phase of Treatment

Once the patient understands that it is possible to change the intensity of his symptoms and the acuteness of the pain has subsided, treatment phase two should be initiated. The primary objective during this phase of management is correction of the previously identified musculoskeletal faults. In myofascial dysfunction, the muscle learns to avoid pain by shortening.[41] The levator scapula of J.K. in case study 1 was shortened as evidenced by restricted forward flexion and (L) rotation of the head. Ice and stretch will quiet an active myofascial trigger point, but active exercise is necessary to maintain a full pain-free ROM of the muscle. To obtain full motion of the head, J.K. actively stretched the muscle to the point of discomfort, maintaining this position for a count of 10 seconds. Initially, all planes of motion were stretched independently of one another; as she progressed, shoulder depression was combined with full forward flexion and (L) rotation of the head. Eventually, these exercises could be performed without the assistance of ice or heat.

During this phase of treatment, it is important that both the therapist and patient realize that treatment will reproduce the patient's symptoms. This symptom reproduction will be the result of either compression of the active trigger point or compression of the taut muscle against the neurovascular structures. I have found that it is beneficial for both the therapist and the patient to agree on the maximum level of discomfort that will be allowed during the course of each day's treatment. Thus, the patient maintains the feeling of control over the intensity of the pain. This concept worked well during L.M.'s second phase of care. Once he learned that the pain could be reduced to a level of one or two after treatment with application of heat, he began to tolerate a pain rating ranging from four to six during treatment.

When the number of musculoskeletal faults seem overwhelming, the examiner should approach treatment in a stepwise fashion and should not try to correct all postural deviations at once. Often, when one area is corrected, the other faults are self-corecting. Although L.M. had extensive shoulder, chest, and neck soft tissue restrictions, the initial treatment was directed only toward the limitations of cervical movement and then toward the shoulder. Because head movement was so restricted, active neck ROM exercises were pursued first in a progressive fashion. The first treatment objective of this phase was to move the head only to the point of discomfort. Several sessions later, movement was taken further into the range of discomfort; the final step was tolerance of more vigorous contract–relax techniques. During this phase, ice continued to precede active exercise, and heat or ultrasound for muscle relaxation followed exercise at the patient's request.

During this phase of treatment, the patient will begin to experience relief and will quite naturally want to pursue long-neglected tasks and activities. To avoid unnecessary setbacks caused by the overzealous patient who carries in a sack of groceries, rakes leaves, shovels snow, vacuums, or tackles a desk full of paper work. It is the therapist's task to frequently remind the patient to remain conscious of symptom producing postures/activities. These reminders should also include guidelines for progressively increasing the patient's level of activity.

Final Phase of Treatment

The final phase of treatment should proceed once the patient has some means of controlling the intensity of symptoms and either has no symptoms or has a pain rating that has plateaued for a period of time so that further treatment is not effective; the specific musculoskeletal faults should be maximally corrected. The patient may not necessarily enter this final phase of treatment symptom-free. It is not at all uncommon for residual low-grade symp-

Table 7-4. General Postural Maintenance Exercises for TIS

Do each exercise ___ times each day.

1. Stand erect with the arms at the sides. (A) Bending the neck to the left, attempt to touch the left ear to the left shoulder without shrugging shoulder. (B) Bending the neck to the right, attempt to touch the right ear to the right shoulder without shrugging the shoulder. (C) Relax and repeat.

2. Stand facing the corner of the room with one hand on each wall, arms at shoulder level, palms forward, elbows bent and abdominal muscles contracted. (A) Slowly let the upper part of the trunk lean forward and press to the chest into the corner. Inhale as the body leans forward. Return to the original position by pushing out with the hands. Exhale with this movement.

3. Stand erect with the arms at the sides, holding in each hand a ___ pound weight. (A) Shrug the shoulders forward and upward. (B) Relax. (C) Shrug the shoulders backward and upward. (D) Relax. (E) Shrug the shoulders upward. (F) Relax and repeat.

4. Stand erect with the arms out straight from the sides at shoulder level; hold a ___ pound weight in each hand (palms should be down). (A) Raise the arms sideways and up until the backs of the hands meet above the head (keep elbows straight). (B) Relax and repeat.

5. Lie face down with (R) arm outstretched overhead with the head turned toward the left. (A) Raise the arm off the supporting surface. Hold this position for a count of three. Inhale as the arm is raised. (B) Exhale and return to original position. (C) Repeat. Do the same with the (L) arm with the head turned toward the right.

6. Lie on the back with arms at the sides, with a rolled towel or small pillow under the upper part of the back between the shoulder blades and no pillow under the head. (A) Inhale slowly and raise the arms upward and backward overhead. (B) Exhale and lower the arms to the sides. Repeat 5 to 20 times.

Clinician should add further exercise specific for patient's needs.

(Adapted from Peet RM, Henriksen JD, Anderson TP, Martin GM: Thoracic Outlet Syndrome: Evaluation of a Therapeutic Exercise Program. Staff Meetings Mayo Clin 31:281, 1956.)

toms to persist; in some cases, these symptoms will gradually subside; other patients may have to learn to accommodate themselves to some symptoms.

Failure of conservative management to provide long-lasting relief for TIS patients is secondary to unsatisfactory completion of this phase of treatment. To maintain the correction of postural faults, the patient must not only continue to be cognizant of the activities/postures which will aggravate symptoms, but must also continue to perform generalized postural exercises to maintain symptom-free status.

The exercises outlined by Peet et al and later adopted by others as the prescribed protocol for the treatment of TIS are quite satisfactory for the purpose of postural maintenance[1,2,33] (Table 7-4). Exercises specific to the patient's particular needs should also supplement this program.

Occasionally, patients will not obtain relief from PT management or will still have severe functional restrictions secondary to their symptoms. In those infrequent cases, if all means of conservative management have been exhausted, the patient's problem may not be one for the physical therapist to manage. If examination provided evidence of neurovascular compression, the therapist should derive satisfaction from the report of McGough et al which showed improved surgical success if the patient had exhausted a long-term PT management before a different type of treatment was considered.[13]

Summary of PT Evaluation and Treatment

The traditional philosophy of those who conservatively manage the TIS patient is that postural faults are responsible for the symptoms. I suggest that successful management of the TIS patient is dependent on both a carefully guided patient interview and a thorough physical examination. It is more important in the interview to gather information about the symptom pattern and occurrence than to determine the cause, since so many of these cases report insidious onset. Physical examination for TIS should proceed only if the upper quarter neurological screen yields negative information for cervical disc and nerve root compression, shoulder dysfunction, and peripheral neuropathies. I suggest a six-part format for examination of the TIS patient, to be supplemented with information obtained from the patient interview. Included in this multipart evaluation format are: (1) a generalized postural examination with attention to the pattern of respiration, (2) evaluation of soft tissue restriction with emphasis on evaluation for taut muscles which might either compress the neurovascular structures or refer pain by myofascial dysfunction, (3) accessory motion testing, (4) an alternative method for use of TIS provocative maneuvers, (5) evaluation of upper extremity and hand sensory involvement with Semmes Weinstein monofilament, and (6) motor testing by individual muscle testing or dynamometer analysis of grip and pinch force.

Once the patient's problem is localized, treatment should follow in three phases. Two case studies have been provided here to serve as examples of a method of management of TIS patients. The purpose of the first phase is to bring the symptoms into control and to assist the patient in gaining awareness in avoiding postures/activities which evoke the symptoms. The second phase of treatment is directed at correction of specific symptom-producing postural faults; continued attention is paid to the goals of the initial phase. The primary purpose of the final phase of care is to prevent symptom recurrence by instructing the patient in generalized postural exercises to be carried out in addition to the exercises specific to the patient's musculoskeletal needs. I believe that this final phase of care is often neglected, which may account for the number of patients who do not achieve long-lasting relief following conservative management of TIS.

REFERENCES

1. Peet RM, Henriksen JD, Anderson TP, Martin GM: Thoracic outlet syndrome: Evaluation of a therapeutic exercise program. Staff meetings Mayo Clin 31:281, 1956

2. Kelly TR: Thoracic outlet syndrome: Current concepts of treatment. Ann Surg 190:657, 1979
3. Roos DB: New concepts of thoracic outlet syndrome that explains etiology, symptoms, diagnosis and treatment. Vasc Surg 13:313, 1979
4. Crawford FA: Thoracic outlet syndrome. Surg Clin North Am 60:947, 1980
5. Dale WA: Thoracic outlet compression syndrome. Arch Surg 117:1437, 1982
6. Warwick R, Williams PL (eds): Gray's Anatomy. 35th British Ed. WB Saunders Co, Philadelphia, 1973
7. Gardner E, Gray DJ, O'Rahilly R: Anatomy: A Regional Study of Human Structure. 4th Ed. WB Saunders Co, Philadelphia, 1975
8. Johnson DA: Posture and cervicobrachial pain syndromes. JAMA 159:1507, 1955
9. Hadler NA: Medical Management of the Regional Musculoskeletal Diseases. Grune & Stratton, Orlando, Fla, 1984
10. Williams HT, Carpenter NH: Surgical treatment of the thoracic outlet compression syndrome. Arch Surg 113:850, 1978
11. Urschel HC, Razzuk MA, Albers JE, et al: Reoperation for recurrent thoracic outlet syndrome. Ann Thorac Surg 21:19, 1979
12. Caldwell JW, Crane CR, Krusen EM: Nerve conduction studies: an aid in the diagnosis of thoracic outlet syndrome. South Med J 64:210, 1971
13. McGough EC, Pearce MB, Byrne JP: Management of thoracic outlet syndrome. J Thorac Cardiovasc Surg 77:169, 1979
14. Raff J: Surgery for cervical rib and scalenus anticus syndrome. JAMA 157:219, 1955
15. Judy KL, Heymann RL: Vascular complications of thoracic outlet syndrome. Am J Surg 123:521, 1972
16. Roos DB: The place for scalenectomy and first-rib resection in thoracic outlet syndrome. Surgery 92:1077, 1982
17. Urschel HC, Razzuk MA: Management of thoracic outlet syndrome. N Engl J Med 285:1140, 1972
18. Pisko-Dubienski ZA, Hollingsworth J: Clinical application of Doppler ultrasonography in the thoracic outlet syndrome. Can J Surg 21:145, 1978
19. Geroudis R, Barnes RW: Thoracic outlet arterial compression: Prevalence in normal persons. Angiography 31:538, 1980
20. Coote H: Pressure on the axillary vessels and nerve by an exostosis from a cervical rib interference with the circulation of the arm. Removal of the rib and exostosis recovery. Med Times Gaz 11:108, 1861
21. Falconer MA, Weddell G: Costoclavicular compression of the subclavian artery and vein. Lancet 2:539, 1943
22. Adson AW, Coffey JR: Cervical rib. Ann Surg 85:839, 1927
23. Roos DB: Congenital anomalies associated with thoracic outlet syndrome. Am J Surg 132:771, 1976
24. Jaeger SH, Read R, Smullens S, Breme P: Thoracic outlet syndrome: Diagnosis and treatment. p. 378. In Hunter J, Mackin E, Bell J, Callahan A (eds): Rehabilitation of the Hand. CV Mosby, St. Louis, 1984
25. Wright IS: The neurovascular syndrome produced by hyperabduction of the arms. Am Heart J 29:1, 1945
26. Sanders RJ, Monsour JW, Gerber WF, Adams WR, Thompson N: Scalenectomy versus first rib resection for the treatment of thoracic outlet syndrome. Surgery 85:109, 1978
27. Stanton PE, McClusky DA, Richardson HD, Lamis PA: Thoracic outlet syndrome: a comprehensive evaluation. South Med J 71:1070, 1978

28. London GW: Normal ulnar nerve conduction velocity across the thoracic outlet: comparison of two measuring techniques. J Neurol Neurosurg Psychol 38:756, 1975

29. Jebsen RH: Motor conduction velocities in the median and ulnar nerves. Arch Phys Med Rehab 48:185, 1967

30. Honet JC, Jebsen RH, Perrin EB: Variability of nerve conduction velocity determinations in normal persons. Arch Phys Med Rehab 49:650, 1968

31. Glover JL, Worth MD, Bendick PJ, et al: Evoked responses in the diagnosis of thoracic outlet syndrome. Surg 89:86–93, 1980

32. Dale WA, Lewis MR: Management of thoracic outlet syndrome. Ann Surg 181::;575, 1975

33. Roos DB: Experience with first rib resection for thoracic outlet syndrome. Ann Surg 173:429, 1971

34. Stopford JS, Telford ED: Compression of the lower trunk of the brachial plexus by a first dorsal rib. Br J Surg 7:168, 1919

35. Spurling RG, Grantham EG: The painful arm and shoulder with especial reference to the problem of scalene neurocirculatory compression. J Miss Med Assoc 38:340, 1941

36. Reichert FL: Compression of the brachial plexus: the scalene anticus syndrome. JAMA 118:294, 1942

37. Haggart GE: Value of conservative management of cervicobrachial pain. JAMA 137:508, 1948

38. McGowen JM, Velinsky M: Costoclavicular compression. Arch Surg 59:62, 1949

39. Raff J: Surgery for cervical rib and scalenus anticuus syndrome. JAMA 157:219, 1955

40. Kendall FP, McCreary EK: Muscle Testing and Function. 3rd Ed. Williams & Wilkins, Baltimore, 1983

41. Travell JG, Simons DG: Myofascial Pain and Dysfunction. Waverly Press, Baltimore, 1983

42. Cyriax J: Rheumatic headache. Br Med J 2:1367, 1938

43. Gorrell RL: Musculofascial pain. JAMA 142:557, 1950

44. Evjenth O, Hamberg J: The spinal column and the temporomandibular joint. Ch. 3. In Muscle Stretching in Manual Therapy. Vol. 2. Alfta Rehab Forlag, Sweden, 1984

45. Smith KF: The thoracic outlet syndrome: a protocol of treatment. J Orth Sport Phys Ther 1:89, 1979

46. Kaplan EB: The "tingling" sign in peripheral nerve lesions. p. 8. In Spinner M (ed): Injuries to the Major Branches of Peripheral Nerves of the Forearm. 2nd Ed. WB Saunders Co, Philadelphia

47. von Frey M, Kiesow F: Uber die Function der Tastkorperchen Yeit. Psychol Physiol Sinnesory 20:126, 1899

48. Moberg E: Objective methods for determining the functional value of sensibility in the hand. JBJS 40:454, 1958

49. Porter J, Snider R, Bardana E, et al: The diagnosis and treatment of Raynaud's phenomenon. Surgery 77:11, 1975

50. Hansson KG: Scalene anticus syndrome. Surg Clin North Am 22:611, 1942

51. Cherington M: Ulnar nerve conduction velocity in thoracic outlet syndrome. N Engl J Med 294:1185, 1976

52. Daube JR: Nerve conduction studies in thoracic outlet syndrome. (Abstract) Neurol 25:347, 1975

8 | Management of Brachial Plexus Lesions and Their Relation to the Shoulder

Robert E. DuVall

Lesions of the brachial plexus and its nerves frequently compromise the neurological integrity and function of the shoulder. The brachial plexus is uniquely susceptible to mechanical lesion due to its superficial topographical location between the mobile cervical spine and the mobile shoulder girdle. It may also be affected by other disorders, including inflammatory, hereditary, toxic, nutritional, metabolic, entrapment, and compression causes. The anatomic basis for the different etiological types of brachial plexus lesions, their clinical features, means of evaluation, and principles of treatment will be presented in this chapter.

Proximal brachial plexus lesions are most commonly seen in children and are usually caused by birth injuries.[1] However, peripheral brachial plexus lesions are a more common result of wartime or athletic participation and are not frequently seen in general medical practices.[1,2] Brachial plexus lesions may result from violent throwing, pulling, or wrenching of the arms or shoulder (see Ch. 10); traumatic blows to or weight on the neck and/or shoulder; surgical operations involving the shoulder-girdle; gunshot wounds, stab wounds, automobile accidents; fractures, subluxations, and dislocations of the neck, shoulder, or head of the humerus (see Ch. 9); tumors of the neck or within the shoulder-girdle; aneurysms of the subclavian artery; infections, toxic and multiple neuritis in the neck and shoulder-girdle region; and the scalenus anticus syndrome, cervical rib syndrome, and hyperabduction syndrome (see Ch. 7).[1,2]

Long-term complications of brachial plexus lesions may include skin blisters, ulceration and secondary infection, muscular contractures, joint stiffness, osteoporosis, reflex sympathetic dystrophy, and causalgia.[2] The definitive analysis of the clinical findings, combined with an electroneuromyographic examination, can lead to precise localization of the lesion, which is essential for clinical decision making regarding therapeutic intervention.

ANATOMY OF BRACHIAL PLEXUS

The brachial plexus is comprised of the anterior primary divisions of spinal segments C5, C6, C7, C8, and T1 (Fig. 8-1).[3,4] Its components are the following:

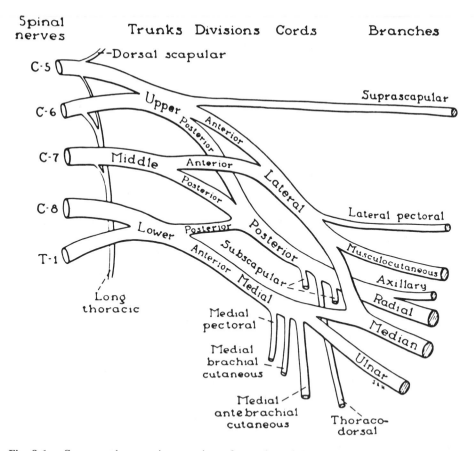

Fig. 8-1. Segmental motor innervation of muscles of the shoulder. (Hollinshead WH: Functional Anatomy of the Limbs and Back. 4th Ed., WB Saunders Co., Philadelphia, 1976.)

1. Undivided anterior primary rami
2. Trunks—upper, middle, lower
3. Divisions of the trunks—anterior and posterior
4. Cords—lateral, posterior, and medial
5. Branches—peripheral nerves derived from the cords

Distributing from the region just distal to the series of intervertebral foramina, the brachial plexus undivided anterior primary rami are situated between the scalene muscles. Anterior primary ramus C5 usually receives an accession from ramus C4, and T1 frequently receives an accession from ramus T2. However, contributions made to the brachial plexus by C4 and T2 are subject to frequent variation.[3] When the branch of C4 is large, the branch from T1 is reduced in size. This constitutes the "prefixed type" of brachial plexus. On the other hand, the branch from C4 may be very small or entirely absent. In that event, the contribution of C5 is reduced in size, but that of T1 is larger and the branch from T2 is always present. This arrangement constitutes the "post-fixed type" of plexus.[2]

From individual primary rami, there arise two nerves of clinical significance: the long thoracic nerve (C5–C7), which descends by a deep course to supply the serratus anterior muscle and the dorsal scapular nerve (C5), is the motor innervation to the rhomboid muscles. A twig from root C5 passes to the phrenic nerve. Additional segmental motor innervation of muscles of the shoulder is identified in Figure 8-2.

The brachial plexus has three trunks: the upper, which contains fibers of segments C4, C5, and C6; the middle, which is a continuation of undivided anterior primary ramus C7; and the lower, which includes fibers from C8 and T1 and sometimes T2. The trunks are positioned mainly in the supraclavicular fossa, all three originating just distal to the scalene muscles. The upper trunk gives origin to the suprascapular nerve (C4–C6) and supplies the supraspinatus and infraspinatus muscles. A nerve extends to the subclavius muscles (C4–C6) from the upper trunks or fifth root.

Fibers of the three trunks are reassembled through the brachial plexus divisions, which are situated deep to the middle third of the clavicle and extend distally to a point just beyond the lateral border of the first rib. Crossing through the anterior divisions are those fibers reaching the ventral parts of the limb, whereas the fibers destined for the limb's dorsal parts extend through the posterior divisions.

Anatomical variations in the pattern of the divisions of the trunks occur with some frequency.[2,3] An additonal anterior division joining the middle trunk to the medial cord is one of the most common variants. The existence of a middle trunk lesion may disable the ulnar nerves field of distribution.

Located in the axilla, the cords of the brachial plexus are formed by the union of brachial plexus divisions. The plexus may be divided into anterior (flexor) and posterior (extensor) positions, corresponding to the flexor and extensor limb muscles.[2,3] The medial and lateral cords of the plexus form the anterior portion and supply the muscles of the pectoral region and all the muscles on the anterior (volar) aspects of the upper arm, forearm, and hand, through

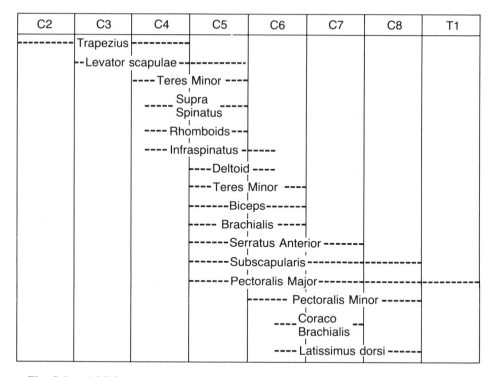

C2	C3	C4	C5	C6	C7	C8	T1

Fig. 8-2. Additional segmental motor innervation of the muscles of the shoulder.

the musculocutaneous, median, and ulnar nerves. The posterior cord supplies most of the muscles of the shoulder and all of the posterior (extensor) muscles in the upper arm and forearm, mainly via the axillary and radial nerves (Fig. 8-3).

The lateral cord is derived from the anterior divisions of the upper and middle trunks, the medial cord from the anterior division of the lower trunk, and frequently also from the middle one; and the posterior cord is derived from the posterior division of all three trunks. The three cords give off the majority of the peripheral nerves. From the lateral cord (flexors) issue the lateral anterior thoracic nerve, the musculocutaneous nerve, and the lateral head of the median nerve; from the medial cord (flexors) issue the medial anterior thoracic nerve, the ulnar nerve, the medial cutaneous nerves of the forearm and arm, the medial head of the median nerve, and a branch to the intercostobrachial nerve; and from the posterior cord (extensors) and axillary issue the radial, the thoracodorsal, and the two subscapular nerves. The medial and lateral anterior thoracic nerves extend from the medial (C8–T1) and lateral (C5–C7) cords, respectively, and are united by a loop. They supply the pectoralis major and pectoralis minor muscles. The three scapular nerves from the posterior cord consist of: (1) the upper (or short) subscapular nerve (C5–C6) to the subscapularis muscle; (2) the middle (long) subscapular or thoracodorsal nerve (C7–C8), which inner-

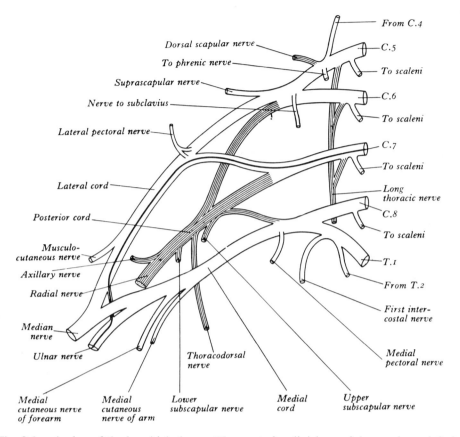

Fig. 8-3. A plan of the brachial plexus. The posterior divisions of the trunks and their derivatives are shaded, representing the extensor nerve supply. The medical and lateral cords, not shaded, represent the flexor supply. (Warwick R, Williams PL: Gray's Anatomy, 35th British Ed. Churchill Livingstone, Edinburgh, 1973.)

vates the latissimus dorsi muscle; and (3) the lower subscapular muscle. Sensory branches of the medial cord (C8–T1) comprise the medial antebrachial cutaneous nerve to the medial surface of the forearm and the medial brachial cutaneous nerve to the medial surface of the arm.

Different components of the plexus are in close relation with blood vessels.[2–5] Located immediately behind the subclavian artery is the lower trunk; each cord approximates the axillary artery. The medial cord lies at first posterior, then medial to the axillary artery; the lateral cord remains lateral to the axillary artery; the posterior cord shifts from a lateral to a posterior position in relation to the axillary artery.

Autonomic sympathetic nerve fibers are present in all parts of the plexus; they consist of postganglionic fibers derived from the sympathetic ganglionated chain.[2,3] The only preganglionic fibers in the brachial plexus are those coursing distally in undivided anterior primary ramus T1.

Topographical Relations of the Brachial Plexus

In the neck, the brachial plexus lies in the posterior triangle in the angle between the clavicle and the lower part of the posterior border of the sternocleidomastoid, being covered by the skin, platysma, and deep fascia.[2–6] The brachial plexus is crossed by the supraclavicular nerves, the nerves of the subclavius, the inferior belly of the omohyoid, the external jugular vein, and the transverse cervical artery. The plexus emerges between the scalenus anterior and scalenus medius; its proximal part is above the third part of the subclavian artery, and the lower part is posterior to the artery; the plexus next passes behind the anterior convexity of the medial two-thirds of the clavicle, the subclavius, and the suprascapular vessels, and lies on the first digitation of the serratus anterior and the subscapularis. In the axilla, the lateral and posterior cords of the plexus are on the lateral side of the first part of the axillary artery and on the medial cord behind it. The cords surround the second part of the axillary artery on three sides, the medial cord lying on the medial side, the posterior cord behind, and the lateral cord on the lateral side of the artery. In the lower part of the axilla, the cords split into the nerves for the upper limb. With the exception of the medial root for the median nerve, the branches of the three cords bear the same relationship to the third part of the axillary artery as the cords from which they spring bear to the second part, i.e., branches from the lateral cord are lateral, branches from the posterior cord are posterior and branches of the medial cord are medial to the artery.

BRACHIAL PLEXUS LESIONS

Brachial plexus lesions that are sustained above the clavicle, the upper and middle trunks, and their emergent nerves are likely to suffer; if such lesions are sustained below the clavicle, the cords and their branches are more subject to damage.[2] The convergence of the brachial plexus as it extends distally makes its trunks more vulnerable to axillary lesions than cervical lesions. Furthermore, with axillary lesions, blood vessels are more subject to damage.

The examination of a patient who has sustained mechanical trauma in the region of the brachial plexus must include identification of such factors as injury of bones, joints, muscles, and blood vessels. If these variables are not identified, the performance of clinical muscle testing may be hindered and/or contrainidicated, making it difficult to assess the degree of damage to nerve trunks. Another factor to consider in the examination of a patient with a traumatic injury to the brachial plexus is that such an injury sometimes leads to transient palsy of the entire limb. Until the period of total paralysis is past, little information as to the components injured will be provided by an examination.[2]

Proximal Brachial Plexus Lesions

Paralysis of serratus anterior, levator scapulae, or the rhomboids may be caused by a lesion either in their respective nerves or in the undivided anterior primary rami through which their fibers course. If the lesion is sustained only by the anterior primary rami, a segmental distribution of the disability, motor as well as sensory, will occur. An interruption in the undivided anterior primary ramus T1 will manifest Horner's syndrome. The reverse of Horner's syndrome (pupillary dilatation, widening of the palpebral fissure, exophtalmous, and disturbance of sweat secretion in the ipsilateral part of the face) occurs if a lesion of this ramus is irritative.[1,2]

Brachial Plexus Trunk Lesions

When a lesion is sustained to the trunks of the brachial plexus, the motor and sensory changes display a segmental distribution. Three types of syndrome may be distinguished: upper, lower, and middle.

The Upper Type (of Duchenne-Erb)

Readily recognizable when well developed, the upper type of brachial plexus palsy affects those muscles innervated by spinal segments C5 and C6 (see Fig. 8-2 for a list of the affected muscles). This syndrome causes severe restriction of movements at the shoulder and elbow joints. The flexion and abduction functions of the deltoid and supraspinatus muscle are greatly inhibited. The infraspinatus and teres minor muscle are unable to rotate the arm laterally when placed in a position of medial (internal) rotation. When the forearm is placed in a pronated position, the supinator muscle fails to supinate the arm. The muscles responsible for bending the forearm at the elbow (biceps, brachialis, and brachioradialis) are unable to perform this movement.

Usually characteristic of the upper type of syndrome is a limb position which is limp at the side, pronated, and medially rotated. The only region of the limb that shows a deficit in sensibility is the deltoid and the area along the course of the musculocutaneous nerve.[1,2]

Whether the plexus is postfixed or prefixed determines the distribution of the disability. The deltoid and spinati muscles are affected most when the plexus is postfixed, whereas the pronator teres and radial extensors are affected in the prefixed plexus.[2,3]

The Lower Type (of Klumpe)

Traumatic movements such as being dragged by the arm or a forceful upward pull of the shoulder during birth may result in the lower type of brachial palsy. Disabilities of finger and wrist movements characterize this syndrome, as the affected muscles are supplied by spinal segments C8 and T1. In the case of lower brachial palsy, a sensory deficit is present along the ulnar side of the arm, forearm, and hand, similar to that of combined ulnar and median palsy.

Horner's syndrome will result if the sympathetic fibers traversing the proximal part of the undivided anterior primary ramus T1 are involved.

As in the upper type of brachial palsy, the distribution of disability in the lower type is determined by whether the plexus is prefixed or postfixed. The small muscles of the hand are only slightly affected in a lesion of the prefixed plexus, whereas a lesion of the postfixed plexus is likely to result in paralysis of the flexors of the hand and forearm. In a prefixed palsy, sensory loss is also evident in the region of T2 and perhaps in a part of T3 as well; the distribution of sensory deficit, however, extends no lower than the level of T1 or C8 in a lesion of the postfixed plexus.[2,3]

The Middle Type

The fibers extending to the radial nerve are chiefly affected by an interruption of the middle trunk or of the corresponding undivided anterior primary ramus. This type of brachial plexus weakens the extensors of the arm and forearm; however, it does not affect the brachioradialis, which is supplied chiefly from spinal segment C6. A minor sensory deficit, usually occurring as a narrow strip of hypoesthesia on the back of the forearm and on the radial aspect of the dorsum of the hand, is characteristic of the middle type.

Brachial Plexus Cord Lesions

The areas affected by cord lesions are dependent on the location of the lesion, as evidenced in Figure 8-3. When the lesion is lateral, the fields of distribution of the musculocutaneous and lateral anterior thoracic nerves as well as of the lateral root of the median (which innervates flexor carpi ulnaris and pronator teres) are implicated, therefore producing weakness of flexion and pronation of the forearm. A medial cord lesion leads to combined ulnar and median palsy, as the ulnar, medial cutaneous nerves of the arm and forearm and the medial root of the median (which innervates the flexors of the fingers) are affected.[7] Commonly noted in medial cord lesions is a loss of sensibility along the medial border of the limb. A posterior cord lesion involves the fields of distribution of radial, axillary, subscapular, and thoracodorsal nerves, thereby causing weakness of the extensors, impairment of medial rotation of the arm at the shoulder, and difficulty in elevating the limb.

Brachial Plexus Nerve Branch Lesions

Long Thoracic Nerve

The long thoracic nerve originates from undivided anterior primary rami C5, C6, and C7 shortly after they emerge from intervertebral foramina. The nerve reaches the serratus anterior muscle by traversing the neck behind the brachial plexus cords, entering the medial aspect of the axilla, and continuing downward on the lateral wall of the thorax (Fig. 8-3). Individual branches of the descending nerve trunk supply the serratus muscle, innervated from spinal segment C5; the middle part of the nerve trunk is innervated from segment C6, and the lower part from segment C7.

Because of the long thoracic nerve's exposed position, straight course, and fixation by the scaleni, it is often the only nerve involved in casual mechanical trauma. Wounds which cause considerable damage to the most proximal part of the brachial plexus may also affect the long thoracic nerve. Isolated palsy of the long thoracic nerve is rarely observed.[2]

In an examination of the shoulder for total palsy of the serratus anterior, the arms should be at rest at the sides of the body.[8] A slight winging of the tip of the scapula will be apparent on careful examination. Also typical of total palsy of the serratus anterior is a minor shift in the shoulder girdle's position. This shift is caused by action of the trapezius, latissimus dorsi, and rhomboids, which normally pull the should girdle back and medially.[8-10] A medial rotation of the scapula so that its inner border, especially the lower part, is closer than usual to the vertebral column and a slight backward displacement of the acromial end of the clavicle are both characteristic of a shift in the shoulder girdle.

Normal movement of the shoulder girdle is created by the perfect synchronization of individual motor and fixation muscles functioning alternately during successive phases of any one movement. Contributing to this synchronization is the serratus anterior muscle, which also holds the shoulder blade closer to the thoracic wall for pushing movements and rotates the inferior angle of the scapula up and forward when the arm is raised. In the case of serratus palsy, the scapular shift produces a striking deformity of the shoulder girdle when either of these two movements is attempted.

When the movement of pushing is attempted in an affected shoulder, the entire scapula, especially its medial half, shifts backward, producing a wing effect. When the arm is raised in flexion, due to the action of the levator scapulae and loss of fixation in the case of serratus palsy, the tip of the shoulder blade moves upward and rotates in such a way that its superior angle is further removed from the spine than its inferior angle. Incomplete palsies may not affect the power of abduction, whereas complete palsies limit abduction to ~90°, as the force of the elevating arm drives the inadequately fixed scapula toward the vertebral column.

Anterior Thoracic, or Pectoral, Nerves

There are two anterior thoracic nerves, the medial and lateral. Derived from spinal segments C8 and T1, the medial anterior thoracic nerve arises from the most proximal part of the medial cord of the plexus. The lateral anterior nerve, from segments C5, C6, and C7 comes off the anterior divisions of the trunks of the plexus (Fig. 8-3). The two nerves descend to the pectoralis major and minor, communicating en route by means of an anastomotic loop which circles the axillary artery.

Joined by anastomotic fibers from the lateral nerve (from segment C7), the medial thoracic nerve is distributed to the pectoralis minor and the more inferior part of the sternocostal portion of the pectoralis major. The lateral anterior thoracic nerve supplies the clavicular and (more superior) sternocostal portion of the pectoralis major but does not reach the pectoralis minor. Thus, segments C7, C8, and T1 innervate the pectoralis minor; segments C5 and C6 innervate the clavicular portion of the pectoralis major; the sternocostal part of the pectoralis major is innervated by C5, C6, C7, C8, and T1.

Because atrophy of the pectoralis major tends to corroborate other localizing signs of lesion to the brachial plexus, the anterior thoracic nerves are of little clinical importance.

Dorsal Scapular Nerve

Also known as the nerve to the rhomboids, the dorsal scapular nerve is one of the few derived from the most proximal part of the brachial plexus (Fig. 8-3). Arising from spinal segment C5 and extending through the corresponding anterior spinal root, the dorsal scapular nerve emerges from the proximal part of the undivided primary ramus and courses downward behind the brachial plexus to reach the medial border of the shoulder blade. As it courses to the shoulder, the nerve supplies the levator scapulae, rhomboid minor, and rhomboid major. The cervical plexus from spinal segments C3 and C4 also innervate the levator scapulae.

Because the levator scapulae receives innervation from both the dorsal scapular nerve and the cervical plexus, the function of the levator scapulae is not appreciably altered in an interruption of the dorsal scapulae nerve. However, the rhomboids are significantly affected by the dorsal scapular nerve's interruption. Although the rhomboids are small muscles, their contraction can be felt as they help to adduct the shoulder when the patient braces the shoulder against resistance. Following interruption of the dorsal scapular nerve, the scapula shifts somewhat laterally, causing the vertebral border, especially the lower part, to separate somewhat from the thoracic cage. This effect is observable when the patient attempts to square the shoulders as the scapula of the affected side takes an oblique position, the upper part of its vertebral border moving medially and the lower part moving laterally.

Suprascapular Nerve

The suprascapular nerve arises from the upper trunk of the brachial plexus after traversing the undivided anterior primary rami C4, C5, and C6 (Fig. 8-3). Situated superficially to the cords of the plexus in the proximal part of its course, the suprascapular nerve proceeds downward, passing through the suprascapular notch and advancing to the back of the shoulder blade. The nerve gives off a branch to the supraspinatus muscle and then passes through the spinoglenoid notch to reach and supply the infraspinatus.

The suprascapular nerve is rarely involved in brachial plexus lesions.[11] When the nerve is affected, motor sensory changes above and below the scapula's position is not altered. The arm can still be abducted by the deltoid despite the loss of function of the supraspinatus.[12] Likewise, the arm's ability to rotate laterally (externally) at the shoulder, a movement involving the infraspinatus, is not greatly affected because of participation of the teres minor.

Most frequently affecting the suprascapular nerve are lesions to the upper plexus involving undivided primary rami segments C5 and C6. Lateral rotation at the shoulder is difficult when lesions occur to the upper plexus, as both the infraspinatus and the teres minor are affected.

Thoracodorsal Nerve

Emerging from the brachial plexus in close association with subscapular nerves is the thoracodorsal nerve, also known as "the long subscapular nerve" or "the nerve to the latissimus dorsi" (Fig. 8-3). It originates from spinal segments C7 and C8 and, frequently, from C6.

The thoracodorsal nerve's fibers reach the posterior cord of the plexus by traversing the plexus' three trunks (upper, middle, and lower) and passing through the posterior divisions of the trunks. From the posterior cord of the plexus, the thoracodorsal nerve passes behind the medial cord and courses downward in the axilla (between the two suprascapular nerves) to reach the latissimus dorsi. Lesions of the posterior cord or more proximal parts of the plexus are usually the cause of interruption of the thoracodorsal nerve.

In latissimus dorsi palsy, there is little change in the shoulder's appearance or ability to function. There may be a winging of the inferior angle of the scapula cause by weakness of the part of the muscle that crosses over the angle, helping to hold it next to the chest.[1,9] The paralysis causes the shoulder to shift upward when the extended arm is pushed forward strongly against a stationary object, as the latissimus dorsi normally tends to lower the shoulder.

Subscapular Nerves

Arising from spinal segments C5 and C6, the fibers of the two subscapular nerves traverse the corresponding anterior roots and undivided anterior primary rami to merge in the upper trunk of the plexus. On reaching the posterior cord, via the posterior division of the upper trunk, the fibers emerge as two separate nerves (Fig. 8-3). The upper subscapular nerve courses downward and innervates the subscapular muscle, whereas the lower subscapular nerve travels laterally to supply chiefly the teres major but also branches to the subscapularis muscle.

Brachial plexus lesions involving the posterior cord of more proximal parts of the plexus, which carry fibers from spinal segments C5 and C6, usually result in subscapular nerve palsies. The ability of the arm to rotate medially (internally) at the shoulder is diminished by the interruption of these nerves. The anterior fibers of the deltoid and, to a lesser degree, the latissimus dorsi and pectoralis major, are also responsible for the medial (internal) rotation of the arm at the shoulder.[10]

Axillary, or Circumflex, Nerve

Originating from segments C5 and C6, the axillary nerve courses to the distal part of the posterior cord of the brachial plexus and advances laterally through the axilla. The nerve then bends around the back of the surgical neck of the humerus to supply the deltoid muscle and the overlying skin. The teres minor muscle also receives innervation from a branch of the axillary nerve (Fig. 8-3).

Trauma, such as the dislocation of the head of the humerus, may cause an isolated axillary nerve palsy; however, the palsy is usually only a part of a wider lesion of the brachial plexus.[12,13] Interruption of the posterior cord will inevitably result in axillary palsy, as will damage of the upper trunk.

Axillary nerve palsy, when well developed, is recognizable on inspection by the flat or slightly concave contour of the normally rounded upper arm, owing to motor interruption of the deltoid. Equally noticeable is the shoulder's disordered movement. In an unaffected shoulder, the arm is abducted to the horizontal plane by the middle fibers of the deltoid; the deltoid's anterior fibers help to bring the arm forward, and the posterior ones aid in drawing the arm backward. The patient with paralysis of the deltoid may be partly successful in attempting to abduct the arm to the horizontal plane with the aid of the supraspinatus, serratus anterior, trapezius, and pectoralis major, which ordinarily give little aid to the deltoid. In the attempt to raise the arm, the patient shrugs the shoulder and tilts the trunk to the other side, thus raising the arm with the help of the rib cage. Compromised to about the same degree is elevation of the arm by forward and backward flexion.

Occasionally, patients with paralysis of the deltoid are able to abduct the arm actively through 90° and through 45° in cases of combined deltoid and supraspinatus palsy.[14] As the patient abducts the arm the head of the humerus is fixed in the glenoid fossa, presumably by the long head of the biceps and coracobrachialis, while the scapula is rotated externally by the trapezius, carrying the arm away from the side. The clinician can detect the manner in which the arm is abducted by observing the lateral motion of the inferior angle of the scapula while palpating the deltoid, supraspinatus, and trapezius for evidence of contraction. If performed in a plane midway between abduction and forward flexion, elevation of the arm in deltoid or in combined deltoid and supraspinatus palsy may be even more successful.

Because the lateral (external) rotation of the arm at the shoulder is aided by other muscles (e.g., infraspinatus), paralysis of the teres minor is not observable clinically.[14] In complete division of the axillary nerve, disturbances of the cutaneous sensibility over the deltoid are almost always encountered.

CLASSIFICATION OF BRACHIAL PLEXUS LESIONS

Attempts have been made to classify the numerous possible types of brachial plexus lesions as radicular, trunk, and cord lesions; upper, middle, and lower types; incomplete and complete types; and supraclavicular and infraclavicular lesions, etc. Meige's diagram (Fig. 8-4) illustrates some of the difficulties of these attempts at classification.[1] While using Meige's diagram, the clinician can systematically test the muscles by electromyography, electrical stimulation, and/or manual muscle testing. Then recording the results opposite the muscle names on the chart (*W* for weak and *P* for paralyzed muscles), the clinician can localize the lesion by tracing into the plexus to the point where the fibers to the affected muscles are most concentrated. The distribution of sensory and tropic disturbances is also considered in localizing the injury.[1] Precise localization of brachial plexus lesions is difficult and time-consuming;

Table 8-1. Etiological Classification of Brachial Plexus Injuries as Related to the Shoulder

Traumatic
  Open injuries
  Closed injuries:
    Obstetric
    Postnatal exogenous
Compression
  Exogenous (sometimes isolated branches)
  Anatomic predisposition (sometimes isolated branches)
  Genetically determined (sometimes isolated branches)
Tumors
  Primary tumors of brachial plexus
  Secondary involvement of plexus by tumors of surrounding tissues
Vascular
  Local vascular processes or lesions
  Participation in generalized vasculopathies (e.g., polyarteritis nodosa and
    lupus erythematosus)
Physical Factors
  Radiotherapy
  Electric shock
Infectious, Inflammatory, and Toxic Processes
  Involvement of local sepsis
  Viral or infectious
Cryptogenic (neuralgic amyotrophy)
  Parainfectious
  Related to serum therapy
  Genetic predisposition
  Cryptogenic

(Modified from Mumenthaler M: Brachial plexus neuropathies. In Dyck PJ, Thomas PK, Lambert EH, Bunge R (eds): Peripheral Neuropathy, Vol. 2. WB Saunders Co, Philadelphia, 1984.)

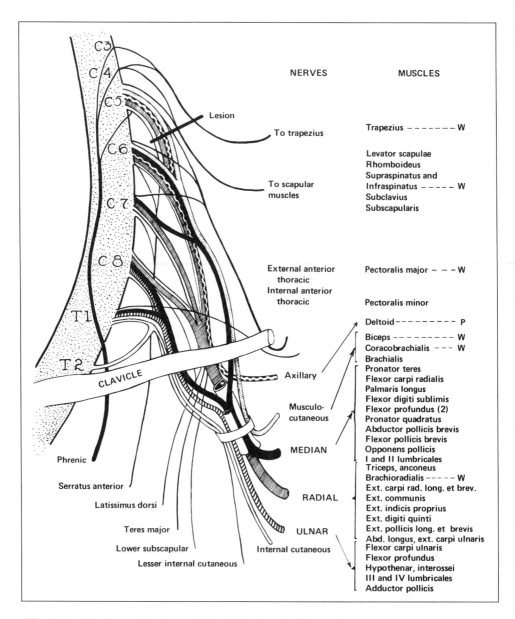

Fig. 8-4. The brachial plexus (after Meige). The illustration shows an example of an injury which produced paralysis of the deltoid and weakness in the supraspinatus and infraspinatus, trapezius, pectoral, biceps, coracobrachialis, and brachioradialis muscles. (Chusid JG: Correlative Neuroanatomy and Functional Neurology, 16th Ed., Lange Medical Publications, Los Altos, CA, 1976.)

Table 8-2. Frequency of Etiological Categories for Brachial Plexus Lesions (1,620 cases in an 11-year period)

	Men	Women	Total	Percentage
Traumatic (upper plexus)	352	106	458	28.2
Traumatic (total or near total)	237	76	313	19.3
Traumatic (lower plexus)	185	76	261	16.1
Neuralgic amyotrophy	175	52	227	14.0
Following radiotherapy	28	67	95	6.0
Tumors	43	26	69	4.2
Thoracic outlet syndromes	51	51	93	6.4
Other compression lesions	17	25	42	2.6
"Brachial Plexus neuritis"	18	10	28	1.7
Unknown cause	15	7	22	1.3
Compression by crutches	2	1	3	0.2
	1123(69.3%)	497(30.7%)		

(Modified from Mumenthaler M: Brachial plexus neuropathies. In Dyck PJ, Thomas PK, Lambert EH, Bunge R (eds): Peripheral Neuropathy, Vol. 2. WB Saunders Co, Philadelphia, 1984.)

however, this process is requisite to effective clinical decision-making regarding therapeutic intervention.

Further attempts to classify brachial plexus lesions have been made by etiologic classification. Mumenthaler[15] summarizes the etiologic categories of brachial plexus lesions as presented in Table 8-1. The frequency of the different etiologies of 1,620 patients from a neurologic outpatient department is shown in Table 8-2.[15]

LABORATORY INVESTIGATION OF BRACHIAL PLEXUS LESIONS

After the clinician has performed the clinical evaluative procedures of motor status testing, sensory status testing, and documentation of tropic changes, further testing may be necessary. Clinical electrophysiological studies have proven to be a valuable means of assessing brachial plexus lesions.[16–19] Electromyography (EMG), motor and sensory nerve conduction studies (NCS), somatosensory evoked potential recordings (SEP), and electrodiagnostic listing (EDX), (strength–duration testing) are useful means of determining not only the localization and severity of a neutral lesion, but also the rate and degree of neuromuscular restoration.

Electromyography

Electromyographic examination is beneficial in the differentiation of motor weakness that may represent either neurogenic or myopathic disorders. Furthermore, motor dysfunction may be identified as either upper or lower motor neuron disorders. This identification is important because conventional muscle testing and sensory examination may be unable to differentiate these disorders.

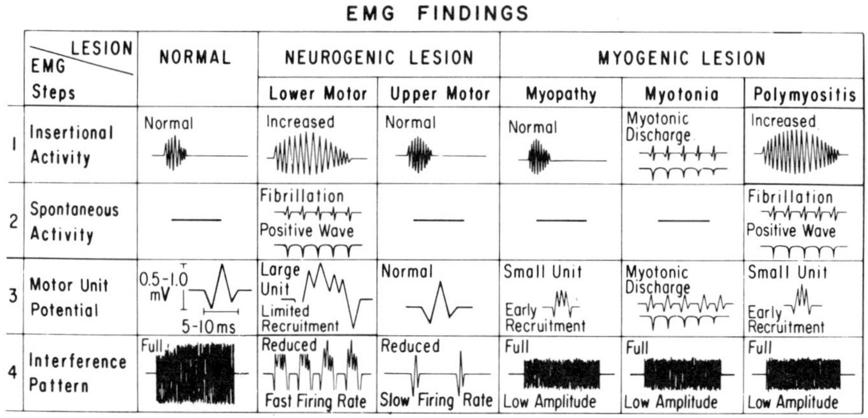

EMG FINDINGS

LESION / EMG Steps	NORMAL	NEUROGENIC LESION		MYOGENIC LESION		
		Lower Motor	Upper Motor	Myopathy	Myotonia	Polymyositis
1 Insertional Activity	Normal	Increased	Normal	Normal	Myotonic Discharge	Increased
2 Spontaneous Activity		Fibrillation / Positive Wave				Fibrillation / Positive Wave
3 Motor Unit Potential	0.5-1.0 mV / 5-10ms	Large Unit / Limited Recruitment	Normal	Small Unit / Early Recruitment	Myotonic Discharge	Small Unit / Early Recruitment
4 Interference Pattern	Full	Reduced / Fast Firing Rate	Reduced / Slow Firing Rate	Full / Low Amplitude	Full / Low Amplitude	Full / Low Amplitude

Fig. 8-5. Typical findings in lower and upper motor neuron disorders and myogenic lesions. (Kimura J: Electrodiagnosis in Diseases of Nerve and Muscle: Principles and Practice, FA Davis Co, Philadelphia, 1983.)

Typical electromyographic findings associated with each disorder are shown diagrammatically in Figure 8-5.

The EMG findings of muscles innervated by a brachial plexus lesion would confirm the presence of a lower motor neuron lesion. The clinician is able to localize the lesion by sampling muscles innervated by different nerves and root levels. Other EMG findings consistent with sampling a muscle innervated by a nerve associated with a brachial plexus lesion would include: increased insertional activity, spontaneous fibrillation and positive wave activity, large polyphasic motor unit potentials, and reduced interference patterns.

Nerve Conduction Studies

A primary use of NCS is the determination of peripheral neuropathies.[16,17,20,21] Nerve conduction studies may be useful in establishing the location of brachial plexus lesions.[20] Numerous neuromuscular conditions can imitate a brachial plexus lesion and thus make identification of the accurate pathology difficult. As an example, frequently there is confusion in differentiating whether shoulder muscular weakness is a result of cervical intervertebral disc protusion, anterior horn cell diseases, or a brachial plexus lesion. Because anterior horn cell diseases and intervertebral disc protrusions do not influence nerve conduction latency, the clinician can be certain that a proximal nerve conduction delay is the result of a brachial plexus lesion.

Another form of NCS used in evaluation of brachial plexus injuries involves F-wave studies. The F-wave is a wave-form response to peripheral mixed-nerve stimulation.[17,21] When a peripheral mixed nerve is electrically stimulated, the stimulus is conducted orthodromically via efferent nerve fibers to the effector muscle. The electrically stimulated muscle contraction is recorded as a muscle action potential or *M* response by recording electrodes placed over or in the effector muscle. The *M* response is the first recorded response to the electrical stimulus. During supramaximal stimulation of the same mixed nerve, the electrical stimulus is transferred both orthodromically and antidromically in the efferent nerve fibers. Orthodromically, an *M* response is recorded. Antidromically, the stimulus is carried to the anterior horn cell, where it is reflected orthodromically back down the efferent fiber to the effector muscle. When this timely process is complete, it is recorded by recording electrodes over the effector muscle as an F-wave.

When a patient is suspected of having a unilateral brachial plexus lesion, bilateral F-wave latency testing can be used to verify a unilateral conduction delay in the efferent system of peripheral mixed nerves. The F-wave conduction study has the unique ability to assess the conduction integrity of the anterior primary rami (the efferent limb of the reflex arc) of spinal segments.

Somatosensory Evoked Potentials

Averaged SEPs are recorded from the intact human scalp during electrical stimulation of skin or nerves in the upper or lower extremities.[19,22] Upper extremity electrical stimulation has been found beneficial in recording evoked sensory potentials when lesions to the brachial plexus have caused motor paralysis and anesthesia due to avulsed spinal roots. Generally, with brachial plexus traction lesions, only the spinal roots are avulsed, leaving the sensory fibers intact with the dorsal root ganglion.[23] However, even though the sensory fibers are intact with the dorsal root ganglion, the patient may experience anesthesia. Somatosensory evoked potentials that are recorded in spite of anesthesia indicate the existence of surviving efferent fibers reaching the central nervous system (CNS). Stimulation that fails to evoke SEPs in the involved limb indicates that sensory fibers have been avulsed distal to the ganglia and that a more severe brachial plexus lesion is the result. The SEPs provide clinically important information regarding the severity and nature of brachial plexus lesions.[22,24]

Electrodiagnostic Testing

Electrodiagnostic testing has unique qualities in the process of identification and quantification of neuromuscular dysfunction. Although EDX results are similar to the more popular EMG and NCS results, EDX has application in cases of traumatic nerve injury when it is necessary to determine (a) what nerves and/or muscles are injured, (b) the degree of denervation (c) where the neuromuscular lesion is located, and (d) the course of recovery.[25] In addition, EDX strength–duration curves may show evidence of denervation following nerve lesion at times when spontaneous fibrillations are difficult to detect.[1]

Electrodiagnostic testing is performed by electrically stimulating a muscle

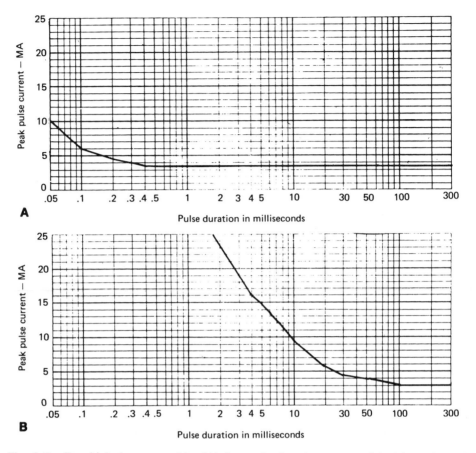

Fig. 8-6. Brachial plexus neuritis. (A) Strength–duration curve, right biceps brachii muscle, 11/25/64; rheobase, 3.5 mA; chronaxie, 0.08 ms. (B) Strength–duration curve, right deltoid muscle, 11/25/84; rheobase 3.0 mA; chronaxie, 19 ms. (Cohen HL, Brumlik J: Manual of Electroneuromyography, 2nd Ed., Harper & Row, Hagerstown, MD, 1976.)

at its motor points with the least amount of current flowing for an infinite period of time to cause minimal contraction of muscle. A strength–duration curve is then plotted consisting of pulse duration (milliseconds) against current (milliamperes) necessary to cause minimal contraction at each of several pulse durations.

Serial strength–duration testing provides the clinician with a graphic display of neuromuscular recovery.

Figure 8-6 illustrates the usage of strength–duration curves on a patient suffering brachial plexus neuritis. The strength–duration curve of the right deltoid muscle showed marked denervation but required more time and current to get a minimal muscular contraction.

PHYSICAL THERAPY MANAGEMENT OF BRACHIAL PLEXUS LESIONS

Presently, there is little information available regarding the direct physical therapy treatment of actual brachial plexus lesions. However, with certain brachial plexus lesions, the physical therapist is able to apply therapeutic measures designed to restore the integrity and function of the pathological components of the brachial plexus. In essence, the therapeutic measures are not geared toward the direct treatment of symptomatology but toward the treatment of the lesion itself. Therapeutic measures that may facilitate the recovery of a brachial plexus lesion include heat, massage, and electrotherapy. In addition, if mechanical compression or traction causes the brachial plexus lesion, physical therapy intervention frequently includes the manual skills of mobilizing, manipulating, or stretching the involved anatomical structures in an effort to remove or change the mechanical compressor or traction.

For many brachial plexus lesions there is no specific physical therapeutic intervention to effect a cure. The most effective approach is prevention—avoidance of those situations in which there is potential for mechanical insult to the brachial plexus adequate and properly designed equipment to protect the brachial plexus during contact athletic endeavors, vaccination for viral diseases, and education to prevent toxic brachial plexus neuropathies.[26] Thus, physical therapy management of brachial plexus lesions is often based on treatment of symptoms.

Symptomatology and Physical Therapeutic Measures

Symptoms that are most likely to occur as a result of a brachial plexus lesion include pain, causalgia, anesthesia, paresthesias, dysesthesias, motor involvement, atrophy, trophic changes, autonomic involvement, and connective tissue tightness.

Pain and Causalgia

Pain frequently is a significant symptom resulting from a brachial plexus lesion. Pain in focal brachial plexus lesions can be experienced in a specific predictable distribution. However, variability of pain distribution frequently results in widely radiating pain, making anatomical localization difficult.[27] Acute brachial plexus lesions may be associated with severe pain and painful paraesthesias. In chronic neuropathies, pain is frequently reported as a continuous deep-seated ache in the limbs. At other times, chronic pain is described as a superficial burning and skin pain. The exact anatomical and physiological mechanisms responsible for pain is uncertain.[28] Pain has been found in conditions in which there is active nerve fiber degeneration and in chronic inactive neuropathies.

Causalgia is a burning pain due to lesion of a peripheral nerve. Frequently, it is accompanied by trophic skin changes. The pain is characteristically aggravated by emotional stimuli. It is more frequently reported following lesions to the lowest trunk of the brachial plexus.[27]

Numerous modes of physical therapy have been reported effective in the management of peripheral neuropathy pain.[26,29] Although the exact scientific mechanism by which pain is decreased in not fully understood, most patients feel relief of pain from therapeutic application of heat, cold, massage, vibration, and electrotherapy.[26,29,30] Whether pain will be diminished can be determined only on an individual trial-by-trial basis.

Anesthesia, Paresthesias, Dysesthesias

A lesion of the brachial plexus always leads to sensory changes except when the lesion is a pure root avulsion involving motor rami only.[2] The nature of sensory disorders varies in patients with brachial plexus lesions. However, plexus lesions usually produce dermatomal or sensory root deficits. Infraclavicular lesions produce complex sensory deficits in either a cord or a peripheral nerve distribution.

Physical therapy management of anesthesia, paresthesia, and dysesthesias as related brachial plexus lesions consists of therapeutic measures designed not to treat the sensory symptoms but to restore the integrity and function of the lesioned plexus parts. The application of any modality should be carefully monitored owing to the patient's impaired sensory feedback mechanisms. Therapeutic measures that may facilitate the recovery of a brachial plexus lesion include heat, massage, vibration, electrotherapy, and manual therapy. In addition, the patient should be educated regarding the exact nature of the sensory deficit and taught alternative means to compensate for the compromised sensory system.

Motor Involvement and Denervation Atrophy

Paralysis of voluntary motor function frequently results from a conduction block in motor nerve fibers or from loss or interruption of the motor axons.[27] If there is a temporary demyelination with preservation of axonal continuity, recovery is rapid and complete. However, interruption of brachial plexus motor axons either from general neuropathy or localized lesion results in paralysis and atrophy of muscle. The onset of paralysis is usually sudden: clinically evident atrophy appears in a few weeks. After 2 to 3 months, denervated human muscle lose muscle fibers. After 3 years of denervation, few muscle fibers remain.[31] Only if reinnervation has developed within 12 months is complete functional restoration possible.[32]

Many physical therapy measures are effective in facilitating the restoration of muscular strength in denervated and partially denervated muscle. Possibly, the most popular means of retardation of atrophy in denervated muscle is the use of electrical stimulation. Numerous studies have verified the positive effect of electrical stimulation in delaying the denervated atrophic process.[33,34] Additional physical therapy treatment may include the reeducation techniques of biofeedback and the many modes of neuromuscular facilitation.[35] After voluntary motor control has been established, the physical therapy program should include conventional strengthening exercises.

Tropic Changes

After denervation owing to a brachial plexus lesion, nutritional or tropic changes may appear in the skin, nails, subcutaneous tissues, muscles, bones, and joints.[1] The once-held concept of specific tropic nerve fibers being involved in the maintenance of the structural integrity of tissues and organs can no longer be upheld.[27] It is now believed that tropic changes result from the effects of disuse, alterations of blood supply, and loss of pain sensation, which expose the tissues to repeated destructive trauma.[27,36,37]

The physical therapy management of tropic changes should include the use of conventional hydrotherapy, thermotherapy, massage, exercise, and electrotherapy. All therapeutic measures should be applied in an effort to enhance the nutritional and structural integrity of involved structures. The application of any physical agent should be carefully monitored because of the patient's impaired sensory feedback mechanisms. In addition, the patient should be carefully educated regarding the impaired sensory mechanisms and taught alternative methods to compensate for the compromised sensory system.

Autonomic Nervous System Involvement

Autonomic nervous system sympathetic nerve fibers are in close proximity to all parts of the brachial plexus. However, the only autonomic involvement resulting from a pure brachial plexus lesion is the result of a lesion affecting the first thoracic nerve root. The resultant condition is called Horner's syndrome, which is characterized by enophthalmos, miosis, and ptosis owing to interruption of sympathetic nerves to the face and eye.

Other autonomic symptoms appear frequently in lesions that effect the brachial plexus and nearby postganglionic fibers derived from the sympathetic ganglionated chain. Among the symptoms are vasomotor disorders including reflex sympathetic dystrophy (RSD). Reflex sympathetic dystrophy is a chronic painful condition characterized by neuromuscular disturbances, vasomotor disturbances, and dystropic changes in skin and bone.

There is little information available regarding the physical therapy treatment of Horner's syndrome. However, with the physical therapy treatment of

RSD, the use of transcutaneous electrical nerve stimulation (TENS) has been used successfully.[38–40] In patients who have suffered peripheral nerve injuries resulting in RSD, TENS application has been found beneficial in resolving pain, hyperesthesia, poor circulation, edema, and dystropic changes.

Connective Tissue Tightness

Connective tissue tightness causing decreased passive ROM at the shoulder may develop as a result of acute or chronic brachial plexus lesions. At the onset of a brachial plexus lesion, certain muscles responsible for moving the shoulder through voluntary ROM are paralyzed. Decreased voluntary shoulder movement results from this neuromuscular paralysis. During immobility, restrictive adhesions may form within joints and the surrounding connective tissue.[41] Subsequently, connective tissue lesions contribute to restrictions in shoulder mobility.

The goal of physical therapy intervention in the management of connective tissue tightness is restoration of normal joint mobility. However, if early intervention is available, preventive ROM exercises should be performed to maintain normal mobility. If connective tissue tightness has developed, stretching techniques should be implemented. Physical therapy therapeutic measures found effective in restoring connective tissue mobility include thermotherapy, cryotherapy, hydrotherapy, massage, exercise, electrotherapy, and manual manipulative and mobilizing therapy.

Orthotics may be used to prevent or correct connective tissue tightness. Mobility-restoring procedures and orthoses should be used to prevent deformity which may result from chronic brachial plexus lesions.

CONCLUSION

Brachial plexus lesions frequently lead to muscle weakness or paralysis and sensory disturbances related to the shoulder. The definitive localization of brachial plexus lesions is a clinical challenge due to the anatomical complexity of the brachial plexus. However, with the use of evaluative techniques presented here, localization of lesions should be efficient. Physical therapy early intervention is an essential component in the management of brachial plexus lesions. Physical therapy treatment is frequently directed toward lessening the severity of brachial plexus lesion symptomatology; however, in certain cases, manual therapy mobilizing or manipulative techniques may be beneficial in removing or changing a mechanical compressor or traction.

REFERENCES

1. Chusid JG: Correlative Neuroanatomy and Functional Neurology. 16th Ed. Lange Medical Publications, Los Altos, Calif, 1976
2. Mumenthaler M, Narakas A, Gilliatt RW: Brachial plexus disorders. p. 1383. In

Dyck PJ, Thomas PK, Lambert EH, Bunge R (eds): Peripheral Neuropathy. Vol. 2. WB Saunders Co, Philadelphia, 1984

3. Warwick R, Williams PL: Gray's Anatomy. 35th British Ed. WB Saunders Co, Philadelphia, 1973
4. Grant JC: An Atlas of Anatomy, 6th Ed., Williams & Wilkins, Baltimore, 1972
5. Bateman JE: Trauma to Nerves in Limbs, WB Saunders Co, Philadelphia, 1962
6. Gibbs RW: A protective collar for cervical radiculopathy. Physician Sports Med 12:139, 1984
7. Krieger AJ: Hyperabduction syndrome. Hosp Med p. 81, July 1983
8. Hoppenfeld S: Physical Examination of the Spine and Extremities. Prentice-Hall, New York, 1976
9. Brunnstrom S: Clinical Kinesiology. FA Davis Co, Philadelphia, 1962
10. Basmajian JV: Muscles-Alive, 2nd Ed. Williams & Wilkins Co, Baltimore, 1967
11. Skurja M, Monlux JH: Case studies: the suprascapular nerve and shoulder dysfunction. J Orthop Sports Phys Ther 6:254, 1985
12. Szabo RM: Peripheral nerve injuries in athletes. Mediguide Orthop 5:1, 1985
13. Delee JC: Traumatic dislocation of the shoulder. Hosp Med p. 47, Sept 1981
14. Kent BE: Functional anatomy of the shoulder complex. J Am Phys Ther Assoc 51:867, 1971
15. Mumenthaler M: Brachial plexus neuropathies. p. 1389. In Dyck PJ, Thomas PK, Lambert EH, Bunge R (eds): Peripheral Neuropathy. Vol. 2. WB Saunders Co, Philadelphia, 1984
16. Schaum HH, Spencer PS, Thomas PK: Disorders of Peripheral Nerves, FA Davis Co, Philadelphia, 1983
17. Kimura J: Nerve conduction studies and electromyography. p. 919. In Dyck PJ, Thomas PK, Lambert EH, Bunge R (eds): Peripheral Neuropathy. Vol. 1. WB Saunders Co, Philadelphia, 1984
18. Buchtal F, Rosenbalck A, Behse F: Sensory potentials of normal and diseased nerves. p. 981 In Dyck PJ, Thomas PK, Lambert EH, Bunge R (eds) Peripheral Neuropathy, Vol 1. WB Saunders Co, Philadelphia, 1984
19. Lehmkuhl LD: Evoked spinal, brain stem, and cerebral potentials. p. 123. In Wolf SL (ed): Electrotherapy. Vol 2. New York, Churchill Livingstone, 1981
20. Smorto MP, Basmajian JV: Clinical Electroneurography. William & Wilkins Co, Baltimore, 1971
21. Echternach JL: The use of conduction velocity measurements as an evaluative tool. p. 73. In Wolf SL, (ed): Electrotherapy. Churchill Livingstone, New York, 1981
22. Desmedt JE: Cerebral evoked potentials. p. 1045. In Dyck PJ, Thomas PK, Lambert EH, Bunge R (eds): Peripheral Neuropathy. Vol. 1. WB Saunders Co, Philadelphia, 1984
23. Drake CG: Diagnoses and treatment of lesions of the brachial plexus and adjacent structures. Clin Neurosurg 11:110, 1964
24. Goodgold J, Eberstein A: Electrodiagnosis of Neuromuscular Diseases. William & Wilkins Co, Baltimore, 1972
25. Cohen HL, Brumlik J: Manual of Electroneuromyography, 2nd Ed. Harper and Row, Hagerstown, Maryland, 1976
26. Johnson EW, Alexander MA: Management of motor unit diseases. p. 679. In Kottke FJ, Stillwell GK, Lehmann JF (eds.) Krusen's Handbook of Physical Medicine and Rehabilitation, WB Saunders Co, Philadelphia, 1982
27. Thomas PK: Clinical features and differential diagnoses. p. 1169 In Dyck PJ, Thomas PK, Lambert EH, Bunge R. (eds), Peripheral Neuropathy. Vol 2. WB Saunders, Philadelphia, 1984

28. Dyck PJ, Lambert EH, O'Brien PC: Pain in peripheral neuropathy related to rate and kind of fiber degeneration. Neurology (Minneap) 26:466, 1976
29. Stillwell GK: Rehabilitative procedures. In Dyck PJ, Thomas PK, Lambert EH, Bunge R (eds): Peripheral Neuropathy. Vol. 2. WB Saunders Co, Philadelphia, 1984
30. Wolf SL (ed): Electrotherapy. Churchill Livingstone, New York, 1981
31. Bowden REM, Gutmann E: Denervation and reinnervation of human voluntary muscle. Brain 67:273, 1944
32. Sunderland S: Capacity of reinnervated muscles to function efficiently after prolonged denervation. Arch Neurol Psychiatry 64:755, 1950
33. Gutmann E, Guttmann L: Effect of electrotherapy on denervated muscles in rabbits. Lancet 1:169, 1942
34. Hatano E et al: Electrical stimulation on denervated skeletal muscles. p. 469. In Goria A (ed): Posttraumatic Peripheral Nerve Regeneration: Experimental Basis and Clinical Implications. Raven Press, New York, 1981
35. Harris FA: Facilitation techniques in therapeutic exercise. In Basmajian JV (ed): Therapeutic Exercise. 3rd Ed. Williams & Wilkins, Baltimore, 1978
36. Lewis T, Pickering GW: Circulatory changes in the fingers in some diseases of the nervous system with special reference to the digital atrophy of peripheral nerve lesions. Clin Sci 2:149, 1936
37. Spillane JD, Wells CEC: Acrodystrophic Neuropathy. London, Oxford Medical Publications, 1969
38. Subbarao J, Stillwell GK: Reflex sympathetic dystrophy of the upper extremity: analysis of total outcome of management of 125 cases. Arch Phys Med Rehabil, 62:549, 1981
39. Owens S, Atkinson ER, Lees DE: Thermographic evidence of reduced sympathetic tone with transcutaneous nerve stimulation. Anesthesiology 50:62, 1979
40. Stilz RJ, Carron H, Sanders DB: Case history 96—reflex sympathetic dystrophy in a 6-year-old: successful treatment by transcutaneous nerve stimulation. Anesth Analg Curr Res 56:438, 1977
41. Akeson WH, Amiel D, Woo SL-Y: Immobility effects of synovial joints: the pathomechanics of joint contracture. Biorheology 17:95, 1980

9 | Current Research of Selected Shoulder Problems

David C. Reid
Linda Saboe
Robert Burnham

SHOULDER PROBLEMS

Although many published series deal with isokinetic parameters in the lower extremity, few data relate to the upper limb.[1,2] The increasing interest in pericapsular problems in swimmers and its relationship to muscle imbalance has made it imperative to have a knowledge of the normal condition of the upper limb.[3-6] Furthermore, the role of immobilization after initial shoulder dislocation is open to review along with the speed of progression of rehabilitation.[7-10] Discussion on the outcome of most shoulder surgery has been based largely on complication rates, redislocation rates, or the examiner's subjective opinions regarding functional improvement.[11-13] This has made it difficult to evaluate data regarding specific treatment regimens and rehabilitation protocols. This chapter discusses a series of studies that we have made relating to these issues. All isokinetic tests were performed using a Cybex II isokinetic dynamometer and standard protocols.[1,14] Abduction and adduction was tested with the subject in a supported sitting position (Fig. 9-1), and external and internal rotation were tested with the subject in standing and lying positions with the arm at the side and abducted to 90°, respectively (Figs. 9-2 and 9-3). All data are reported for 60° per second using the best of three trials. Some of the data are preliminary but are reported here for completeness.

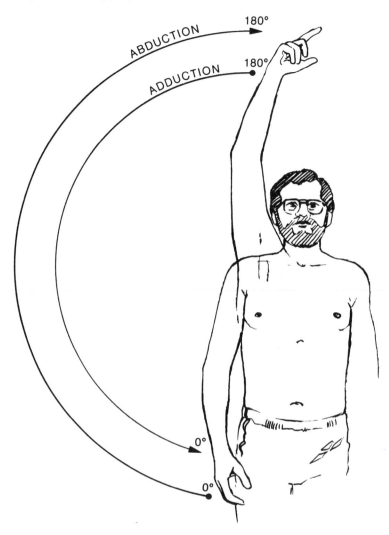

Fig. 9-1.   Abduction and adduction both designated at 0° with the arm at the side.

Normal Subjects

The normal subjects were 40 moderately fit athletic individuals tested for a total of 80 shoulders. For all movements tested, men were approximately twice as strong as women (Fig. 9-4). There was no significant difference between dominant and nondominant arms. The strongest muscle group was the adductors, being about twice as strong as the abductors. If the adductors, being the strongest, are considered as 100 percent, the abductors are ~50 percent. The internal rotators were ~45 percent of the adductors and the external rotators were ~30 percent of the adductors when the arm is at 90° and 45 percent

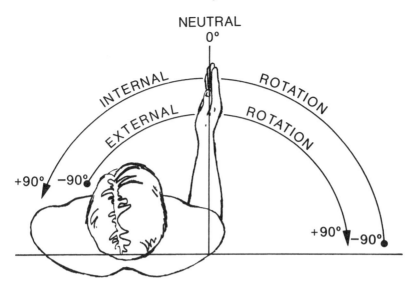

Fig. 9-2. Internal and external rotation with the upper arm held at the side. The neutral position is illustrated and positive and negative ranges are marked. (●── Starting range; ──▶ Finishing range)

when in neutral position. The external to internal rotation ratio was ~80 percent. A similar study was completed by Fowler, who agreed with the ratios for internal and external rotation at 90° abduction, but reported a ratio of 65 percent with the arm in neutral.[15] These ratios represent a normal healthy population and can be used as treatment goals for rehabilitation in much the same way as ratios are used for the quadriceps and hamstrings at the knee.

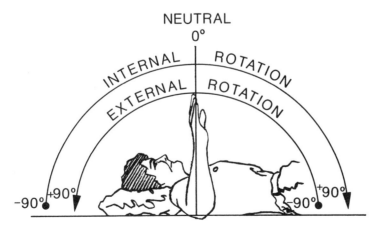

Fig. 9-3. Internal and external rotation with the arm abducted to 90°. The neutral position for each movement is marked. (●── Starting range; ──▶ Finishing range)

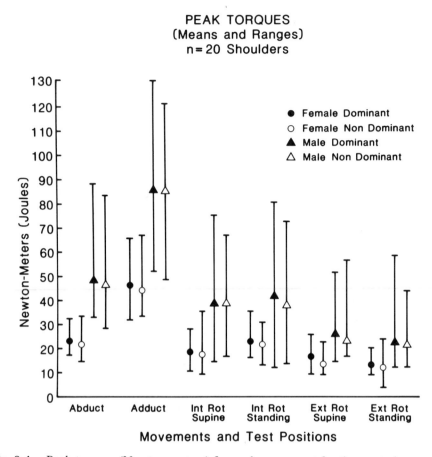

Fig. 9-4. Peak torques (Newton-meters) for each movement for the control or normal group are shown.

Swimmers

The incidence of shoulder pain is probably higher in swimmers than in those who participate in any other sport, constituting ~50 to 60 percent of all problems in highly competitive swimmers. This incidence is a marked increase over the 3 percent figure reported by Kennedy and Fowler in 1974 and reflects the more intensive training at an increasingly young age.[6,16]

The traditional concept of swimmer's shoulder is an anterior impingement syndrome involving mainly the supraspinatus or biceps tendon under the coracoacromial arch.[4] This is obviously an overuse syndrome. The contributing facts are anatomic impingement, impairment of the microcirculation, anatomic variations in the size of the bicipital groove, and muscle imbalance.[4,5,17,18] This last factor is significant in that it points to a potentially treatable entity by relatively simple means, namely exercise. There is also a suggestion that a second constellation of signs and symptoms is present, particularly in swimmers

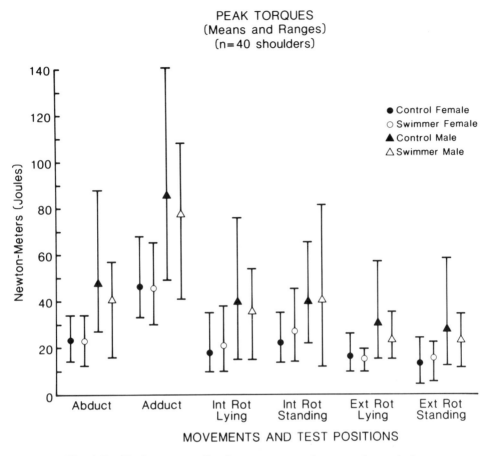

Fig. 9-5. Peak torques of swimmers versus the control population.

who use the back and butterfly strokes, and involves a hypermobility syndrome with a tendency to painful subluxation.[19–21]

We assessed 40 swimmers, 75 percent of whom had reached a national level of competition. Fifty percent of these swimmers had a past history of shoulder pain, reflecting the endurance or distance training of most swimmers with its repetitive abduction and circumduction maneuvers. Indeed, even swimming 10,000 meters a day, a nominal distance for many swimmers, would require that the athlete put each arm through at least 10,000 to 11,000 strokes a week.[1,6] It is important to recall that the upper extremities are the prime movers in swimming, with the lower extremities adding only a small percentage to speed, perhaps as little as 10 percent in the crawl stroke and a little more in breast stroke.[1,22–24] Therefore, as training intensity increases, the stresses on the shoulder increase. Surprisingly, for the most part, the peak torques for swimmers were not significantly higher than for the fit athletic controls (Fig. 9-5). Female swimmers were the exception, having an upper limb strength of ~60 percent of that of males, reflecting the increased upper limb work of female swimmers over that of the general female athletic population. These findings have several implications.

First, isokinetic testing in stereotyped positions may not reflect the swimming stroke and hence may not provide a true assessment of the swimmer's power. Nevertheless, the importance of dry land training in strengthening the shoulder girdle area is sometimes neglected.

Second, swimming (even the so-called sprint events) is essentially an endurance sport when assessed from a metabolic viewpoint.[25,26] This concept is further supported by review of muscle biopsies taken from the deltoid area of swimmers which show a larger preponderance of type I fibers than do those of controls.[1] Dry land training should reflect this need, and high repetition work should form a large part of the strengthening program. Futhermore, future testing should include an endurance component so that a realistic assessment can be made of the swimmers' total power.

Last, the tests reported here were made at 60° per second, and testing at higher rates may be more sensitive to the differences among the swimming population.

In terms of practical advice, however, while conceding that dry land training is important, we believe that any swimmer with a history of shoulder pain or one who is recovering from shoulder symptoms should avoid resisted movements above shoulder level. Declined bench work and modified arm positions will give the desired strengthening effect without increasing the symptoms from impingement.

Because of the suggestion of muscle imbalance in the rotator group, special emphasis was given to data relating to internal-external rotation ratios.[1] In our study, the internal rotators were stronger than the controls by ~10 percent; this is anticipated inasmuch as internal rotator strength correlates well with success in 100-meter freestyle swimming. Our results were not as dramatic as those of Fowler, who reported that external-internal rotation ratio in abduction was 62 percent in swimmers as opposed to 78 percent in control subjects.[15] In the neutral position, this difference was less remarkable, namely 66 percent in controls and 53 percent in swimmers. Both of these studies reflect a slight proportionate weakness of the external rotation, and it is suggested that specific external rotator strengthening should form part of the treatment protocol for swimmers' shoulder. Naturally, muscle strengthening is combined with stroke modification. A swimmer in the acute phase of shoulder pain, may have to discontinue swimming, or perhaps use only the breast stroke for several weeks, until the symptoms are resolved. Even then, the crawl or back stroke should be resumed cautiously.

Muscle tightness, particularly in the pectorals and anterior shoulder group may be present in many young swimmers, and attention to this is mandatory for any treatment protocol.[27] However, stretching should be specific and directed at restoring normal range. Mobility of the swimmers' shoulder should be adequate to allow sufficient range of motion (ROM) for a comfortable stroke pattern. There is very little to be gained from excessive mobility. On the contrary, perverse stretching maneuvers may serve to produce functional instability. This is particularly true for those individuals with a tendency toward hypermobility. Preseason testing by team therapists should seek to identify swimmers with evidence of either local laxity of the shoulder or general ligament laxity and to protect them from excessive stretching. Often the first clue to trouble is pain during turning or during the catch or entry phase of the back stroke. Although pain secondary to hypermobility or minor subluxation is difficult to treat, it responds to protection and slow steady strengthening of the rotator groups. More dramatic hypermobility and frank subluxation rarely if ever respond to nonoperative treatment, and the swimmers may have to switch strokes to the crawl or breast stroke.

RECURRENT DISLOCATION

Recurrent anterior dislocation of the glenohumeral joint is a common phenomenon accounting for >80 percent of dislocations of the upper extremity.[13] In some individuals, the dislocation is predictable and can be avoided for the most part by modification of activity. In others, the unpredictability makes this an extremely disabling problem. The usual mechanism of dislocation, in day-to-day activities, is external rotation in the abducted position. However, in sporting activities, another situation is frequently described which involves simply abduction and adduction. For the volleyball player it may occur during spiking or blocking, for the swimmer during touching for the turn, and for the tennis player it may occur during the serve. Little discussion has related to this particular mechanism. Furthermore, the role and efficacy of exercise in the prevention of dislocation is poorly understood.

By isokinetic testing we evaluated 40 subjects who had dislocated a shoulder a minimum of three times. They all had symptoms sufficient to cause them to consider operative repairs. As would be anticipated, these subjects could not start to generate significant torque in the position of the apprehension test, namely external rotation in abduction. However, surprisingly, the abductor and adductor groups reflected most weakness throughout the range, more so than the rotators.

Some persons dislocated shoulders while testing, not during rotation but during forced adduction with the arm straight and externally rotated. In other words, as they contracted their adductors to bring their arm down, their shoulders dislocated. This may explain the mechanism of dislocation so frequently seen in sport. Furthermore, it emphasizes the concept that once someone has developed sufficient capsular laxity to allow recurrent dislocation, muscle strengthening will do little to alleviate the situation. Indeed, the very muscles that keep the humeral head securely in place, in the so-called safe positions of the joint, actively dislocate the head from the glenoid in the abducted position. That is, dislocation tends to be an active process, not simply a passive phenomenon accompanying abduction with external rotation.

These statements do not deny the usefulness of shoulder rehabilitation when muscle weakness exists but explain why muscle strengthening will not prevent redislocation if there is sufficient capsular laxity.

TREATMENT OF INITIAL DISLOCATION

The orthopedic literature reflects confusion as to the correct management of first dislocations.[7,8,13] The length of strict immobilization after reduction varies considerably, from 2 days to 8 weeks.[7-10] The result of these haphazard approaches is reflected in the subsequent redislocation rate which is between 80 percent to 90 percent in persons <20 years of age at the time of their first dislocation,[13] ~60 percent for persons 20 to 30 years of age, and between 20 to 40 percent for those who are >40 years of age.[13] These figures have left most persons with a feeling of inevitability; hence, many physicians and therapists feel that since there is a great chance of redislocation whatever the treatment, it is better to opt for early mobilization, early strengthening, and rapid return to sport, activity, or occupation—a rather fatalistic approach, based on poor control of early treatment, low patient compliance, and inadequate therapy.

A more careful review of the literature reveals an important underlying concept, first suggested by Watson-Jones in 1956,[28] that the initial period of immobilization is important in prevention of recurrences. This perspective has been adopted by several groups recently and is gaining momentum. In 50 individuals <30 years of age, the recurrence rate was reduced to <20 percent with treatment of 6 weeks of strict immobilization. Early isometric exercises are taught to the individual by the therapist while the arm is immobilized in a sling and swath and are performed twice daily for the first 3 weeks. Axillary hygiene is performed with the arm strictly by the side, and the elbow is removed from the sling several times a day to allow flexion and extension, which assists comfort and prevents stiffness. Care is taken to avoid all external rotation. For the second 3-week period, gentle pendular exercises are given, mainly with the arm in a sling, and external rotation is allowed just short of neutral with the arm kept adducted against the body. External rotation is not permitted with the arm away from the side. Abduction with the arm internally rotated is permitted to 45°. Following this period, from 6 weeks on, the emphasis is on strengthening for about 4 weeks, allowing ROM to resume with gentle active motion. After this time, ROM can be actively pursued and becomes a major rehabilitation goal. Passive stretching should be avoided in the first 12 weeks after dislocation. In a few instances in which the shoulder appears particularly stiff, mobilization can be pursued more aggressively and slightly earlier, but only 6 weeks after dislocation.

Kariyama in 1984, gave us a better insight as to the pathology of anterior dislocations by performing arthrograms on 143 first dislocations.[11] His group noticed that there were two main types of dislocations. Two thirds of them were capsular tears, that is, the humeral head ripped out through the capsule. One third were capsular detachments, that is, the glenoid labrum or adjacent capsule was detached from the glenoid margin. The importance of this observation is that capsular tears have a great propensity for healing, which is not so obvious with the labrum detachments. This concept is reinforced by the fact that of those shoulders which later redislocated, 90 percent were of the capsular detachment type—the danger group for redislocation. More important, those persons who were strictly immobilized for 3 weeks had a redislocation rate that was amazingly low: 3.4 percent versus 47.7 percent for those who were immobilized for a shorter period.[11]

Furthermore, Kuriyama showed, with follow-up arthrograms, that capsular healing and rebuilding could be demonstrated at 3 weeks but not before.[11] This underlines the importance of early immobilization during this vulnerable 3-week period.

With these data as a background, every effort should be made to obtain patient compliance for early immobilization with a sling and swath, supplemented by carefully taught isometric exercises. The previously outlined regimen will provide excellent functional outcomes and reduce the devastatingly high redislocation rate that has become to be accepted as inevitable.

FUNCTIONAL OUTCOME OF SHOULDER REPAIRS

The three commonly used surgical techniques for stabilizing recurrent dislocating shoulders are the Magnuson-Stack, the Putti-Platt, and the Bristow repair. These three repairs represent three different principles.

The Magnuson-Stack type of repair is a simple procedure, taking all layers, capsule, cuff, and subscapularis tendon, and overlapping all layers as one, and frequently fixing it with a staple, taking care to avoid the long head of biceps.[29,30]

The Putti-Platt is a more involved procedure, taking the capsule in one layer and the subscapularis tendon in another, and separately plicating each layer.[13] It tends to give a very tight repair, limiting external rotation, hence, it may be less than ideal for the treatment of athletes in some sports.

The Bristow repair is based around transfer of the tip of the coracoid process with the conjoint tendon of biceps and coracobrachialis to the neck of the scapula. As such, a dynamic sling is formed in the position of abduction and external rotation when these tendons tighten across the front of the neck of the scapula.[31,32] Although there is some debate as to whether the bone block forms a static impediment to dislocation, in many cases it is able to do so, sitting as it does in the fossa that may be occupied by a dislocating humeral head. It is the preferred operation for athletes because of the possibility of early restoration of nearly full ROM. The decision for one operation over another has largely been based on complication and redislocation rates, and there is little information about functional outcomes.[13] Our data are incomplete but examine the functional endpoint of these three classes of operations. Our study so far includes 40 patients with Putti-Platts and a preliminary series with the other procedures, with patients followed from 1 to 11 years with a mean of 6 years.

Present information indicates that adequate rehabilitation provides normal strength on the operated side with all repairs. Furthermore, full ROM, or very minimally limited external rotation and abduction is also possible. Occasionally, a person with a Putti-Platt repair may have an unacceptable range for a few selected sports. The incidence of this is very low. ROM is more rapidly achieved with the Bristow repair.

Based on this information, the type of operation should be selected based on the surgeon's skill and experience in performing that procedure and its known complication rates. Furthermore, all the procedures will be more compatible with early return to full function if coupled with an adequate rehabilitation protocol.

The known complications include redislocation, pain, vascular and neural compromise, loose or migrating internal fixation devices, interference with the biceps tendon, infection and, in the Bristow repair, possible non-union. Most of these complications are uncommon with the exception of redislocation rates. A literative review reveals that after the Magnuson-Stack procedure, there is a redislocation rate of 0 to 17 percent with an average of ~4 percent. The Putti-Platt has a redislocation rate of between 0 to 8 percent with an average of 4 percent; finally, the Bristow procedure is reported as having an average of slightly more than 2 percent redislocation, with a range of 0 to 3 percent.[10,13,31,32]

With care taken to obtain an adequate bone block and good screw fixation, and with well-planned therapy, the Bristow procedure is likely to give the earliest return to normal function and the lowest redislocation rate.

Rehabilitation includes isometric exercises for the first 3 weeks after surgery, with pendular and gentle active exercises for the next 3 weeks. No resistance is given; abduction is limited to 45° and external rotation to neutral. At 6 weeks, it is assumed that bone healing is well underway and that the capsular repair is sound. Subsequent rehabilitation is guided by pain. Heavy resisted work and forced external rotation are delayed until postoperative week 12.

SUMMARY

Isokinetic data has been presented in relation to several problems of the shoulder, after initial establishment of normal values. These normal values are offered as treatment goals for a healthy athletic population. There is still a need for normal values to be established for older persons as well as for children before and after their growth spurts.

Swimmers' shoulder, an anterior impingement syndrome, has its basis in overuse, but the disproportionate strength of internal over external rotators may be a contributing factor and should be corrected during therapy for this condition. It is conceded that adequate ROM is essential for good swimming, but overstretching can bring problems of its own. Particular care should be taken to identify those persons who have a basic tendency to loose joints and to protect them adequately from perverse overstretching. Once developed, functional instability of the shoulder is very difficult to treat in swimmers and may necessitate a change in stroke, with elimination of the butterfly and back strokes.

In a study of persons with recurrent dislocations, the role of the adductor muscle group in precipitating dislocation has been described, explaining the failure of muscle-strengthening routines to prevent redislocations. Nevertheless, the importance of restoring normal muscle power, where wasting is present, is undeniable.

The incidence of recurrent dislocation can be directly linked to inadequate immobilization and progressive rehabilitation of the first traumatic dislocation. With correct treatment, an 80 percent redislocation rate is not inevitable, even in a young age group.

Of the frequently used surgical repairs for recurrent dislocation of the shoulder, the Bristow procedure appears to give the earliest return to activity and function as well as the potentially lowest redislocation rate, making it the preferred operation for most athletes.

With the glenohumeral joint having so little bony structural stability, dynamic mechanisms for movement and control are paramount. Much of the muscle action is indirect, through force couples. As such, small alterations in balance of power and neural control can profoundly affect function. It is little wonder then that rehabilitation plays a pivotal role in all of the common orthopedic problems in the shoulder area. The data presented in this chapter emphasize this fact.

REFERENCES

1. Elsner RC, Pedegana LR, Lang J: Protocol for strength testing as rehabilitation of the upper extremity. J Orthop Sports Phys Ther 4:229, 1983
2. McMurray DL: Determination of the isokinetic peak torques of the external and internal rotator muscles of the shoulder in a normal adult female population. M Sc Thesis. University of Alabama. Birmingham, Alabama, 1983
3. Marino M: Profiling swimmers. Clin Sports Med 3:211, 1984. WB Saunders Co, Toronto.
4. Domingrez RH: Shoulder pain in swimmers. Phys Sports Med 8:37, 1980
5. Kennedy JD, Hawkins RJ: Swimmer's shoulder. Phys Sports Med 2:34, 1979
6. Foster CR: Multidirectional instability of the shoulder in the athlete. Clin Sports Med 2:355, 1983. WB Saunders Co, Toronto.
7. Rowe CR: Factors related to recurrences of anterior dislocation of the shoulder. Clin Orthop 20:21, 1961
8. Hastings DE: Recurrent subluxation of the glenohumeral joint. Am J Sports Med 9:352, 1981
9. Aroneu JG: Decreasing the incidence of first time anterior shoulder dislocations with rehabilitation. Am J Sports Med 12:283, 1984

10. Simonet WT, Cofield RH: Prognosis in anterior shoulder dislocation. Am J Sports Med 12:19, 1984
11. Kuriyama S, Fujimaki E, Katagiri T, Uemura S: Anterior dislocation of the shoulder joint sustained through skiing. Am J Sports Med 12:339, 1984
12. Pappas AM: Symptomatic shoulder instability due to lesions of the glenoid labrum. Am J Sports Med 11:279, 1983
13. Rockwood CA: Dislocations about the shoulder. In Rockwood CA and Green DP (eds): Fractures, JB Lippincott, Philadelphia, 1975
14. Cybex, Division of Lumex Corp: Isolated Joint Testing and Exercise. A Handbook for Using the Cybex II and the UBXT Bayshore, New York, 1980
15. Fowler P: Unpublished data. University of Western Ontario, London, Ontario, 1985.
16. Fowler P: Swimmer problems. Am J Sports Med 7:141, 1979
17. O'Donoghue DH: Subluxing biceps tendon in the athlete. J Sports Med 13:28, 1973
18. Hitchcock HH, Bechtol CO: Painful shoulders. J Bone Joint Surg (Am) 30:267, 1948
19. Strauss MB, Wrobel LJ, Neft RS, Cady GW: The shrugged-off shoulder: a comparison of patients with recurrent subluxations and dislocations, Physician Sports Med 11:85, 1983
20. Hastings DE, Coughlin LP: Recurrent subluxation of the glenohumeral joint. Am J Sports Med 9:352, 1981
21. Mathews LS, Oueida SJ: Glenohumeral instability in athletes. Spectrum, diagnosis and treatment. Adv Orthop Surg 8:236, 1985
22. Jopke T: Training swimmers. How coaches get results. Physician Sports Med 10:161, 1982
23. Sharp RL, Troop JP, Costil DL: Relationship between power and sprint free style swimming. Med Sci Sport Exerc 14:53, 1982
24. Rodeo S: Swimming breast stroke: A kinesiological analysis and considerations for strength training. NSCA J 4–8 Aug. and Sept., 1984
25. Costill DL, Fink WJ, Hargreaves M, King DS, Thomas R, Fielding R: Metabolic characteristics of skeletal muscle during detraining from competitive swimming. Med Sci Sports Exerc 17:339, 1985
26. Magel JR, Andersen KL: Pulmonary diffusing capacity and cardiac output in young trained Norwegian swimmers and undetermined subjects. Med Sci Sports 1:131, 1969
27. Hovelius L, Eriksson K, Fredin H: Recurrences after initial dislocation for the shoulder. J Bone Joint Surg 65A:343, 1983
28. Watson-Jones R: Fractures and Joint Injuries. E & S Livingstone, Edinburgh, 1976
29. Aamoth GM, O'Phalen EH: Recurrent anterior dislocation of the shoulder: A review of 40 athletes treated by subscapularis transfer. Am J Sports Med 8:188, 1977
30. Miller LS, Donahue JR, Good RP, Staerk AJ: The Magnuson-Stack procedure for treatment of recurrent glenohumeral dislocations. Am J Sports Med 12:133, 1984
31. Halley DK, Olix MD: A review of the Bristow operation for recurrent anterior shoulder dislocation in athletes. Clin Orthop 106:175, 1979
32. Braly WG, Tullos H: A modification of the Bristow procedure for recurrent anterior dislocation of the shoulder. Am J Sports Med 13:81, 1985

10 | Throwing Injuries to the Shoulder

Turner A. Blackburn, Jr.

Why has the understanding of the throwing act and the injuries associated with it lagged behind that of the study of the knee and ankle? After all, baseball is "America's Pastime." Could it be that the overwhelming number of ankle and knee injuries predisposed more intensive study of these joints? Because knee and ankle injuries occur in almost all sports but throwing injuries only occur in throwers, could the emphasis of research have ignored them? Has the small "clique-ish" world of professional baseball disallowed changes or research that may be of benefit?

Unless there is a dislocation, separation, complete rotator cuff tear, or fracture, it is difficult to diagnose a pitcher's or thrower's complaint about an ache, pain, or overuse injury involving the shoulder. Examination techniques, history taking with an *understanding* of throwing, and an actual ability to see the injury without disabling the athlete with surgery have only recently been developed.

The advent of the arthroscopic diagnostic examination of the shoulder has allowed the correlation of physical examination and history with pathology. Three puncture holes in the shoulder capsule do not preclude the athlete's throwing again. Open procedures on the shoulder almost always produced sufficient scar tissue to prevent full form and flexibility, therefore also preventing a return to full function.

Because the arthroscope is generating more interest in throwers, the biomechanist is now studying the pitching act with much more enthusiasm. An understanding of the pitching act means a better understanding of the pitching injury. Many times, an adjustment in the biomechanics of the form of the thrower will be all that is needed to treat an injury.

The addition of specific exercises applied to the pitching act to recreate concentric or eccentric contractions which occur in specific positions has greatly enhanced the progress the athlete can make in recovering from an injury.

The goals and objectives of this chapter are to familiarize readers with the mechanics of throwing and injuries that occur when overuse or poor mechanics occur, and to provide insight into diagnosis and treatment of injuries. Specific injuries will be discussed with emphasis on soft tissue problems. Arthroscopic surgery will be discussed as surgical intervention. Rehabilitation techniques will be explored extensively with emphasis on proper form for exercise and a return to throwing outline.

MECHANISMS OF THROWING

The act of overhead throwing is a series of rotational movements that include the thrower getting the hand and thus the ball moving at speeds up to 100 mph. This orchestrated and coordinated movement requires skill and athletic ability as well as strength and flexibility. It requires input from all areas of the body including legs, abdomen, back, shoulder, elbow, and wrist. The rotational movements actually allow a "whipping" motion to occur throughout the chain from foot to hand propelling the ball.

As injuries occur in the throwing act, it becomes apparent that the shoulder takes its fair share of the load. The overhead toss calls for the elevation of the humerus which obviously calls for proximal stabilization at the glenohumeral joint and the scapulothoracic joint. Raising the arm overhead uses the much-discussed scapulohumeral rhythm described by Codman.[1] The coordinated movement has a ratio of glenohumeral movement to scapular movement of 3:2.[2] The scapula is controlled by a balance of forces of the various portions of the trapezius, levator scapulae, and serratus anterior. There are associated movements at the acromioclavicular joint and sternoclavicular joint.[3] There is rotation of the clavicle along with retraction and protraction of the shoulder complex occurring at the sternoclavicular joint during the pitching act.

Windup

The pitching act begins with the windup. This phase of pitching will vary with every pitcher and the condition of the game as far as base runners. No injuries occur during this phase, but it is a very important part of throwing because it begins a series of events that puts the body into motion. Windup occurs from the beginning movements to the point where the ball hand and gloved hand separate.

This phase gets the arms up overhead after a downward swing. Body weight is first shifted forward on the right foot (for right-handed pitchers; weight shifts first to the left foot for left-handed pitchers) and then back to the left foot. As in most sports that require propelling of an object, the shift of body weight begins the real power move. Rotation begins in this phase as the shoulder turns 90° to the plate. The left knee is lifted and pulled upward and to the right as the hips also turn nearly 90°. The weight is now shifted forward slightly to the right foot, but the center of balance does not shift over the middle of the body yet. The body is coiled in rotation of right leg, hips, and trunk. The "scapulothoracic rhythm" has the arm position up and away from the body. The individual may show many variations in this movement, especially with knee lift height and rotation.

Cocking

As in any whipping type of action, activities do not occur at the same time along the "chain." The cocking phase describes the positioning of the glenohumeral joint. The point where the hands break to maximal external rotation is described as the cocking phase. At the same time that the hands break, the center of balance of the body moves forward. The left leg extends forward and plants with the foot pointed toward the plate. Once the center of balance is forward, the right leg with foot pointed perpendicular to the line of throw drives the body weight forward. At about the time of left foot plant, the arm is at its fullest external rotation. The left hand and arm are propelled into extension and horizontal abduction to help speed the rotation of the trunk to the left.

The glenohumeral joint is brought to an external rotation of ~140° to 160°. Slow-motion analysis shows that this occurs at the glenohumeral joint and the scapulothoracic joint. The humerus is abducted to 90°. Indeed, the descriptions of a pitcher as throwing "overhand," "three-quarters," or "sidearm" are misnomers. Most of these pitchers have their humerus at 90° but their body lean to right or left gives them the appearance of being in these various positions. Trunk rotation brings the humerus back behind the frontal plane. As the left foot plants and begins the first deceleration of the body's frontal motion, the "whipping" action begins that puts the humerus into 30° of horizontal abduction. Thus, the glenohumeral joint leads the forward frontal horizontal adduction of the humerus. Anterior structures of the glenohumeral joint are under great stress at this point. The internal rotators of the humerus are put under maximum stress and stretch.

During the cocking phase, the posterior deltoid brings the humerus back into horizontal adduction. The supraspinatus, infraspinatus, and teres minor must aid in pulling the arm back as well as stabilizing the humeral head. The subscapularis, as well as other internal rotators such as the pectoralis major and latissimus dorsi, fires in late cocking to stop the posterior movement of the humerus. But because of the whipping chain effect that occurs, the pectoralis major, latissimus dorsi, and subscapularis begin to contract and start pulling the arm forward before the humerus is at full external rotation. Because acceleration occurs once the ball moves forward, these activities have already occurred in the "acceleration" muscles.[4] During this movement, the proximal stabilizers near the scapula are firing to maintain a solid base for the movement of the humerus. The elbow is flexed at 90°, with co-contraction in the triceps and biceps. The forearm is at neutral, and the wrist is slightly extended.

Acceleration

The acceleration phase starts with the forward motion of the ball until it is released. We must not forget that the ball is the last thing to be moving. The thrower's left foot is already planted and the hips have rotated back to the left. The trunk is rotating to the left. The humerus moves in a horizontal adduction direction for 40 ms and the ball comes forward in internal rotation for ~40 ms.

The elbow moves from 90° flexion to 25° to 30° extension. There is tremendous force across the anterior shoulder and the medial side of the elbow. The humeral head has forces that are trying to pull it anteriorly out of the socket. In this brief 80 ms, very high forces occur.

The scapular stabilizers continue to function during this stage. The rotator cuff muscles are active as stabilizers of the humeral head but do not show a high degree of activity.[5] The pectoralis major and latissimus dorsi have done their job by now and, though active, are not doing as much as during the cocking phase. The triceps work extremely hard in accelerating the elbow into extension. The point of ball release is somewhere near the ear level. The hand is moving as fast as the ball (as much as 90 to 95 mph).

Ball Release

The ball release is a very nebulous event. The fastest cameras have a difficult time discerning exactly when the ball leaves the fingertips. Just prior to the 6 to 7-ms event, the pronators of the forearm are controlling the type of pitch. The pitcher applies force to the ball through the fingers. All pitchers go into a relative amount of pronation. The wrist may be slightly flexed at release.

Deceleration

Once the ball is released, the body must slow down the hand and therefore the arm. The foot strike of the left foot starts this deceleration of the body. At ball release, it has been estimated that there may be 300 lb of force trying to pull the arm forward out of the socket.

The forces that occur during the first 40 ms after the ball release are the highest and most difficult to control. The rotator cuff, posteriorly, must accomplish this deceleration. The cuff fires at extremely high levels of EMG activity.[5] Deceleration is accomplished through an eccentric contraction of the posterior cuff. Again, the scapular stabilizers must also do their job to allow the cuff to do its job. The bicep contracts violently, slowing the elbow extension. This force is transmitted across the humeral head for stabilization.

Follow-Through

After the first 40 ms of activity of deceleration, the follow-through phase allows the rest of the absorption of the throwing energy to occur. It also puts the thrower in a position to protect himself from balls that may be hit back toward him. There is a stretch of the posterior shoulder structure as well as a diminished activity in the posterior cuff muscle.

INJURY MECHANICS

The American Medical Association's Standard Nomenclature of Athletic Injuries,[6] describes the classifications of musculotendinous injuries that occur at the shoulder in throwing.

Grade I muscle strain:
   a. Mild
   b. No tearing
   c. Minimal symptoms
   d. Heal quickly
Grade II muscle strain:
   a. Moderate
   b. Tearing fibers
   c. Swelling
   d. Functional disability
   e. May take 6 weeks to heal
Grade III muscle strain:
   a. Severe
   b. Complete tear or rupture
   c. Severe loss of function
   d. Much time loss

Some type of overloading occurs at the shoulder joint during the pitching motion for injury to occur. This overload may be intrinsic or extrinsic. It may come from forces produced by the body itself intrinsically through muscle contractions such as in the acceleration phase when the anterior muscles contract and pull the arm forward. It may occur when the ball is released and the arm is out of control, which produces higher forces than are usually found with concentric contractions during the acceleration phase. This extrinsic force produced when the ball is released must be controlled through eccentric contractions of the posterior cuff. Because most injuries occur during the acceleration and deceleration phases, the intrinsic–extrinsic concept helps one correlate the pitching motion with the injury.

During acceleration, the movements of horizontal adduction and internal rotation produce a grinding force on the glenoid labrum. The acceleration muscles are trying to pull the humerus anteriorly over the labrum and out of the socket. Movement of the humeral head may damage the labrum anteriorly and superiorly. If the posterior stabilizing muscles (i.e., posterior rotator cuff) are weaker, the anterior force may succeed in damaging the anterior labrum. The forces during acceleration are high, but the rate remains relatively constant, so muscles rarely tear. During deceleration, forces are high and the rate of deceleration is increasing, thereby producing much higher forces on the posterior cuff muscles. This extrinsic loading causes tissue tearing in the posterior rotator cuff.

Overuse causes an inflammatory response to microtrauma, leaving the athlete sore. Early mild injuries such as this respond quickly to rest, exercises, and modalities. When these overuse situations are pushed, they become chronic and severe. Usually the overuse situation causes a change in throwing biomechanics, and insult is added to injury. As weakness occurs because of abnormal biomechanics, more stress is put on structures that when damaged cause more severe damage, such as the rotator cuff. Poor mechanics may even put stress on the suprascapular nerve which is sometimes injured in the throwing athlete.

The force that the bicep produces when slowing the elbow during deceleration is also applied across the anterior humerus. The long head of the biceps has an intimate attachment to the glenoid labrum. These high forces may help tear the biceps partially. Biceps tendinitis occurs in many throwing overuse syndromes. Rarely is the biceps at fault, but it is representative of other problems about the shoulder.

Because the arm is only taken to 90° of abduction in throwing, impingement syndromes in the pure sense of the word do not occur as in swimming when the arm is taken overhead >90°. Extrinsic overload at the posterior rotator cuff causes tissue tearing at the superior cuff area. This will present itself as an impingement pain on examination when the arm is brought up >90°.

Of course poor pitching mechanics can cause undue stress (i.e., decreased external rotation, horizontal abduction, or full horizontal adduction) during throwing. The most common combination seen is weakness in the posterior cuff muscle and a lack of full external rotation.

Anterior pain can usually be associated with opening up too soon. This means the pitcher tries to whip the arm by rotating the body away from the pitching arm sooner and faster than he should to create more arm speed. Injuries resulting in this situation are mild and respond to conservative measures quickly. Proper instruction in pitching technique is important to prevent injury. Exercise strengthens the shoulder.

EXAMINATION

The usual history of a thrower with a partial rotator cuff tear or labrum tear is one of 12 to 18 months of symptoms that come and go. Symptoms usually improve with rest. Return to play usually exacerbates them again. Many times players are told to rest and not to throw, and are given no exercises. Then they are asked to pitch in a game after 10 days. Naturally, reinjury occurs.

Those throwers with an anterior-superior labrum tear have problems at ball release when they describe they cannot "let the ball go." The partial rotator cuff lesion athlete has pain on trying to increase the intensity of the pitching act, but may be able to throw with no pain at lesser intensity.

Many athletes go home during the off-season months and "rest" the injury and then come back to spring training and have a difficult time. Young pitchers who just make a club may come to spring camp trying to impress the coaches, throwing harder and more times than they ever have. They are injured and say nothing, afraid they will be cut from the team, and end up hurting their careers.

The physical examination must be systematic and precise so that nothing is omitted. With the athlete sitting up straight a visual inspection will reveal atrophy in the upper quadrant in both anterior and posterior positions. This may occur in the supraspinatus, infraspinatus, teres minor, deltoid, and sometimes the pectoralis major. Chronic problems in the shoulder area will show deltoid atrophy much as the quadricep will demonstrate atrophy with a knee problem. Supraspinatus nerve lesions are demonstrated by posterior cuff weakness.

The coordination of scapulothoracic involvement can be observed when the arm is raised overhead. The throwing side of the athlete will be hyperatrophied and may show abnormal positioning of the scapula.

Palpation of the shoulder can also be accomplished with the athlete in the sitting position. The coracoid process, where the short head of the bicep attaches as well as the shoulder depressors, may be sore. The long head of the biceps can be palpated next. The sternoclavicular joint, the acromioclavicular joint, the deltoid, the subdeltoid bursae, the trapezius, and the levator scapula insertion can all be palpated with the athlete in a sitting position.

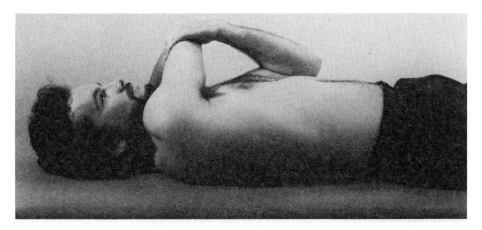

Fig. 10-1. Horizontal adduction flexibility.

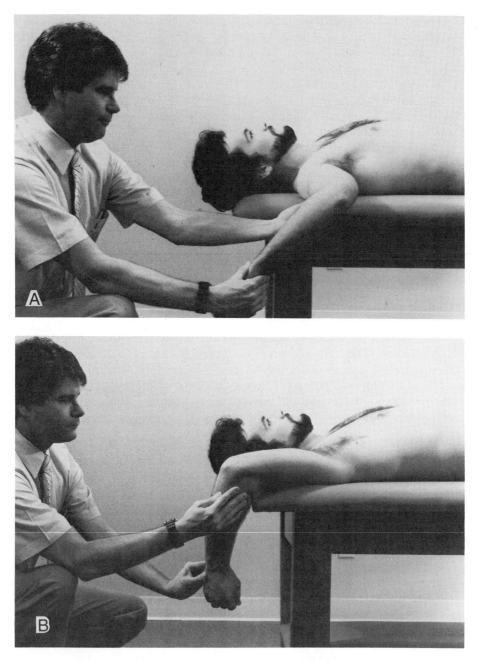

Fig. 10-2. (A) External rotation at 90° abduction. (B) External rotation at 135° abduction (Figure continued.)

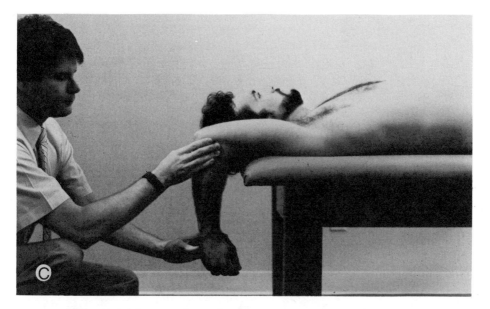

Fig. 10-2 (*Continued*).   (C) External rotation at full abduction.

With the athlete supine and the humerus in neutral position, the long head of the biceps can be examined. With the humerus externally rotated, the subscapular tendon can be checked. With the humerus internally rotated, the supraspinatus insertion can be palpated for tenderness. With the athlete prone and the arm hanging off the table, the examiner's fingers can work under the posterior deltoid and palpate the posterior cuff.

Passive flexibility of the shoulder is now ascertained. When the athlete is sitting, a passive horizontal adduction (Fig. 10-1) maneuver indicates the tightness of the posterior structures. It is important to follow through with this motion. When the athlete is supine, external rotation of the shoulder is checked at 90°, 135°, and full abduction (Fig. 10-2A, 2 B and 2C). Passively, it should reach well into the 140° to 160° range. There should be no pain. Internal rotation will be reduced to as much as 45°, which appears normal in baseball pitchers. Pure abduction without winging of the scapula should be evident (Fig. 10-3). The shoulder should be able to reach 30° of horizontal abduction.

Several manual muscle tests give clues about specific injuries about the shoulder. Jobe has taught us that the supraspinatus is isolated best in the standing position with the arm abducted to 90° and horizontally abducted to 30°. The humerus is internally rotated fully.[7] (Fig. 10-4). Weakness here represents the supraspinatus. Baseball players with an otherwise normal shoulder will have pain in this test. The deltoid atrophies with injury and should be tested in flexion and abduction. External rotation is tested with the humerus at 90° abduction, 45° external rotation (Fig. 10-5). This represents the strength of the posterior cuff in the throwing position. The external rotation test at 0° of humeral

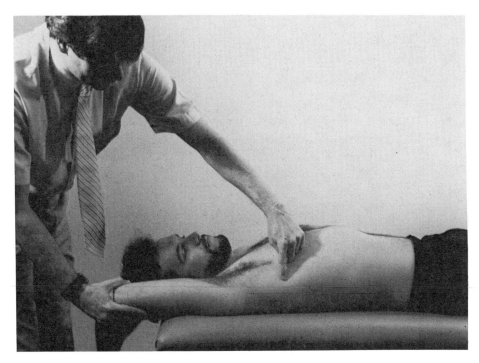

Fig. 10-3.   Pure abduction with winging of scapula.

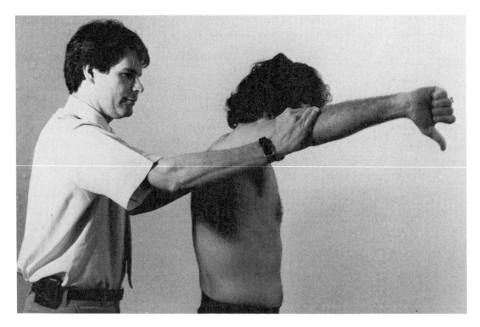

Fig. 10-4.   Supraspinatus position.

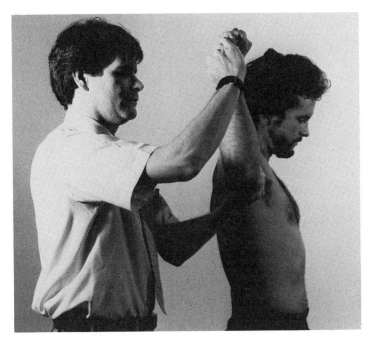

Fig. 10-5. External rotation manual muscle test at 90°.

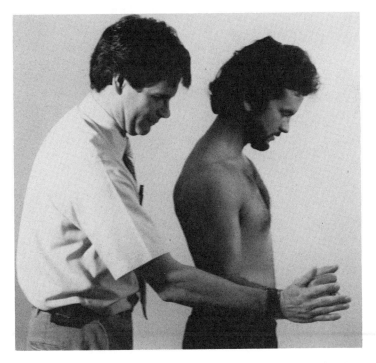

Fig. 10-6. External rotation manual muscle test at 0°.

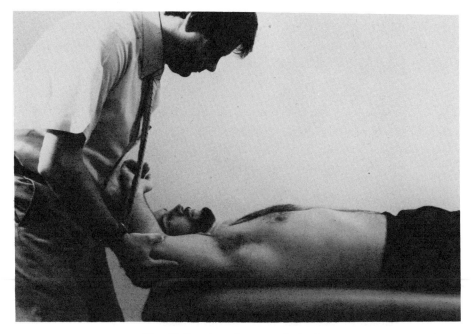

Fig. 10-7.   Anterior capsule laxity.

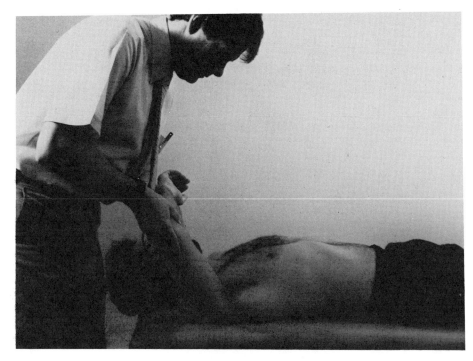

Fig. 10-8.   Posterior capsule laxity.

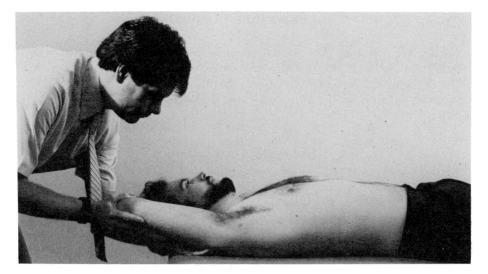

Fig. 10-9. Glenoid labrum grind test.

abduction with the elbow at 90° tests the infraspinatus and teres minor (Fig. 10-6). The posterior musculature can be checked with the athlete prone and the arm horizontally abducted at 90°.

Joint testing involves several maneuvers. Laxity of the capsule can be elicited with the patient supine by manually trying to slide the humerus anteriorly (Fig. 10-7) and posteriorly (Fig. 10-8). During this maneuver, the popping of a torn labrum may be elicited (Fig. 10-9) by bringing the arm into full abduction and circumduction.

COMMON INJURIES

Deltoid

A deltoid strain can cause anterior pain. Grade I and II strains may slow the athlete down but usually heal quickly. Conservative measures including ice, moist heat, ultrasound, and electrical stimulation are of benefit. Exercises for the anterior deltoid are most important. In chronic shoulder problems, the anterior deltoid atrophies. It is a most important structure, especially in the acceleration phase of throwing.

Subdeltoid Bursitis

This inflammatory process can occur in the thrower. It is found by direct palpation of the bursa. It is usually associated with pain during the acceleration phase of throwing. Again conservative measures apply. A steroid injection may be considered only in the stubborn cases and only if there is no rotator cuff injury.

Subdeltoid Adhesions

If there are frequent repeated episodes of subdeltoid bursitis, a chronic inflammatory process will develop. This can lead to adhesions in the bursal sac. The player will have a reduction in range of motion (ROM) with a painful arch of movement. Other tests will prove negative for other problems. An injection of 0.5 percent bupivacaine (morcaine) and early light throwing can break up these adhesions. Chronic adhesions may have to be excised surgically.

Subscapular Tendonitis

During the acceleration phase, the subscapularis is very active in throwing. This muscle can develop tendonitis. Palpation will elicit this pain, and conservative measures and exercise should help it to heal.

Pectoralis Major Muscle Ruptures

A very rare injury is the rupture of the pectoralis major. It is usually seen in the throwing of heavy objects such as a javelin or discus. It also occurs in weight lifters. It occurs during the acceleration phase of throwing. Many times, it occurs at the sternal and clavicular origin of the pectoralis major. There may be a history of extrinsic overload and soreness locally. The pectoralis muscle belly can rupture by intrinsic overloading in the midphase of acceleration.

Latissimus Dorsi Muscle Rupture

These injuries are about as common as pectoralis major ruptures. They occur when internal rotation forces are applied during the throwing act.

Biceps Tendonitis

Tendinitis of the long head of the biceps as it passes through the bicepital groove is overdiagnosed in the throwing athlete. Many times it is associated with other pathology. The biceps tendon long head has an important stabilization function in the throwing act. If other stabilizers (i.e., posterior rotator cuff) are weakened, the bicep must carry more of the load. The tendon is sore through excursion through the bicepital groove. Modalities and exercise remedy this problem.

Recurrent Subluxation of the Long Head of the Biceps

The long head of the biceps can sublux during the cocking and early acceleration phase, especially in athletes who have shallow bicepital grooves. The long head has a 30° posterior angle where it attaches to the superior portion of the glenoid rim. This can cause subluxation when the humerus goes from external rotation to internal rotation. This subluxation can be produced by externally and internally rotating the humerus and palpating the subluxation with the finger tips.

Biceps Tendon Ruptures

The long head of the biceps may partially avulse at this insertion along the superior rim of the glenoid fossa. During acceleration and deceleration, the bicep is active and the high forces may partially tear the tendon and the glenoid labrum. This is an intraarticular problem and can be seen with the arthroscope.

Glenoid Labrum Tears

The anterior glenoid labrum can tear by the shoulder grinding factor or by subluxation of the humeral head. The biceps long head can also pull a portion of it. The examiner can make it pop when checking for laxity of the anterior capsule. The thrower complains of a pain on acceleration of the arm. If the tear propagates anteriorly and inferiorly, the subluxation of the humeral head can be a problem. Arthroscopic surgery easily removes this joint irritant.

Subluxation of the Humerus

Most throwers have a loose-jointed shoulder. It is rare that a pitcher will dislocate while throwing. The anterior and posterior capsule can be tested and found to be loose, but this is specific to the activity. If there is a subluxation problem, it is difficult to decide in what direction it occurs during the act of pitching because both can happen in cocking, acceleration, and deceleration. An athlete with an anterior subluxation will have an anterior inferior labrum tear; one with a posterior subluxation usually has a midposterior labrum tear. These can be treated arthroscopically, and the patient can be rehabilitated to full function.

Rotator Cuff Tears

Most throwers who injure the rotator cuff do not tear it completely. A partial tear develops in the thickness of the cuff. Deceleration of the throwing arm causes this pathology. If the cuff becomes fatigued, the microtrauma to the tendon begins to develop. Over time, an incomplete tear develops within the supraspinatus tendon insertion. This occurs on the undersurface of the cuff intraarticularly. Impingement syndromes do not tear the tendon, or the lesion would be external to the cuff.

An athlete who has pain on deceleration of the throwing arm cannot get back to usual speed and ends up continuing to reinjure the arm. The athlete slowly develops weakness throughout the shoulder during this process.

Arthroscopic debridement can stimulate healing. With proper exercise, the athlete may return to full pitching in 6 months. Athletes with complete tears of the rotator cuff have a much smaller chance of returning to play.

SURGERY

A scar on the shoulder of a thrower usually spelled doom for the aspiring player. The advent of the arthroscope changed all this. Because very little scar tissue develops with arthroscopic puncture holes, the athlete achieves full ROM and can get into the throwing position. The arthroscope has allowed visualization of injuries that for so long have been hidden.

Three major problems can be handled with arthroscopic surgery. The torn glenoid labrum in the anterior superior quadrant can be easily debrided. If the biceps tendon is frayed intraarticularily, debridement can reduce pain and instability. The necrotic tissue of a partial rotator cuff tear can be debrided and the "healing pump" started with increased blood supply caused by the surgery.

CONSERVATIVE CARE

Most injuries to the throwing shoulder do not result in surgery. Most are treated conservatively with modalities, anti-inflammatories, exercise, and a gradual return to throwing. These athletes usually do not have "frozen shoulders" or other shoulder conditions that make the evaluation difficult. The arthroscope has allowed a correlation of physical findings and history to actual injury.

Modality use can be beneficial. Use of moist heat before throwing and ice after throwing is the usual routine. Ultrasound with or without anti-inflammatory gel delivers its properties deep into the rotator cuff or other structures. High-voltage stimulators also aid in healing and pain relief. Transcutaneous electrical nerve stimulation (TENS) will help to control pain postoperatively.

The most difficult situation is determining rotator cuff irritation. Early in the development of rotator cuff problems, the athlete can recover quickly from symptoms, but because of continued high-pressure throwing, the injury exacerbates. Rest and exercise and a graduated return to throwing program allows the problem to heal without reinjury.

The glenoid labrum tear can be discovered on examination. The shoulder must be strengthened to prevent abnormal forces from causing further damage. As with a torn meniscus in the knee, the glenoid labrum tear is not an emergency situation. The athlete may continue to throw. The lesion will not heal; therefore, surgery will probably result.

Both the postoperative rotator cuff debridement and labrum excision follow the same rehabilitation program. Both are usually done as outpatient procedures. The patient usually uses a sling for 1 or 2 days for comfort. Postoperative dressings are removed at day 3, and bandages are used over the puncture holes until they heal.

At postoperative day 1, ROM and strengthening exercises begin. They are done to the patient's tolerance but are pushed along quickly, especially because of the need for full ROM. Codman exercises are effective early for mobilization of the glenohumeral joint. Supine flexion and abduction used with a wand allows the athlete to work these motions at least 25 times, 3 to 5 times daily. Often the athlete develops a contracture between the scapula and humerus inferiorly at the glenohumeral joint. Manual stretching may be indicated by stabilizing the scapula and allowing for stretching of the humerus overhead. Putting a pad under the scapula raises the body and allows for more ROM work when the athlete must work alone and increase shoulder retraction.

External rotation stretching is by far one of the most important motions to perform. This motion applies graduated controlled stress to the healing and scarring area, allowing collagen to form in a much more organized fashion and keeping scar formation small and smooth so that impingement problems are prevented. The athlete performs the actively assisted external rotation stretch at 90°, 135°, and full abduction. The goal is development of more than normal external rotation and a pain-free ROM end.

Other ROM must be exercised including internal rotation. The follow-through phase requires good posterior flexibility and is accomplished by the horizontal adduction stretch.

For strengthening, a high-repetition, low-weight program appears to be the most therapeutic. Five sets of 10 repetitions and no weight, with progress up to 5 lb, is usually all that is required during the first 6 weeks. This program increases strength to the point where the manual muscle test will be normal in all positions and not irritate the joint. All lifts require a dead stop at their extreme and are done at a measured pace. The athlete may work higher as this gets easier, but never with >10 lb. The athlete generally does not work with weight machines until capable of throwing normally.

Shoulder shrugs are done with scapular adduction and shoulder retraction. Forward flexion and pure abduction are done with the humerus externally rotated and the thumb up. The supraspinatus is exercised with the arm at 30° in forward flexion with the humerus internally rotated fully. The hand is lifted to eye level. The posterior shoulder structures are strengthened with prone horizontal abduction, with the glenohumeral joint at 100° and the arm externally rotated fully. Prone external rotation is done with the humerus supported on the exercise table. Side-lying external rotation is performed for infraspinatus and teres minor strengthening. The bicep curl and tricep extension or french curl increase strength in those important throwing muscles. The sitting push-up or dip strengthens the internal rotators, shoulder depressors, and triceps and is the only internal rotation strengthening that is done. An imbalance of weaker posterior muscles versus anterior muscles may lead to injury. Appendix 10-1 is a shoulder exercise program that can be individualized for each patient.

At 4 weeks for the labrum tear, and at 6 weeks for the partial rotator cuff tear, the athlete is expected to have full ROM with very little pain at extremes and a G+ to N manual muscle test for the shoulder. The interval throwing program (Appendix 10-2), another patient exercise program, should be started, allowing the athlete to condition the arm slowly. The original injury most likely occurred because of fatigue. The muscles of the arm are strong but the tendon and joint structures are not ready for the high stresses of 90 mph fast balls. A thrower who now overworks the arm will reinjure the area.

The interval is 5 minutes of long toss and 5 minutes of short toss (Appendix 10-2). The athlete warms up with moist heat and stretching, then tosses the ball for several minutes at 30 ft, gradually building up to 90 ft. This is the long toss, which allows the pitcher to work on good form at low intensity. The pitcher then tosses the ball at 30 ft and throws at half speed or as tolerated. The thrower should rest for 30 minutes, do the prescribed exercises and then repeat the sequence. The thrower will have accomplished 20 minutes of throwing but will not fatigue the arm. The long toss progresses by 30 ft to 250 ft. The short toss progresses from 30 ft at half speed to 60 ft at half speed, then to three-quarter speed, three-quarter speed from mound, three-quarter speed from mound and curve balls, and finally works up to full speed. As the athlete gets stronger, he may reach plateaus that cannot be worked through; an additional few minutes or another interval may be of benefit. The athlete must listen to his body and not force progress too fast. It usually takes 3 months to recover from a labrum excision to full participation and 6 months for the partial rotator cuff tear. Speed gun testing will help the athlete determine progress. The athlete should continue the exercises vigorously. Because every athlete is different, progress will be individual.

PREVENTION

A player should not be sent home during the off season without a program, injured or not. A player who expects to throw the next season should have the arm conditioned all year by throwing a ball for 15 minutes three times weekly. A maintenance weight program centered around the supraspinatus lift, the prone horizontal abduction, prone external rotation, and external rotation stretching will help the shoulder stay strong. A pitcher never "rests."

Biomechanical analysis through high-speed video will become a reality as technology improves. Kodak now has a camera that can shoot video at 2,000 frames per second. Film can work faster but is harder to work with and cannot be shown immediately. The coach and the athlete can observe biomechanical abnormalities and correct them.

The physician, therapist, trainer, and coach must work together in close harmony to assure the progress of the injured thrower. Exercise, rest, modalities, proper medication, and a graduated return to throwing program will enhance a player's return to throwing activity.

APPENDIX 10-1

SHOULDER EXERCISE PROGRAM

1. Circumduction
   Lean over with opposite arm on table. Let involved arm hang straight down. *Be relaxed.* Move body and let arm swing in circle clockwise, counterclockwise, forward and backward, and side to side. Do at least 1 minute every hour you are awake (Fig. 10-10).

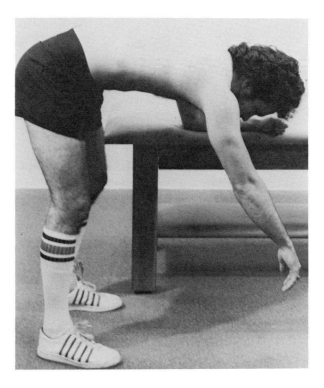

Fig. 10-10. Circumduction.

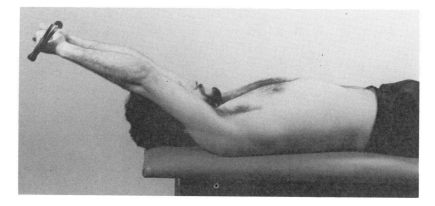

Fig. 10-11.   Supine flexion.

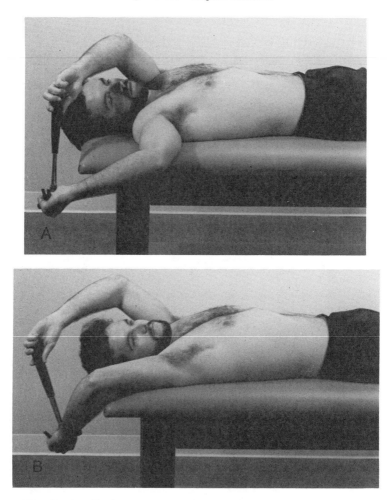

Fig. 10-12.   Supine external rotation (A, B). (Figure continued.)

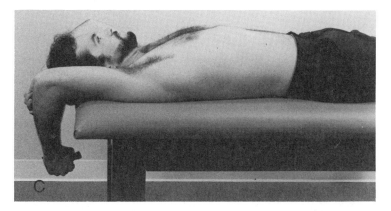

Fig. 10-12 (*Continued*).   (C) Supine external rotation.

2. Supine Flexion
    Lie on back. Grip hammer in both hands with elbow straight, take both arms over head as far as possible and hold for count of 5. Return to starting position. Repeat ____ times ____ times per day (Fig. 10-11).
3. Supine External Rotation
    Lie on back with involved arm out to side at 90° and elbow at 90°. Use the hammer to push the arm straight back into external rotation. Hold for a count of 5. Relax and repeat ____ times ____ times daily. Repeat this at 90° abduction, at 135°, and full abduction (Fig. 10-12).
4. Supine Internal Rotation
    Lie on back with involved arm out to side at 90° and elbow at 90°. Use hammer to push the arm straight into internal rotation. Hold for a count of 5. Relax and repeat ____ times ____ times per day (Fig. 10-13).

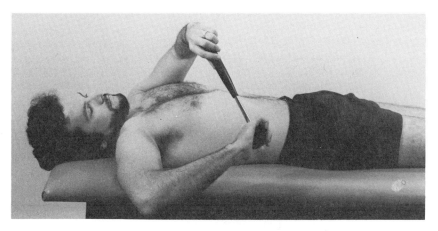

Fig. 10-13.   Supine internal rotation.

5.   Supine Abduction
      Lie on back with involved arm out to side as far as possible and arm
      externally rotated as far as possible. Slide arm *along floor* as close to
      ear as possible. Use hammer or hand to help pull. Hold for a count of
      5. Relax and repeat ____ times, ____ times daily (Fig. 10-14).

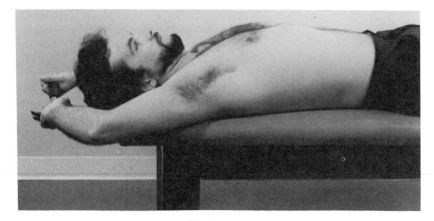

Fig. 10-14.   Supine abduction.

6.   Rope and Pulley
      Rope and pulley should be in doorway with pulley in one corner of the
      door jamb. Sit in a chair with back against door jamb under pulley.
      Clasp handles of pulley.
      A.   With elbow straight, raise arm out to front using your muscle. When
            you have it as high as possible, then assist by pulling on the rope.
            Take arm as high as possible, hold for a count of 5, then lower the
            arm using as much muscle power as possible. Repeat ____ times,
            ____ times daily.
      B.   With elbow straight and arm out to side, palm facing upward. Re-
            peat ____ times, ____ times per day.
7.   Shoulder Shrugs
      Stand with arms by your side. Lift shoulders straight up to your ear,
      hold for a 2 count, then pull shoulders back and pinch shoulder blades
      and hold for a count of 2. Relax shoulder. Repeat ____ times, ____ times
      per day. Progress up to ____ pounds held in your hands (Fig. 10-15).
8.   Shoulder Flexion
      Stand. Raise arm out to front of body as high as possible. Hold this for
      a count of 2, then lower. Do ____ times, ____ times daily. Start with
      ____ pounds and progress to ____ pounds (Fig. 10-16).
9A.   Shoulder Abduction
      Stand. Raise arm out to side of body as high as possible while rotating
      arm externally. Hold for a count of 2, then lower. Do ____ times, ____

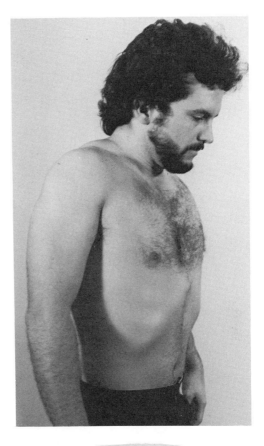

Fig. 10-15. Shoulder shrugs.

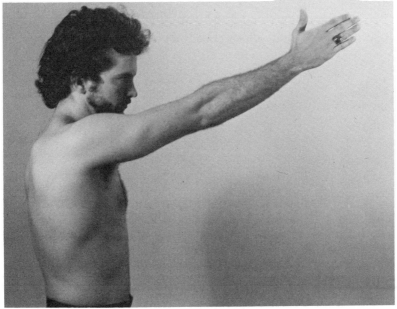

Fig. 10-16. Shoulder flexion.

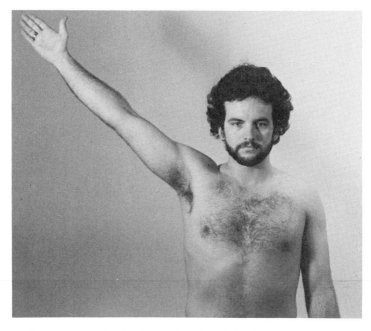

Fig. 10-17.   Shoulder abduction.

times daily. Start with ____ pounds and progress to ____ pounds (Fig. 10-17).

9B.   Supraspinatus
Raise the arm out to the side in front of body 30° with arm internally rotated. Hold thumb down. Lift to eye level (Fig. 10-18).

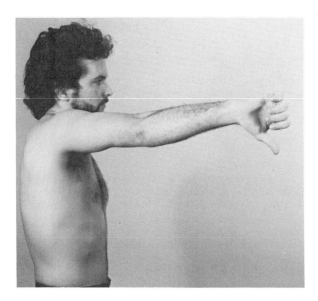

Fig. 10-18.   Supraspinatus.

10. Prone Horizontal Abduction
    Lie on table on stomach with involved arm hanging straight to the floor,
    thumb up. Hand should be at eye level. Raise arm out to side. Hold for
    a count of 2, lower and relax. Do ____ times, ____ times daily. Start
    with ____ pounds and work up to ____ pounds (Fig. 10-19).

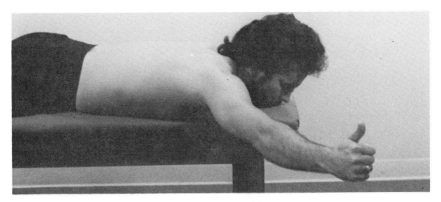

Fig. 10-19.   Prone horizontal abduction.

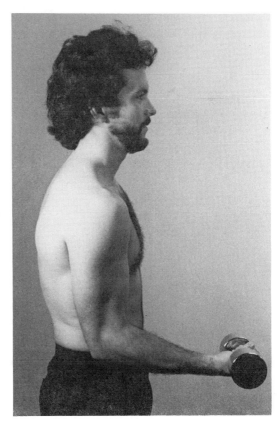

Fig. 10-20.   Biceps curl.

11. Biceps Curl

    Support arm on opposite hand. Bend elbow to full flexion, then straighten arm completely. Repeat ____ times, ____ times daily. Start with ____ pounds and work to ____ pounds (Fig. 10-20).

12. French Curl

    Raise arm overhead. Take opposite hand and give support at elbow. Straighten arm overhead, hold for a count of 2. Relax. Repeat ____ times, ____ times daily. Start with ____ pounds and work to ____ pounds (Fig. 10-21).

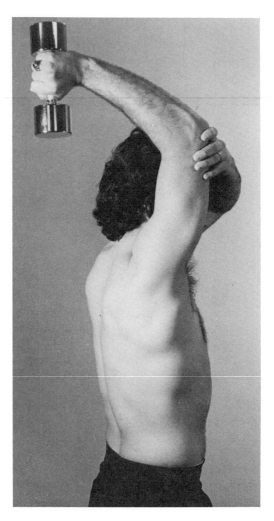

Fig. 10-21.   French curl.

13. Sitting Dip
   Sitting on edge of chair with hands by your side, lift buttocks off surface.
   Hold for a count of 2, then relax. Start with ____ times. Work up to
   ____ repetitions (Fig. 10-22).

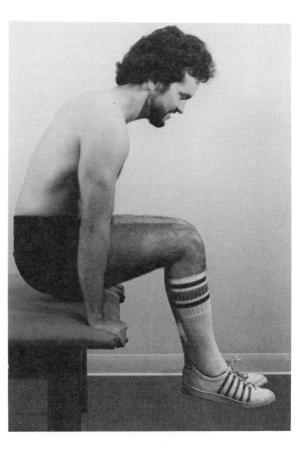

Fig. 10-22. Sitting dip.

14. Hanging
   Hang from chin-up bar, feet on floor, bend knees and absorb a comfortable amount of weight. Perform for 1 minute, three times daily.
15A. External Rotation
   Lie prone with arm supported at the elbow. Lift weight into external
   rotation. Hold for a count of 2. Relax. Perform ____ times, ____ times
   daily. Start with ____ pounds and work up to ____ pounds (Fig. 10-23).
15B. External Rotation Side-Lying
   Lie on opposite side, arm resting on side and elbow flexed at 90°. Rotate
   arm upward (Fig. 10-24).

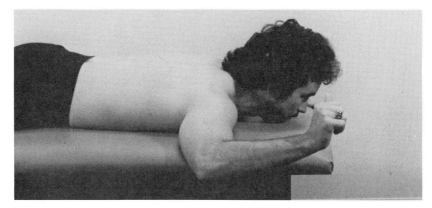

Fig. 10-23. External rotation prone.

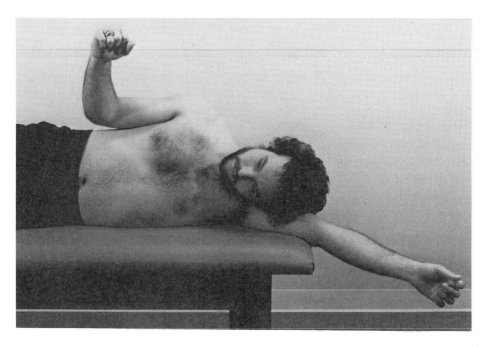

Fig. 10-24. External rotation side-lying.

16. Progressive Push-up
    Start with push-up into the wall. Gradually progress to table-top and eventually to floor. Do as tolerated. (Fig. 10-25).

17. Horizontal Adduction Stretch
    Grasp elbow of involved arm with opposite hand and pull arm across front of chest. Hold for a count of five. Relax. Repeat ＿＿ times, ＿＿ times daily (Fig. 10-26).

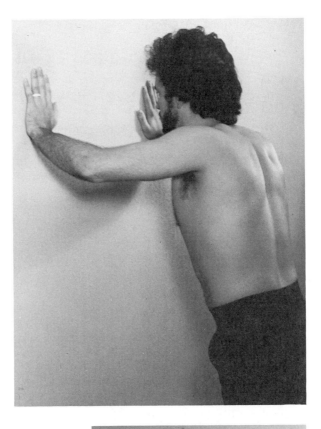

Fig. 10-25. Progressive push-up.

Fig. 10-26. Horizontal adduction stretch.

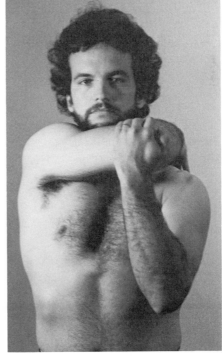

APPENDIX 10-2

INTERVAL THROWING PROGRAM

The interval throwing program is designed to allow you to work several times a day at a submaximal level, never trying to fatigue the arm, but to get a light workout. This will enable the arm to gradually become stronger and more conditioned to the throwing act. The program should begin with a thorough stretching of the throwing extremity and application of moist heat. It should be followed by ice, if appropriate. Even though you could throw at a more intense level, that is not the idea of this program. It is the slow build-up and conditioning of the arm that will allow you to progress and not reinjure yourself. Throw ____ (2) days and rest ____ (1) days. One interval equals one long toss and one short toss.

Begin each throwing session with several minutes of 30-ft tossing to get the arm warm for long toss. You may gradually work to your long-toss distance. You do not have to start at the set distance.

Your long toss may start with throws that will just roll to your partner and graduate to one hop and then the fly.

The long-toss and short-toss intervals may progress independently of each other.

Progress may not be in a straight line. There will be advances and regressions. Ease off when you hurt. Do not advance a phase until you are completely comfortable at your present phase. *Expect some soreness.*

PHASE I   ____ Interval/day (2)*
            ____ Rest between (15–30)

Long toss			Short toss		
Feet	____ (90')		Feet	____ (30')	
Minutes	____ (5)		Minutes	____ (5)	
Throws	____ (25)		Throws	____ (50)	
Intensity	____ (to tolerance)		Intensity	____ (Work to $\frac{1}{2}$ speed)	

PHASE II ____ Interval/day (2)
           ____ Rest between (15–30)

Long toss			Short toss		
Feet	____ (120')		Feet	____ (60')	
Minutes	____ (5)		Minutes	____ (5)	
Throws	____ (25)		Throws	____ (50)	
Intensity	____ (to tolerance)		Intensity	____ (work to $\frac{1}{2}$ speed)	

PHASE III ____ Interval/day (2)
            ____ Rest between (15–30)

Long toss			Short toss		
Feet	____ (150')		Feet	____ (60')	
Minutes	____ (5)		Minutes	____ (5)	
Throws	____ (25)		Throws	____ (50)	
Intensity	____ (to tolerance)		Intensity	____ (work to $\frac{3}{4}$ speed)	

PHASE IV ____ Interval/day (2)
             ____ Rest between (15–30)

Long toss			Short toss		
Feet	____	(180′)	Feet	____	(60′)
Minutes	____	(5)	Minutes	____	(5)
Throws	____	(25)	Throws	____	(50)
Intensity	____	(to tolerance)	Intensity	____	(work to $\frac{3}{4}$ speed, mound)

PHASE V ____ Interval/day (2)
            ____ Rest between (15–30)

Long toss			Short toss		
Feet	____	(210′)	Feet	____	(60′)
Minutes	____	(5)	Minutes	____	(5)
Throws	____	(25)	Throws	____	(50)
Intensity	____	(to tolerance)	Intensity	____	($\frac{1}{2}$ to $\frac{3}{4}$ speed, mound breaking ball)

PHASE VI ____Interval/day (20)
             ____ Rest between (15–30)

Long toss			Short toss		
Feet	____	(250′)	Feet	____	(60′ +)
Minutes	____	(5)	Minutes	____	(5)
Throws	____	(25)	Throws	____	(50)
Intensity	____	(to tolerance)	Intensity	____	($\frac{3}{4}$—full speed, mound, breaking ball)

---

* Numbers in parentheses are suggestions.

REFERENCES

1. Codman EA: The Shoulder. Thomas Todd Co, Boston, 1934
2. Freedman L, Munro RR: Abduction of the arm in the scapular plane: scapular and glenohumeral movements. J Bone Joint Surg 48A:1503, 1966
3. Inman UT, Saunders JB de CM, Abbott LC: Observations on the function of the shoulder joint. J Bone Joint Surg 26:1, 1944
4. Jobe FW, Moyers DR, Tibone JE, et al: AM EMG injury of the shoulder in pitching: a second report. Am J Sports Med 12:218, 1984
5. Jobe FW, Perry JB, Perry T, et al: An EMG analysis of the shoulder in throwing and pitching: a preliminary report. AMF Sports Med 11:3, 1983
6. American Medical Association. Standard Nomenclature of Athletic Injuries, 1975, Chicago, 99
7. Jobe FW, Moyers DR: Delineation of diagnostic critera and rehabilitation program for rotator cuff injuries. AMF Sports Med 10:336, 1982

11 | Mobilization of the Shoulder

Robert Donatelli

In the past decade, mobilization has been demonstrated clinically to be an important part of rehabilitation and assessment of restricted joint movement. Clinical application is based on an understanding of joint mechanics, connective tissue histology, and muscle function. Mobilization has developed into a clinical science, requiring the therapist to understand anatomical and histological characteristics of synovial joints. Significant advancements have been made in describing the benefits of passive movement. Thanks to the hard work and dedication of such researchers as Akeson, Woo, Amiel, and Peacock,[9,11,14] we have a better understanding of joint stiffness and wound healing. As clinicians, we can take this knowledge and apply our mobilization techniques during critical stages of wound healing to influence the extensibility of scar tissue and reduce the development of restrictive adhesions. We can also use this knowledge to prevent and treat joint stiffness by applying the appropriate stress to the muscles and connective tissue, promoting homeostasis.[1] It is through an understanding of normal tissue function, tissue changes during immobilization, and the structure of scar tissue, that we can establish the criteria for mobilization.

This chapter will discuss mobilization from a basic science approach. The mobilization techniques for the shoulder will be described, with emphasis on the mechanical and neurophysiological effects.

DEFINITION

Several terms must be defined when mobilization is discussed. Articulation, oscillation, distractions, manipulation, and mobilization all describe a specialized type of passive movement.

241

Articulatory techniques are derived from the osteopathic literature. They are defined as passive movement applied in a smooth rhythmic fashion to stretch contracted muscles, ligaments, and capsules gradually.[2] They include gentle techniques designed to stretch the joint in each of the planes of movement normal to it.[2] The force used during articulatory techniques is usually a prolonged stretch into the restriction or tissue limitation.

Oscillatory techniques are best defined by Maitland, who describes oscillations as passive movements to the joint, which can be of a small or large amplitude and applied anywhere in a range of movement, and which can be performed while the joint surfaces are held distracted or compressed.[3] There are four grades of oscillations. Grade 1 is a small amplitude movement performed at the beginning of range. Grade 2 is a large amplitude movement performed within the range but not reaching the limit of the range. Grade 3 is a large amplitude movement up to the limit of range. Grade 4 is a small amplitude movement performed at the limit of range.[3] Grades 1 and 2 are used for the neurophysiological effects, and grades 3 and 4 are designed to initiate mechanical changes in the tissue.

Distraction is defined as "separation of surfaces of a joint by extension without injury or dislocation of the parts."[4] Distractive techniques are designed to separate the joint surfaces attempting to stress the capsule.

Manipulation is defined by *Dorland's Medical Dictionary* as "skillful or dextrous treatment by the hand. In physical therapy, the forceful passive movement of a joint beyond its active limit of motion."[5] Maitland describes two manipulative procedures. Manipulation is a sudden movement or thrust, of small amplitude, performed at a speed which renders the patient powerless to prevent it.[3] Manipulation under anesthesia is a medical procedure used to restore normal joint movement by breaking adhesions.

Mobilization is defined as, "the making of a fixed or ankylosed part movable. Restoration of motion to a joint."[4,5] To the clinician, mobilization is passive movement which is designed to improve soft tissue and joint mobility. It can include oscillations, articulations, distractions, or manipulations.

Mobilization, in this chapter, is defined as a specialized passive movement, attempting to restore the arthrokinematics and osteokinematics of joint movement. It includes articulations, oscillations, distractions, and thrust techniques. The techniques are built on active and passive joint mechanics. They are directed at the periarticular structures that have become restricted secondary to trauma and immobilization. These same techniques can be effective tools in the evaluation of joint movement.

ROLE OF MOBILIZATION

The major goal of the physical therapist is to restore normal function. The normal mechanics of synovial joints include a combination of arthrokinematics (the intimate mechanics of joint surfaces), osteokinematics (the movement of bones), and muscle function.[6]

Gray's Anatomy describes the intimate joint mechanics as roll, spin, and slide (as noted in Chapter 1). These movements occur during active movement between articular surfaces.[6] In addition to the active movements, there are accessory movements, two types of which are described in *Gray's Anatomy*. The first type occurs only when resistance is encountered during active movement; e.g., metacarpophalangeal joint rotation can only occur when a solid object is grasped by the hand.[6] The second type of accessory movement is purely a passive motion produced by an outside force[6]; e.g., if muscles surrounding the shoulder joint are relaxed a distractive force can separate the head of the humerus from the glenoid cavity.

The combination of the active movements of roll, spin, and slide plus the accessory movements constitute joint mobility. For example, as the glenohumeral joint externally rotates in the adducted position, the humerus slides anteriorly, rolls posteriorly, and spins into external rotation. The activity of the rotator cuff muscles are largely responsible for this action. The muscle can not produce the normal active range if joint mobility is limited. The goal of mobilization is to restore joint mobility.

EFFECTS OF PASSIVE MOVEMENT

Normal joint motion includes a dynamic combination of arthrokinematics, sufficient periarticular tissue extensibility, osteokinematics, and normal muscle function. Joint stiffness results from a loss or change in one or all of the components of joint mobility. Passive movement has its most therapeutic effect in the treatment of joint stiffness secondary to immobilization and trauma. Continuous passive movement has been demonstrated to be effective in reducing wound edema and joint effusion, eliminating joint restrictions following trauma.[1] Coutts and associates found that continuous passive movement resulted in increased patient comfort and shorter hospital stays.[1] Passive movement has been shown to provide proprioceptive feedback to the central nervous system (CNS) by maintaining tension in the muscle.[1] It has also been hypothesized that stimulation of the proprioceptors interferes with transmission of pain through the CNS.[1] The nociceptive afferents (pain fibers) have a much higher threshold of excitation than do the mechanoreceptor afferents,[7,8] and there is evidence that the stimulation of peripheral mechanoreceptors blocks the transmission of pain to the brain.[7] Wyke explains this phenomenon as a direct release of inhibitory transmitters within the basal spinal nucleus, inhibiting the onward flow of incoming nociceptive afferent activity.[7] Mobilization is one method of enhancing the frequency of discharge from the mechanoreceptors, thereby diminishing the intensity of many types of pain. If the mechanoreceptor stimulation is of high enough frequency and is maintained long enough, the pain may be abolished.[7]

An important aspect of passive movement is in the prevention and treatment of the complications resulting from immobilization. The lack of stress to connective tissue results in changes in normal joint mobility. The periarticular tissue and muscles surrounding the joint demonstrate significant changes after periods of immobilization. Akeson et al have substantiated a decrease in water and glycosaminoglycans (GAG, the fibrous tissue lubricant), and increase in fatty fibrous infiltrates (which may form adhesions as they mature into scar), an increase in abnormally placed collagen cross-links (which may contribute to the inhibition of collagen fiber gliding), and the loss of fiber orientation within ligaments, which significant reduces their strength.[1,9] Passive movement or stress to the tissues can help to prevent these changes by maintaining tissue homeostasis.[1] The exact mechanisms of prevention are uncertain.

EFFECTS OF PASSIVE MOVEMENT ON SCAR TISSUE: INDICATIONS AND CONTRAINDICATIONS FOR MOBILIZATION

Research indicates that mobilization is most effective in reversing the changes that occur in connective tissue following immobilization.[1] Conversely, mobilization after trauma must be carefully analyzed. When is it safe to apply stress to scar tissue? How much stress should be applied to the scar in order to promote remodeling? In what direction should the stress be applied? These important questions must be answered before we can determine the indications for mobilization of scar tissue.

Research has demonstrated that stress applied early to healing wounds is important in establishing the characteristics of scar tissue. The production of scar tissue begins on the fourth day of wound healing and increases rapidly during the first 3 weeks.[10,11] Peacock has substantiated this peak production of scar by the increased quantities of hydroxyproline.[11] Hydroxyproline is a byproduct of collagen synthesis.[11,12] New collagen is deposited in the scar, at a rate higher than normal connective tissue, for up to 4 months. Research indicates that early stress to scar tissue influences the remodeling process. The collagen fibers are initially deposited within the scar in a random fashion. This random order changes as the tissue begins to remodel. The new collagen fibers align with the preexisting fibers, and the assimilation of the new fibers is part of the remodeling process. Scar tissue begins to resemble the previous normal tissues by the process of maturation.[10,11] Another important aspect of remodeling is the ability of the collagen fibers to glide. If this does not occur, the scar tissue can cause limitations in the mobility of the normal tissue.

The collagen fibril in its early stages is very weak. Intermolecular and intramolecular cross-linking of collagen molecules develop, designed to resist tensile forces.[11,12] The tensile strength of the collagen fibers continues to develop linearly for at least 3 months.[10,11] Arem and Madden demonstrated that after 14 weeks of scar maturation, elongation of the scar was no longer possible.[13] In contrast, the 3-week old scar was significantly lengthened when subjected to tension.[13] It is evident that as scar tissue matures it develops the capability to resist tensile forces. Peacock hypothesizes that the mechanism by which the length of the scar is increased becomes critical for the restoration of the gliding mechanism.[11] Stretching or an increase in length of the scar is a result of straightening or reorientation of the collagen fibers, without a change in their dimensions.[11] For this to occur, the collagen fibers must glide on each other. This gliding mechanism is hampered in unstressed scar tissue by the development of abnormally placed cross-links and a random orientation of the newly synthesized collagen fibrils.[9] Clinically, this can mean limited joint movement.

Joint stiffness results from immobilization and/or trauma. The limitations in movement result from the changes that occur in the periarticular tissues as described above. Mobilization is indicated when the lack of extensibility of the periarticular structures limits the arthrokinematic movement of joint surfaces. This limitation will produce compensations in normal motion and changes in muscle function. The patient experiences pain and limited movement of the involved joint. The therapeutic effects of mobilization on scar and immobilized tissue is important in reestablishing normal active range of motion (ROM). Mobilization of the immobilized tissue stimulates the production of GAGs which is important for lubrication and maintaining a critical distance between collagen fibers to allow for the gliding mechanism to occur.[9,14] It also assures an orderly deposition of nem collagen fibrils, thereby preventing abnormal cross-link formation.[9,14] Enneking and Horowitz[15] and Evans et al[16] document that forceful manipulation breaks intracapsular fibrofatty adhesions that may have formed within the joint during immobilization.

As previously mentioned, early stress to scar tissue determines the tissue flexibility. Arem and Madden advocate stressing the tissue, as early as the third week of scar tissue production.[13] Tissue flexibility is enhanced by passive movement of the young scar, and this is accomplished by promoting alignment of new collagen fibers with preexisting fibers, preventing the development of obstructive adhesions and enhancing fiber glide. The direction, velocity, duration, and magnitude of the stress to scar tissue needs further investigation. The exact effects mobilization has on the remodeling process have not been determined. The forces applied during application of the mobilization techniques are controlled by the pain tolerance of the patient and tissue resistance. The direction of stress applied to connective tissue should be determined in the evaluation by the location of tissue resistance and assessment of joint mobility. Mobilization techniques are built on active and passive joint mechanics.

It is easier to understand the contraindications of mobilization by becoming aware of the common abuses of passive movement. The abuses of passive movement can be broken down into two categories, creation of excessive trauma to the tissues and the causing of "undesired" or abnormal mobility.[1]

Improper techniques, such as extreme force, poor direction of stress, and excessive velocity, may result in serious secondary injury or damage to the tissues surrounding the joint that is mobilized. In addition, mobilization to joints that are moving normally or that are hypermobile can create and/or increase joint instabilities.

Controlled stress to scar tissue can be beneficial to the healing process. Too much stress to the young scar can be harmful. The tensile strength of the scar takes several weeks to develop. If the magnitude of the force is excessive, it can easily disrupt the scar.

Ultimately, selection of a specific technique will determine contraindications. For example, the very gentle grade 1 oscillations, as described by Maitland, rarely have contraindications. These techniques are mainly used to block pain. They are of small amplitude and controlled velocity. In contrast, manipulative techniques have many contraindications. Halderman describes the following conditions as major contraindications for thrust techniques; arthritides, dislocation, hypermobility, trauma of recent occurrence, bone weakness and destructive disease, circulatory disturbances, neurological dysfunction, and infectious disease.[17]

PRINCIPLES OF MOBILIZATION TECHNIQUES

If the goal of the physical therapist is to reestablish normal joint mobility, it is critical for the therapist to understand the normal joint mechanics as described in the section on mechanics of the shoulder girdle (Chapter 1). This section will attempt to emphasize several biomechanical principals that are important to the application of techniques.

When forces are applied to the glenohumeral joint, the major goal is to reproduce the normal forces encountered by the joint structures during movement. The intricate movements of the humerus are critical to normal joint mobility. For example, Poppen and Walker have established that during the first 30° to 60° of shoulder elevation, the head of the humerus moves upward approximately 3 mm. Thereafter, it moves 1 or 2 mm upward and downward between each successive position.[18] The earlier works of Saha demonstrate the movements of roll, spin, and slide of the humeral head during elevation of the shoulder.[19] Poppen and Walker verify the significance of external rotation of the humerus resulting from the above kinematics of the humeral head.[18]

In addition to the movement of the humerus, the glenoid is also moving to ensure proper joint congruity. The scapula must rotate externally (a counter-clockwise rotation with the superior angle of the scapula moving away from the body wall and the inferior angle moving into the body wall) to position the glenoid during shoulder elevation.[18] Mobilization techniques emphasizing the above intimate joint mechanics are used to reestablish the normal movements of the humerus and scapula.

What specific portions of the glenohumeral joint capsule should mobilization techniques stress? Elevation of the shoulder stresses the glenohumeral joint capsule. Different stages of shoulder elevation will stress certain parts of the glenohumeral capsule more than others. For example, as the humerus moves into abduction, the inferior aspect of the capsule begins to unfold. Maximum extensibility of the inferior aspect of the capsule is critical for full abduction to occur.[20] External rotation of the humerus stresses the anterior aspect of the capsule. It has been substantiated through arthrogram studies that loss of external rotation is evident when dye does not fill the anterior recess of the glenohumeral capsule.[20]

In summary, several principles of the normal joint mechanics are important to remember when mobilization techniques are applied. The following pages illustrate the application of mobilization techniques to the shoulder girdle. The techniques attempt to restore the mechanical principles previously discussed. They emphasize general and specific application of stress.

MOBILIZATION TECHNIQUES

The mobilization techniques are designed to restore intimate joint mechanics. Several general principals should be remembered during application of the techniques.

Hand Position

The mobilization hand should be placed as close as possible to the joint surfaces, and the forces applied should be directed at the periarticular tissues. The stabilization hand counteracts the movement of the mobilizing hand by applying an equal but opposite force or by preventing movement at surrounding joints.

Direction of Movement

The direction of forces to the joint should be away from pain and into resistance. The resistance represents the direction of limitation in the joint. Movement into the restriction is an attempt to make mechanical changes within the capsule and its surrounding tissue. The mechanical changes can include breaking up of adhesions, realignment of collagen, or increasing fiber glide. The direction of the movement should not exceed the normal limits of the joint. The therapist must be aware of the joint's movement within the body planes (degrees of freedom) and the contour of the joint surfaces when applying the mobilization techniques. The glenohumeral joint has three degrees of freedom, or it is capable of moving in all three body planes (frontal, sagittal, and transverse).[6] The scapula movements are of a gliding nature around the chest wall. They can be described as elevation, depression, forward and backward movement around the chest wall, and rotation forward or upward, using the inferior angle as the reference point.[6] The movement of the scapula is dependent on the associated movements at the acromioclavicular (AC) and sternoclavicular joints (SC). Movement of the AC and SC is essential for rotation of the scapula on the clavicle during shoulder elevation. In addition to the degrees of freedom, the contour of the joint surface must be considered when the direction for forces is determined. The arthrokinematic movements of roll and slide occur in opposite directions with movement of a convex joint surface. Conversely, the roll and slide occur in the same direction with a concave joint surface movement. A more detailed analysis of shoulder joint movement is reviewed in Chapter 1. To determine the direction of forces, the therapist must understand the specifics of joint movement.

Body Mechanics

It is important for the therapist to maintain good body mechanics during the application of mobilization techniques. The therapist should stand as close as possible to the patient. The therapist's hands and arms should be positioned to act as fulcrums and levers and the therapist's position should allow for the most efficient application of techniques.

Duration and Amplitude

Several studies have been performed to determine the most effective technique for obtaining permanent elongation of collagenous tissue, using different loads and loading time. The studies used rat tendons to demonstrate the elongation of tissue under varied loads. The treatments included low-load and a long duration using 5 g and stretch for 15 minutes. High-load, short duration treatment used 105 to 165 g for 5 minutes.[21,22] The results indicated that low-load, long duration stretch was more effective in obtaining a permanent elongation of the tissue. Several studies also indicated further improvement with the use of heat before or during the stretch and ice immediately afterwards.[23,24]

GLENOHUMERAL JOINT TECHNIQUES

Figure 11-1: Inferior Glide of the Humerus

Patient position: supine with the involved extremity close to the edge of the table. A strap stabilizes the scapula. The extremity is abducted to the desired range.

Therapist position: facing the lateral side of the upper arm. Left hand is into the axilla as close as possible to the joint line. The web space of the right hand is over the superior humeral head as close as possible to the acromion. The left hand maintains the abducted position while applying a distractive force. The right hand pushes the head of the humerus inferiorly attempting to stress the axillary pouch or inferior portion of the glenohumeral capsule. Oscillatory techniques using grades 3 and 4 are effective. For more aggressive stretching

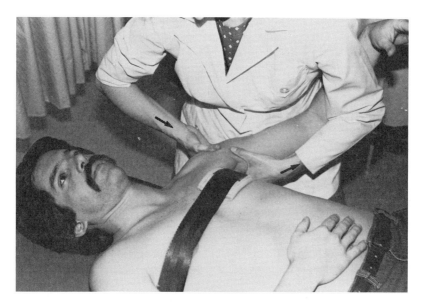

Fig. 11-1.

to the inferior capsule, a prolonged stretch and manipulations are effective with the patient's arm held in 60° of abduction or less.

Figure 11-2: Longitudinal Distraction—Inferior Glide of the Humerus

Patient position: supine with the involved extremity as close as possible to the edge of the table.

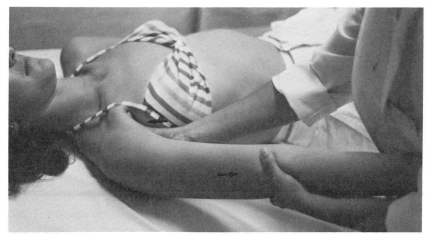

Fig. 11-2.

Therapist position: facing the joint with right hand into the axilla attempting to hold the glenoid. The left hand grips the epicondyles of the humerus, applying a downward traction on the humerus, stressing the inferior capsule. A prolonged stretch is effective with this technique.

Figure 11-3: Caudal Glide of the Humerus

Patient position: supine with the involved extremity flexed to 90° at the shoulder.

Therapist position: as close as possible to the involved extemity with both hands grasping the humerus as close as possible to the head of the humerus. The hands pull the humerus inferiorly, stressing the inferior aspect of the glenohumeral capsule. A prolonged stretch is most effective.

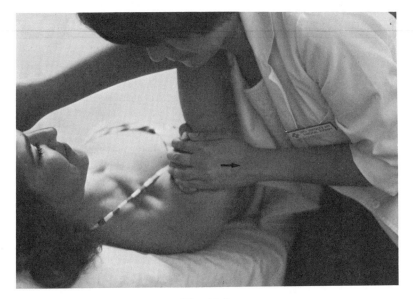

Fig. 11-3.

Figure 11-4: Posterior Glide of the Humerus

Patient position: patient is supine, with the involved extremity as close as possible to the edge of the table. A wedge is placed under the dorsal scapula. The extremity is flexed and horizontally adducted to the desired range. The elbow is flexed.

Therapist position: faces cranially, with right hand maintaining the flexed and adducted position and the left hand over the elbow with the forearm parallel

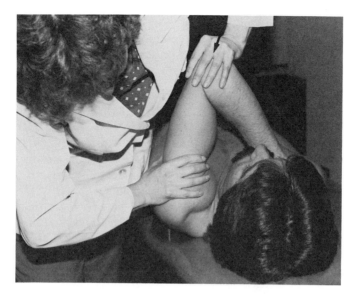

to the patient's forearm. The force is applyed through the elbow, pushing the humerus posteriorly and stressing the posterior aspect of the glenohumeral capsule and the tendinous portion of the subscapularis. A prolonged stress or oscillatory techniques are useful.

Figure 11-5: Lateral Distraction of the Humerus

Patient position: patient as close as possible to the edge of the table, with the involved extremity flexed at the elbow and glenohumeral joint. The extremity rests on the therapist's shoulder. A strap stabilizes the scapula.

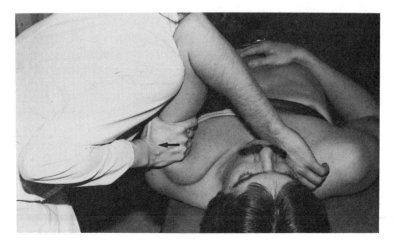

Fig. 11-5.

Therapist position: facing laterally, both hands grasp the humerus as close as possible to the joint. The force is a lateral pull to the humerus stressing the anterior, posterior, superior, and inferior aspect of the capsule. A prolonged stretch is most effective.

Figure 11-6: Anterior Glide of the Humerus

Patient position: prone with the involved extremity as close as possible to the edge of the table. The head of the humerus must be off the table. A wedge is placed just medial to the joint line under the coracoid process. The extremity is abducted in the plane of the scapula.

Therapist position: distal to the abducted part facing cranially. The left hand applies an inferior pull to the humerus. The right hand moves the head of the humerus anteriorly, stressing the anterior recess and capsule. The tendinous portion of the subscapularis is also stressed with this technique. A prolonged stretch with oscillations at the end of the available range is very effective.

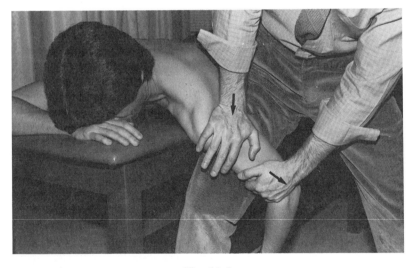

Fig. 11-6.

Figure 11-7: Anterior Glide of the Head of the Humerus

Patient position: supine with the involved extremity as close as possible to the edge of the table. A strap may be used to stabilize the scapula. (See Fig. 11-5.)

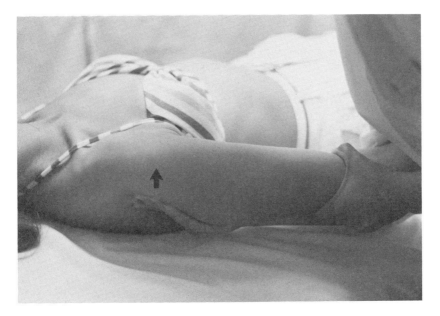

Fig. 11-7.

Therapist position: facing cranially, with the right hand holding the head of the humerus as close as possible to the joint line. The left hand stabilizes the distal humerus, applying a slight distractive force. The force of the right hand moves the head of the humerus in an anterior direction stretching the anterior capsular structures and the tendinous portion of the subscapularis. A prolonged stretch is most effective.

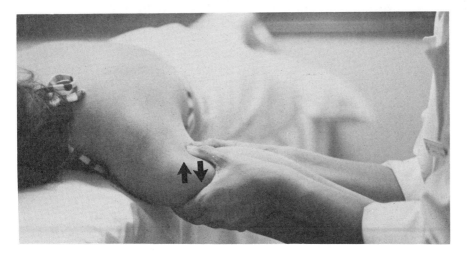

Fig. 11-8.

Figure 11-8: Anterior/Posterior Glide of the Head of the Humerus

Patient position: prone with the involved extremity over the edge of the table abducted to the desired range. A strap may be used to stabilize the scapula.

Therapist position: facing laterally in a sitting position with the forearm of the involved extremity held between the therapist's knees. Both hands grasp the head of the humerus and apply an up-and-down movement, oscillating the head of the humerus. Grades 1 and 2 are mainly used with this technique to stimulate mechanoreceptor activity.

Figure 11-9: Anterior/Posterior Glide of the Head of the Humerus

Patient position: supine with the involved extremity supported by the table. A towel roll or wedge is placed under the elbow to hold the arm in the plane of the scapula (abduction anterior to the frontal plane).

Therapist position: facing laterally in a sitting position. The fingertips hold the head of the humerus while a gentle up-and-down movement is applied. This technique is used with grade 1 and 2 oscillations.

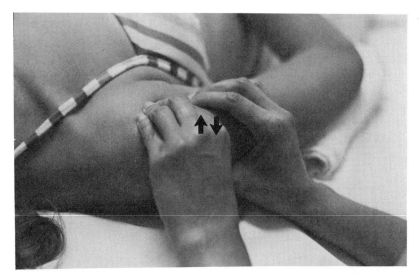

Fig. 11-9.

Figure 11-10: External Rotation of the Humerus

Patient position: supine with the involved extremity supported by the table. The arm is held in the plane of the scapula.

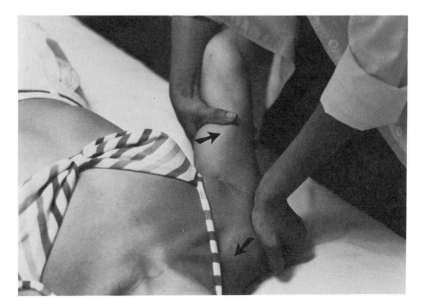

Fig. 11-10.

Therapist position: facing laterally with the right hand grasping the distal humerus; the heel of the left hand is placed over the lateral aspect of the head of the humerus. The force is applied through both hands. The right externally rotates the humerus. The left pushes on the most lateral aspect of the humeral head in a posterior direction, promoting external rotation of the humerus. A long-axis distractive force is applied during this technique. Graded oscillations or a thrust technique can be used.

Figure 11-11: External Rotation/Abduction/Inferior Glide of the Humerus

Patient position: supine with the involved extremity supported by the table. The arm is abducted in the plane of the scapula.

Therapist position: facing laterally with the right hand holding the distal humerus and the heel of the left hand over the head of the humerus. The forces are applied simultaneously. The right hand abducts the arm and externally rotates the humerus while maintaining the plane of the scapula position. The left hand is pushing the head of the humerus into external rotation and an inferior glide. The force applied can be a thrust or a prolonged stretch both occurring at the end of the available range.

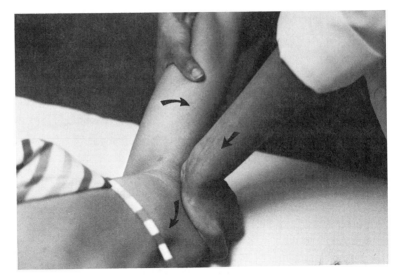

Fig. 11-11.

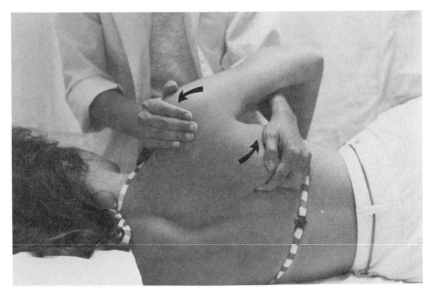

Fig. 11-12.

Scapulo/Thoracic Techniques

A prolonged stretch is used with all the scapulo/thoracic techniques.

Figure 11-12: Scapula External Rotation

Patient position: side lying with the involved extremity accessible to the therapist.

Therapist position: facing the patient, with the left arm under the involved extremity through the axillary area. This allows the left hand to grasp the inferior angle of the scapula. The right hand holds the superior aspect of the scapula. The force is applied simultaneously producing an external rotation of the scapula.

Figure 11-13: Scapula Distraction

Patient position: same as in Fig. 11-12.

Therapist position: facing the patient with the left hand grasping the inferior angle of the scapula, the right hand grasping the vertebral border of the scapula. Both hands pull the scapula up and away from the thoracic wall.

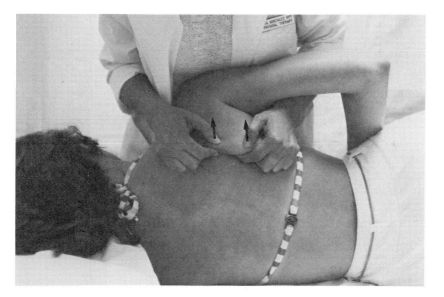

Fig. 11-13.

Figure 11-14: Inferior Glide of the Scapula

Patient positions: same as Fig. 11-12.

Therapist position: facing the patient with the left web space surrounding the inferior angle of the scapula. The right hand holds the superior aspect of

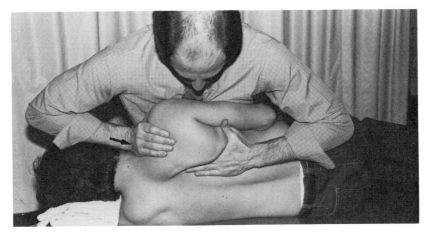

Fig. 11-14.

the scapula with a lumbrical grip. The right hand pushes in a caudal direction while the left hand moves under the inferior angle of the scapula.

Figure 11-15: Scapula Distraction, Prone

Patient position: prone with the involved extremity supported by the table.
Therapist position: facing cranially with the left hand under the head of the humerus and the right web space under the inferior angle of the scapula.

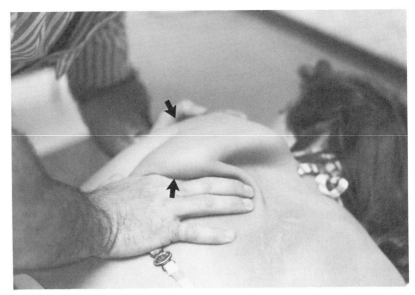

Fig. 11-15.

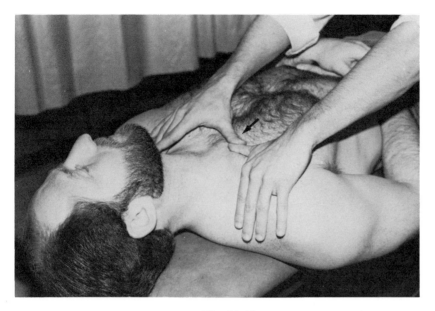

Fig. 11-16.

The forces are applied simultaneously. The left hand lifts the humerus while the right web space moves under the inferior angle of the scapula.

STERNOCLAVICULAR AND ACROMIOCLAVICULAR TECHNIQUES

Figure 11-16: Superior Glide of the SC Joint

Patient position: supine with the involved extremity close to the edge of the table.

Therapist position: facing cranially. The volar surface of the left thumb pad is placed over the inferior surface of the most medial aspect of the clavicle. Right thumb reinforces the dorsal aspect of the left thumb. Both thumbs push the clavicle superiorly. The graded oscillations are most successful with this technique.

Figure 11-17: Anterior Glide of the AC Joint

Patient position: supine at a diagonal to allow the involved acromioclavicular joint to be over the edge of the table.

Therapist position: with the dorsal surface of the thumbs together, the therapist places the distal tips of the thumbs posteriorly to the most lateral

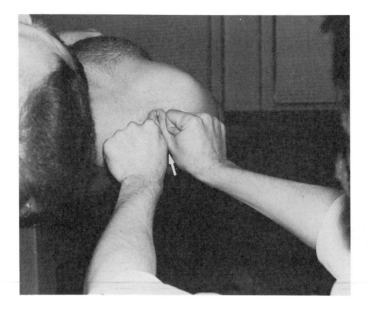

Fig. 11-17.

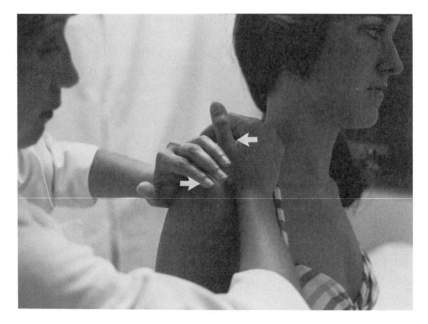

Fig. 11-18.

edge of the clavicle. Both thumbs push the clavicle anterior. The graded oscillations are mainly used with this technique.

Figure 11-18: Gapping of the AC Joint

Patient position: sitting close to the edge of the table.

Therapist position: facing laterally with the heel of the left hand over the spine of the scapula and the thenar eminence of the right hand over the distal clavicle. The force is applied simultaneously. Both hands push the bones in opposite directions, obtaining a general stretch to the capsular structures of the AC joint. Oscillations or a prolonged stretch are used with this technique.

The duration and amplitude of force suggested with each technique is based on my clinical experience.

SUMMARY

This chapter has reviewed several important mechanical, histologic, and neurophysiologic effects of mobilization. The shoulder joint is a complex organ. Mobilization is one aspect of treatment. The application of the mobilization techniques for the shoulder are dependent on the evaluation and assessment of the therapist. The indications and contraindications must be based on an understanding of the histology of immobilized and traumatized connective tissue. Remodeling of scar tissue is far more difficult than reversing the effects of short periods of immobilization. The most recent research indicates that early passive movement is important in the rehabilitation of joint restrictions. However, the velocity, amplitude, duration, and direction of force needed to produce a therapeutic effect requires further investigation. The role of mobilization in the future will be determined by the clinical research performed over the next decade.

ACKNOWLEDGMENTS

I would like to thank William Boissonnault M.S., R.P.T., Steve Janos, R.P.T., Zita Gonzalez R.P.T., and Amy Sowinski for their assistance with the technique pictures, and extend special thanks to Christy Moran for her assistance in editing this chapter.

REFERENCES

1. Franks C, Akeson WH, Woo S, et al: Physiology and therapeutic value of passive joint motion. Clin Orthop 185:113, 1984
2. Stoddard A: Manual of Osteopathic Technique. Hutchinson, London, 1959

3. Maitland GD: Peripheral Manipulation. Butterworths, London, 1970
4. Clayton L (ed): Taber's Cyclopedic Medical Dictionary, FA Davis Co, Philadelphia, 1977
5. Friel J (ed): Dorland's Illustrated Medical Dictionary. 25th Ed. WB Saunders Co, Philadelphia, 1974
6. Warwick R, Williams P (ed): Gray's Anatomy 35th British ED. WB Saunders Co, Philadelphia, 1973
7. Wyke BD: The neurology of joints. Ann R Coll Surg Engl 41:25, 1966
8. Wyke BD: Neurological aspects of pain therapy: a review of some current concepts. p. 1. In Swerdlow M (ed): The Therapy of Pain. MTP Press Ltd. Lancaster, England, 1981
9. Akeson WH, Amiel D, Woo SL-Y: Immobility effects on synovial joints. the pathomechanics of joint contracture. Biorheology 17:95, 1980
10. Kelly M, Madden JW: Hand surgery and wound healing, p. 49. In Wolfort FG (ed): Acute Hand Injuries, a Multispeciality Approach. Little, Brown and Co, Boston, 1980
11. Peacock EE Jr: Wound Repair. 3rd Ed. WB Saunders Co, Philadelphia, 1984
12. Cohen KI, McCoy BJ, Diegelmann RF: An update on wound healing. p. 264. Annals of Plastic Surgery, Vol. 3. No. 3. 1979
13. Arem AJ, Madden JW: Effects of stress on healing wounds: intermittent noncyclical tension. J Surg Res 20:93, 1976
14. Woo S, Matthews JV, Akeson WH, et al: Connective tissue response to immobility: correlative study of biomechanical and biochemical measurements of normal and immobilized rabbit knees. Arthritis Rheum 18:257, 1975
15. Enneking W, Horowitz M: The inter-articular effects of immobilization on the human knee. J Bone Joint Surg 54-A:973, 1972
16. Evans E, Eggers G, Butler J, Blumel J: Immobilization and remobilization of rats' knee joints. J Bone Joint Surg 42-A:737, 1960
17. Haldeman S: Modern Developments in the Principles and Practice of Chiropractic. Appleton-Century-Crofts, E. Norwalk, Conn, 1980
18. Poppen NK, Walker PS: Normal and abnormal motion of the shoulder. J Bone Joint Surg 58A:195, 1976
19. Saha AK: Theory of Shoulder Mechanism: Descriptive and Applied. Charles C Thomas, Springfield, Ill, 1961
20. Kummel BM: Spectrum of lesion of the anterior capsule mechanism of the shoulder. Am J Sports Med 7:111, 1979
21. Light LE, Nuzik S, Personius W, Barstrom A: Low-load prolonged stretch vs. high-load brief stretch in treating knee contractures. Phys Ther 64:330, 1984
22. Warren CG, Lehman JF, Koblanski JN: Elongation of rat tail tendon: effects of load and temperature. Arch Phys Med Rehabil 52:465, 1971
23. Warren CG, Lehman JF, Koblanski JN: Heat and stretch tech-procedure: an evaluation using rat tail tendon. Arch Phys Med Rehabil 57:122, 1976
24. Lehman JF, Masock AJ, Warren CG, Koblanski JN: Effects of therapeutic temperatures on tendon extensibility. Arch Phys Med Rehabil 51:481, 1970

12

Management of Myofascial Dysfunction of the Shoulder

Patricia Scagnelli

Myofascial trigger points are often overlooked as a source of musculo-skeletal dysfunction. Trigger points occur frequently in the shoulder girdle musculature secondary to the many mechanical stresses directed to this region of the body. When a patient's complaint is of pain in the region of the shoulder, with or without restricted motion, the muscles of the shoulder girdle may be the origin of that pain.

Kellgren[1] concluded that pain referred from skeletal muscle usually followed spinal segmental patterns that were not dermatomal, but he noted many exceptions. Travell and Rinzler[2] showed that muscles referred pain extrasegmentally in characteristic patterns specific to each muscle. Travell and Simons[3] have done further work and produced detailed documentation on myofascial pain and dysfunction.

This chapter focuses on trigger points and myofascial pain as a primary source of dysfunction. Clinically, the patient may have several factors causing dysfunction, only one of which is myofascial pain. Each patient should be given a thorough musculoskeletal evaluation, and the appropriate treatments should be rendered.

A generalized discussion of myofascial pain syndrome and its characteristics follows. Treatment is discussed in terms of techniques and modalities which have been most effective. The musculature of the shoulder girdle and their referred pain patterns is then reviewed.

NATURE AND MECHANISM

A myofascial trigger point is a hyperirritable focus within a taut band of skeletal muscle located in the muscular tissue and/or its associated fascia. The point is painful on compression and can evoke characteristic referred pain and autonomic phenomena. The pain referred from the trigger point does not follow a simple segmental pattern, but is characteristic for each specific muscle.[2,3]

The literature on myofascial pain is confusing, and contains a profusion of terms, all attempting to describe muscle pain syndromes. Many of the terms have multiple meanings, depending on the author. The following terms are sometimes synonymous with myofascial pain and trigger points: myalgia,[4,5] myositis,[4,5] fibrositis,[4–6] fibromyositis,[4,5] myofibrositis,[4] fascitis,[4,5] myofascitis,[4,5,7] muscular rheumatism,[4,5] muscular strain,[4] nonarticular rheumatism,[6] myogelosis,[8] interstitial myofibrositis.[9,10]

There is little information on the trigger point's exact histologic makeup and neurophysiologic mechanism. In a review of the literature, the term fibrositis is initially used at the turn of the century to explain tender muscles. Inflammatory changes in the fibrous structures of the muscles, nerves, and fascia were believed to be the cause of the pain.[6] Histologic investigation has failed to confirm this theory. The term fibrositis then became associated with nonspecific muscle pain that lacked abnormal x-ray and laboratory findings,[6] and without implication of pathogenesis.[5]

Other authors continued to attempt to define the mechanism of the trigger point. In 1927, Albee[7] introduced the term myofascitis. He described a toxic condition of the blood caused by the colon with local manifestations in the muscle and fascia. Copeman and Ackerman[11] identified herniations of fatty tissue through their fibrous fascial compartments which caused painful tension. They postulated that the production of pain at the trigger point took place in the fibrofatty tissue and not in the muscle.

Localized muscle spasm[12–14] was believed to be the cause of the palpable band or trigger point until the 1960s. Electromyographic studies performed by Kraft et al[6] in 1968 demonstrated that the area of "muscle spasm" was electrically silent. The concept of "spasm-pain-spasm" and the use of ethyl chloride spray or heat to "relax the spasm" was deemed not credible. Kraft et al[6] proposed that altered kinin production in the skin could explain the palpable changes seen in the fibrositic muscles, the associated dermatographia, as well as the marked response to painful stimuli. Kinins are a group of polypeptides capable of inciting pain, causing vasodilation, and increasing capillary permeability.[6]

The term interstitial myofibrositis[9,10] gained popularity with several authors who believed that the disorder was inflammatory and involved the interstitial connective tissue elements of the muscle. The findings of Ibrahim et al[10] suggested that the pattern of serum and muscle isoenzymes in patients with myofibrositis are similar to those in patients with some connective tissue diseases. Brendstrup et al[15] in 1957 and Awad[9] in 1973 took biopsies of fibrositic nodules and found local edema and interfascicular deposition of acid mucopolysaccharides in connective tissue of the muscle. Brendstrup[15] proposed that the pain from the fibrositic muscles might be secondary to the resultant distention of the connective tissue of the muscle caused by interstitial edema.

A few authors have demonstrated that the histological findings of the muscle fibers are unspecific, but indicate that the muscle fibers are abnormal. Miehlke and Schuke[16–18] and associates found histologic changes, including fatty infiltration, increased number of fibrocytic and sarcolemmal nuclei, and loss of cross-striations of the muscle fibers. Henriksson et al[19] found a moth-eaten appearance of fibers evenly distributed over the whole cross-section and affecting only type I fibers. He also noted mitochondrial abnormalities, and an abnormal relationship that existed between the mitochondria and the myofibrils. Energy metabolites and glycogen were also decreased significantly in these patients. Henriksson et al[19] postulated a primary metabolic disturbance or an overload myopathy secondary to a more or less continuous increase in muscle tension. A recent study by Hagberg and Kvarnström[20] demonstrated that the electromyographic endurance time was short for muscles affected with myofascial syndrome, but normal in relation to electromyographic fatigue changes. Hagberg and Kvarnström[20] believed that the increased localized muscle fatigue possibly was caused by the decrease in mitochondria reported by Henriksson et al.[19]

Simons and Stolov[21] believed that the band-like induration could be caused by circumscribed transient muscle contraction rather than histologically demonstrable structural changes. Travell and Simons[3] have further developed this theory, proposing that the palpable band can probably be explained as a physiological contracture of muscle fibers (a contraction without action potentials[3]). A contracture of muscle fibers in the band would make it feel hard and tense as compared with the surrounding fibers in the muscle. They propose that the initial activation of the trigger point starts with trauma which damages the sarcoplasmic reticulum. The sarcomeres are exposed to calcium which initiates contractile activity. The sarcomeres that are exposed to calcium for an extended period would then maintain contractile activity as long as their ATP energy supply lasted. A sustained contractile force creates tension, and the contraction of these fibers results in a palpable band. The contractile force stops if the muscle is stretched and the sarcomere is elongated enough to separate the myosin heads from the reactive portion of the actin filaments.

Hyperirritability of the trigger point may be explained by the sensitization of the muscle afferent nerve endings.[3,9] Awad[9] found nerve-sensitizing substances released from platelets (serotonin) and degranulating cells (histamine) in the area of the trigger point. The kinins reported by Kraft et al[6] could also act as sensitizing agents.[3]

It is apparent that many discrepancies exist regarding the nature of trigger points. Some authors reported normal histological findings whereas others reported unspecific abnormal findings in the muscle fibers. Travell and Simons[3] postulated that this could be a result of an acute versus chronic or dystrophic phase in the trigger point. In the acute phase, there would be no demonstrable histological findings whereas, in the dystrophic phase, abnormal histological findings would be present in the muscle fibers.

Melzack et al[22] believe that trigger points and acupuncture points represent the same phenomena. Pressure at certain points is associated with particular pain patterns, and brief intense stimulation of these points sometimes produces prolonged relief of pain.[22] In a study correlating spatial distribution and associated pain patterns, Melzack et al[22] found 71 percent correspondence between trigger points and acupuncture points. The referred pain from both the trigger point and the acupuncture point can be explained as the result of mechanisms understood in terms of the "Gate Control Theory" described by Melzack et al.[22] Further discussion of this topic is beyond the scope of this chapter, but may be found in Melzack's work.[22]

CLINICAL CHARACTERISTICS

There are different classifications of trigger points. An active trigger point causes pain and decreased extensibility of a muscle. A latent trigger point is clinically silent with respect to pain, but may cause decreased extensibility and weakness of that muscle. The patient may not be aware of the latent trigger point until the clinician compresses it and the patient experiences the local and/or referred pain. Satellite trigger points may form in the referred pain region whereas secondary trigger points may form in adjacent muscles owing to increased stresses placed upon them from the primary muscle's hypersensitivity, shortened position, and weakness.[3]

Trigger points can be activated directly or indirectly. Direct activation occurs by acute overload, sustained muscle contraction, direct trauma, and chilling.[3] Indirect activation can result from other trigger points, visceral disease, arthritic joints, and emotional distress.[3]

Any sex or age group can develop trigger points, but the sedentary middle-aged woman is the most vulnerable.[3,6] The likelihood of developing active trigger points increases with age through the middle active years.[3] In the later years when there is less strenuous activity, the trigger points may become latent and be exhibited primarily as stiffness and restricted motion.[3]

The patient's complaints are usually of stiffness at rest and a deep aching pain if allowed to stay in a prolonged position. Some relief is felt after the patient first changes position or moves. The patient usually reports that a moderate amount of activity causes increased aching as well as fatigue. Cold, damp weather as well as emotional stress or tension aggravate the symptoms. Complaints of weakness and stiffness in the involved muscle are common. Muscular strength can become unreliable and the patient with shoulder girdle trigger points may report unexpected dropping of objects.

Symptoms and complaints relate to the most active trigger point. When treatment has begun and this trigger point has been eliminated, the pain pattern may shift to that of an earlier or less active trigger point.[3] This explains why many patients may report pain/symptoms shifting in location or from one side to the other.

The more hypersensitive the trigger point, the more intense and constant the referred pain and the more extensive its distribution.[1,3] The size of the muscle is not important.[1,3]

Phenomena other than pain are often caused by the trigger points.[3] Many autonomic symptoms such as localized vasoconstriction, sweating, lacrimation, coryza, salivation, and pilomotor activity can occur in the referred pain region. Proprioceptive disturbances such as imbalance, dizziness, and tinnitus also occur.

Travell and Simons[3] formulated a list of the general clinical characteristics of trigger points:

1. When an active trigger point is present, passive or active stretching of the affected muscle increases the pain.

2. The stretch range of motion of the particular muscle is restricted.

3. The pain is increased when the affected muscle is strongly contracted against resistance.

4. The maximum contractile force of the affected muscle is weakened and is not associated with atrophy or pain unless the patient uses significant effort.

5. Deep tenderness and dysesthesia is referred by active trigger points to the referred pain region.

6. Autonomic disturbances sometimes occur in the referred pain region.

7. Muscles in the vicinity of the trigger point feel tense to palpation.

8. The trigger point is found in a palpable band as a sharply circumscribed spot of exquisite tenderness.

9. Digital pressure applied to an active trigger point causes the patient to jump and cry out.

10. Snapping palpation of the trigger point frequently evokes a local twitch response.

11. Moderately sustained pressure on an irritable trigger point causes or intensifies pain in the referred pain pattern of that trigger point.

12. The skin of some patients displays dermatographia (whealing) and panniculosis ("orange-peel" effect).

PERPETUATING FACTORS

Management of the many perpetuating factors of myofascial pain syndrome is necessary for the patient to get optimum relief. The shoulder girdle is especially vulnerable because its anatomic relationships make it susceptible to fatigue. There are three kinds of mechanical stresses which can perpetuate a trigger point within the shoulder girdle[3]: postural stresses, constriction of muscles, and structural inadequacies.

The postural stresses refer to poor body mechanics, immobility, and poor posture. In the shoulder girdle, poor posture has been clinically referred to as the forward head posture. The ways in which this altered head, neck, and shoulder girdle relationship can cause or perpetuate dysfunction are described in Chapter 4.

Prolonged pressure on a muscle or constriction of a portion of a muscle can occur often in the shoulder girdle. Tight upper body clothing such as a tight bra strap can create enough constriction to perpetuate dysfunction. The strap of a heavy purse hung on the shoulder may also cause constriction.[3]

Structural inadequacies refer to body asymmetries.[3] The asymmetry must be compensated for, resulting in altered movement patterns. The change in normal function results in continual stress to the musculoskeletal system, and this abnormal stress can perpetuate trigger points.

PHYSICAL THERAPY TREATMENT

The treatments discussed here pertain only to trigger points. The clinician should be aware that often myofascial pain is only a part of the patient's dysfunction and other treatments are warranted as well.

Around a trigger point, the subcutaneous tissues are thickened and congested.[3] The skin becomes adherent to the underlying superficial fascia and loses its movement and elasticity. This is called panniculosis. The skin and superficial fascia should be checked for mobility in all directions. If an area of restriction is found, stroking techniques into the area of restriction should be used on the skin and superficial fascia.

Skin Rolling

Skin rolling is a technique frequently used when panniculosis is evident.[23] The skin and superficial fascia are picked up between the thumb and fingers, and is rolled backward over the advancing thumbs which keep up the pressure behind the roll all the time. No lubricant is used, and when the area of the trigger point is reached, there is an "orange-peel" effect as well as an increase in pain.

Pressure

Sustained pressure or ischemic compression over a trigger point appears to block noxious impulses from the muscles and produces relief of pain as well as relaxation.[3,23] The relaxed muscle is stretched to the verge of discomfort and a thumb or strong finger is pressed directly on the trigger point to create a painful sustained pressure. The pressure should be tolerable. This pressure is gradually increased and continued for ~1 minute.[3,23]

Massage

Massage techniques are used often in the treatment of myofascial pain. Massage has a mechanical effect of helping return venous blood, lymph, and catabolites into the mainstream of the circulation.[23] It aids the absorption of substances within the tissues.[3] Perhaps it produces an effect by washing out the sensitizing substances that are reported in the literature to accumulate around trigger points.[3] Williams and Elkins[24] advocate a firm, heavy friction type of massage rather than a kneading or stroking type in the treatment of their patients. Friction massage, which rubs the most superficial tissues over underlying structures, is often used to the tolerance of the patient. Travell and Simons[3] feel that a vigorous massage of hyperirritable trigger points can cause an adverse reaction with a marked increase in pain. Zohn and Mennell[23] advocate a firm kneading (length or across) or stretching massage.

In general, many clinicians find success by starting the treatment with the superficial fascial techniques and then progressing to light stroking techniques, adding more pressure gradually. The friction massage and deep, firm techniques are much more tolerable to the patient if the tissues are gradually prepared. In acute stages, firm massage cannot be used in many cases.

Stretching

Stretching techniques are the hallmark of the treatment program in a patient with myofascial pain dysfunction. The reasoning behind this lies in the theory mentioned earlier about the sarcomere's exposure to calcium, which produces a contractile force. The contractile force stops if the muscle is stretched and the sarcomere is elongated enough to separate the myosin heads from the reactive portion of the actin filaments. To inactivate the trigger point fully, the muscle must be extended to its full normal length.[3] The stretching should be on the verge of causing pain but should evoke only local discomfort and not referred pain.[3] Optimal tension is about two-thirds of the muscle's normal stretch range of motion (ROM).[3]

Stretching in itself may cause pain and a reflex spasm to develop in a muscle with a very irritable trigger point. When this occurs, a vapocoolant spray can be used. Flouri-methane* spray is the vapocoolant frequently used. In the spray and stretch method, the jet stream of the vapocoolant is applied once to cover the length of the muscle before the stretch is applied. The muscle is slowly stretched with a steady increase in force, as described previously, and the spray is directed in parallel lines from the trigger point over the muscle and through the area of referred pain. After a full stretch is completed, the return must be smooth and gradual.

The vapocoolant acts as a counterirritant.[12] Intense stimulation on the skin by the cold is transmitted by larger afferents faster than the noxious pain impulses from the muscle,[23] creating a refractory period during which reception of the noxious impulses is blocked. During this period, the muscle can be relaxed and stretched to a normal resting length.[12,23] When the normal resting length is obtained, the normal tonic reflexes are restored and the muscle is capable of normal, pain-free function.[23] There is also some degree of direct

---

* Gebauer Chemical Co, Cleveland, OH 44104.

depression of cutaneous receptors by cooling.[12] The vapocoolant spray also has effects similar to those of a light stroking massage.[12]

Recently activated, acute, single muscle trigger point syndromes may respond to passive stretch and hot packs without vapocooling whereas more chronic cases require both stretch and spray.[3] If the condition becomes chronic, the vapocoolant's effect may be significantly diminished.[12] As pain decreases, stiffness with a decrease in ROM is the chief complaint. The muscles during this stage are less responsive to stretch and spray.[3]

The Lewit and Simons[3,25] technique places the muscle to be stretched on a manually resisted isometric contraction followed by relaxation. The clinician passively stretches the involved muscle to a point just short of pain or onset of resistance to further movement. The patient exerts a prolonged, gentle isometric contraction against minimal resistance for ~10 seconds and then relaxes. When there is full relaxation, the clinician instructs the patient to take a deep breath and exhale completely. During exhalation, the muscle is stretched further, but only as far as muscle relaxation allows (slight resistance from the new position). The procedure is repeated. A set of three to five repetitions usually provides as much progress as could be obtained in one session.[25] If increased stretch ROM is not obtained after isometric contraction, the contraction time is increased to 30 seconds.[25] The technique itself can be taught to the patient and can be used as a home stretching exercise.

The Lewit technique is successful because the stretch equalizes the lengths of the sarcomeres throughout each involved muscle fiber and thereby normalizes the function of the contractile elements of the muscle.[25] Therefore, the most important factor in success of this technique is precision in aligning the stretch to the involved muscle fibers.

Zohn and Mennell[23] advocate that ice massage be used if vapocoolant is not available. The ice cube is held by the edge of a small towel which is also used to wipe up the water from the melted ice, keeping the skin dry. The ice is applied out from the trigger point and over its referred pain pattern in parallel lines. Once the skin gets cold and red in a histamine-like response, the patient becomes conscious of a tender mass over the site of maximum pain.[23] When this sensation disappears, the pain is usually relieved and the treated part is cold and numb. Stretching is then begun.

Ultrasound

Ultrasound has been used with some success as an adjunct to the therapy. One technique starts with a setting of 0.5 W/cm^2 with a circular motion that completes one circle in 2 or 3 seconds.[23] The circle is tight enough to overlap the trigger point. Many other clinicians use ultrasound at a setting of 1.0 to 2.0 W/cm^2 in a circular motion as described above.

The literature on the effects of ultrasound on muscle reports an alteration of cell permeability, producing changes in isometric tension, decreased membrane potentials, and retardation of the deterioration of specific muscle proteins.[26,27] Because the nature of trigger points remains in dispute, it is difficult to draw conclusions as to specific benefits of ultrasound. If the trigger point does indeed have a dystrophic phase as suggested previously by Travell and Simons[3], ultrasound effects would appear to be beneficial in reversing or retarding the process. The mechanical action of the sound waves may help to prevent or reverse symptoms arising from adhesions within the interstitial tissue.[23] A recent study by Klemp[28] reported that ultrasound decreased the muscle blood flow in muscles with trigger points. It was generally believed that treatment of trigger points with ultrasound increased the muscle blood flow.

Ultrasound in combination with electrical stimulation has also demonstrated some therapeutic results.[3,23,29] The mechanical pumping by the electrical stimulation probably dissipates the products of increased metabolism or edema away from the muscle being treated and restores its physiological state to near normal.[23]

Heat

Heat in the form of hot packs is effective as an adjunct to therapy. Dry heat is not as effective as wet heat. Application of a hot pack after stretching helps reduce posttreatment muscle soreness.[3] The wet heat promotes further reduction of muscle tension.[3]

SUMMARY

Trigger points occur frequently in the shoulder girdle musculature due to the many mechanical stresses directed to this region of the body. A trigger point is a hyperirritable focus within a taut band of skeletal muscle located in the muscular tissue and/or its associated fascia. The trigger point is painful on compression and can evoke characteristic referred pain specific to each muscle as well as autonomic phenomena.

More research is needed to determine the nature and mechanism of the trigger point. Some authors report normal histologic findings, whereas others report unspecific abnormal findings of the muscle fibers. This may be a result of an acute versus chronic phase in the trigger point. A recent explanation for the taut band or trigger point is that it is a physiological contracture of muscle fibers.

Because of the uncertain nature and mechanism of the trigger point, speculation exists as to why some treatments are beneficial in the treatment of myofascial pain dysfunction. The most important aspect of treatment centers around proper stretching of the involved muscle. Stretching may elongate the sarcomere enough to separate the myosin heads from the reactive portion of the actin filaments and interrupt the physiological contracture. Vapocoolant spray and icing coupled with stretching give additional benefits. Massage, ultrasound, and heat have also been beneficial.

SHOULDER-GIRDLE MUSCLES

An overview of some of the shoulder girdle musculature that refers pain to the region of the shoulder will follow. A brief discussion on referred pain, common patient complaints, findings on evaluation, trigger point locations, and stretch techniques for each particular muscle will be provided. I refer the reader to the bibliography for more detailed information on each particular muscle.

Subscapularis

The subscapularis muscle refers pain mainly to the posterior aspect of the shoulder and posterior arm down to the elbow.[2,3] There is also a strap-like area of referred pain and tenderness around the wrist with the dorsum of the wrist usually more painful and tender than the volar.[2,3]

The patient usually presents with restriction of movement in shoulder abduction and external rotation. Resisted shoulder adduction and internal rotation may be weak and painful. Pain is present at rest and with motion.

Many times the patient has been diagnosed as having adhesive capsulitis or frozen shoulder when Travell and Simons[3] believe that the trigger points in the subscapularis may be the original culprit. They feel that the subscapularis trigger points may sensitize the other shoulder girdle musculature into developing secondary and satellite trigger points. This could lead to a full-blown restriction in glenohumeral motion.

Trigger points are in the scapular fossa along the axillary border of the scapula[2,3] and occasionally more medially toward the superior angle of the scapula.[3]

For stretch position, see Figure 12-1.

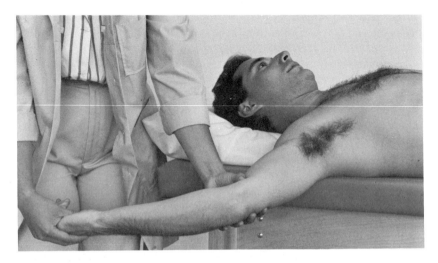

Fig. 12-1.   Stretch for subscapularis.

Supraspinatus

The supraspinatus muscle's referred pain causes a deep ache around the shoulder,[30] especially in the middle deltoid region. It extends down the arm and forearm, sometimes focusing at the lateral epicondyle of the elbow.[2,3]

The patient's chief complaint is pain, especially during abduction of the shoulder, and a dull ache at rest. Snapping and clicking sounds occur around the shoulder due to the tautness of the supraspinatus fibers interfering with the normal glide of the humeral head.[3] Resisted abduction and sometimes resisted external rotation of the shoulder are weak and painful. The patient may be unable to abduct the arm fully.

Two trigger points lie in the supraspinatus fossa of the scapula.[2,3]

For stretch position, see Figure 12-2.

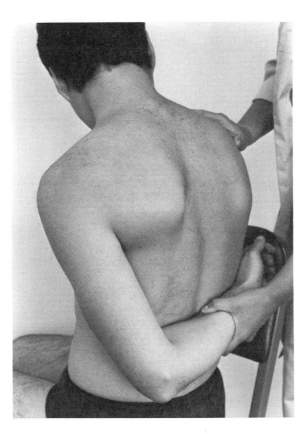

Fig. 12-2. Stretch for supraspinatus.

Infraspinatus

The infraspinatus muscle refers pain to the anterior shoulder/deltoid region,[1-3,13,14,31,32] down the anterolateral aspect of the arm to the lateral fore-

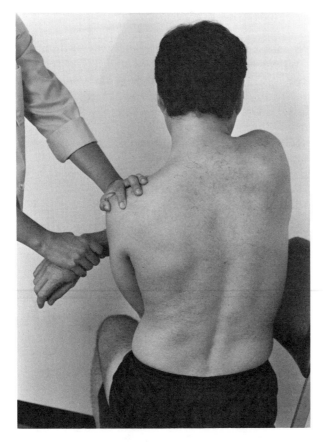

Fig. 12-3. Stretch for infraspinatus.

arm,[1–3,13,14,31] the radial aspect of the hand,[1–3,13,31,32] and occasionally the fingers.[2,3,13]

The patient may complain of shoulder girdle fatigue, weakness of grip, and loss of mobility at the shoulder.[31] A restriction in simultaneous internal rotation and adduction of the shoulder is often present.[3] Difficulty in lying on the same side or supine at night can occur due to the compression and stimulation of the trigger point by the weight of the thorax.[3] Resisted external rotation and adduction may be painful and weak while passive abduction and internal rotation may be painful and restricted.

There are three trigger points, all located in the infraspinatus fossa of the scapula.[2,3]

For stretch position, see Figure 12-3.

Teres Minor

The teres minor muscle refers pain in the posterior deltoid muscle region.[3]

The patient's complaint is more of pain than of restricted motion. Resisted external rotation of the shoulder may be painful and weak. Resisted adduction of the shoulder is occasionally painful.

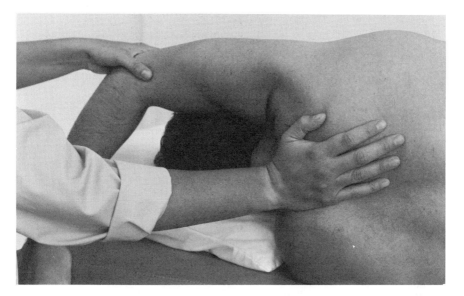

Fig. 12-4. Stretch for teres minor.

The trigger point is found on the lateral edge of the scapula between the infraspinatus above and the teres minor below.[3]

For stretch position, see Figure 12-4.

Teres Major

The teres major muscle refers pain to the posterior deltoid region and over the long head of the triceps brachii.[3,30] It may refer pain into the shoulder joint

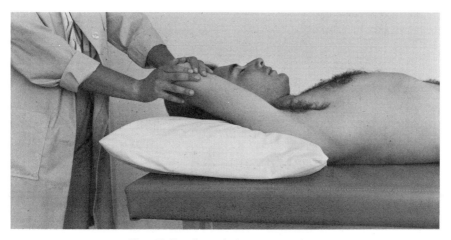

Fig. 12-5. Stretch for teres major.

posteriorly and occasionally to the dorsal forearm, but rarely to the scapula or elbow.[3]

The patient complains of pain on motion or reaching overhead. Rest pain is mild.[3] Resisted internal rotation, resisted extension, and resisted adduction of the shoulder all may be painful and weak. Passive abduction and external rotation of the shoulder may be restricted.

The trigger points are located medially overlying the posterior surface of the scapula and laterally in the posterior axillary fold.[3]

For stretch position, see Figure 12-5.

Deltoid

The deltoid has no distal projection of referred pain. The anterior deltoid refers pain to the anterior middle deltoid region.[2,3,23] The posterior deltoid refers pain to the middle and posterior deltoid region.[2,3,23]

The patient will report experiencing pain deep in the deltoid region with motion of the shoulder, especially with abduction and extension movements of the shoulder combined. Resisted abduction and flexion of the shoulder are painful and weak, with involvement of the anterior deltoid; resisted abduction and extension are painful and weak, with involvement of the posterior deltoid.

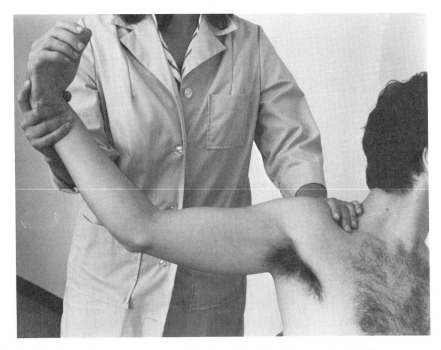

Fig. 12-6.   Stretch for anterior deltoid and coracobrachialis.

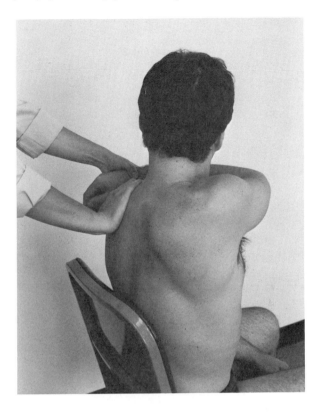

Fig. 12-7. Stretch for posterior deltoid.

Trigger points are located in the anterior portion of the shoulder for the anterior deltoid[3] and more distally along the posterior margin of the muscle for the posterior deltoid.[3]

For stretch position, see Figures 12-6 and 12-7.

Latissimus Dorsi

The latissimus dorsi muscle refers pain to the inferior angle of the scapula and midthoracic region.[1,3] It may also extend to the back of the shoulder, down the medial aspect of the arm, forearm and hand, including the ring and little fingers.[3]

The patient will complain that reaching forward and upward with the arm causes pain. Resisted shoulder internal rotation and extension are painful and sometimes weak. Passive shoulder flexion with external rotation may be painful and restricted.

The trigger points are located in the axillary portion of the muscles.[3]

For stretch position, see Figure 12-8.

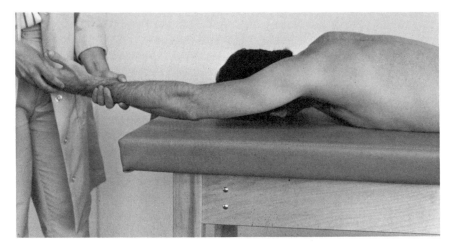

Fig. 12-8.   Stretch for latissimus dorsi.

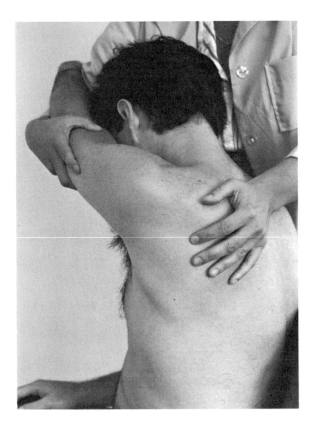

Fig. 12-9.   Stretch for levator scapula.

Levator Scapula

The levator scapula muscle refers pain to the neck and back of the head,[2,3,31] the vertebral border of the scapula[2,3] and the posterior shoulder.[2,3,31]

The patient will report stiffness at the base of the neck.[3,31] There will be some restriction in cervical rotation to the same side as the involved muscle. There may also be an elevated scapula or shoulder shrug on the involved side.

Trigger points are located at the angle of the neck[3] and at the superior angle of the scapula.[2,3]

For stretch position, see Figure 12-9.

Rhomboid Major and Minor

The rhomboid major and minor muscles refer pain to the vertebral border of the scapula[3] and may spread up over the supraspinatus portion of the scapula.[1,3]

Snapping and crunching noises during movement of the scapula may be due to trigger points in the rhomboid muscles.[3] Motion of the glenohumeral joint does not aggravate the symptoms.

Trigger points are located along the scapular vertebral border.[3,32]

For stretch position, see Figure 12-10.

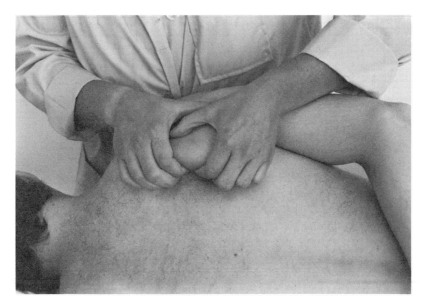

Fig. 12-10. Stretch for rhomboid major and minor.

Pectoralis Major

The pectoralis major muscle refers pain substernally,[3] to the anterior chest and breast,[2,3] the anterior shoulder,[2,3] and the ulnar aspect of the arm to the fourth and fifth fingers.[2,3]

Generally, a patient will complain of pain in the anterior shoulder and subclavicular region.[3] Breast pain and diffuse soreness may also be a complaint.[3] Symptoms similar to cardiac pain may also be present.[3]

Examination of the patient reveals a protracted shoulder on the involved side. Resisted horizontal adduction and internal rotation of the shoulder may be painful and weak. Passive stretch of the shoulder into horizontal abduction with external rotation is restricted and painful.

Trigger points are found throughout all portions of the muscle.[3]

For stretch position, see Figure 12-11.

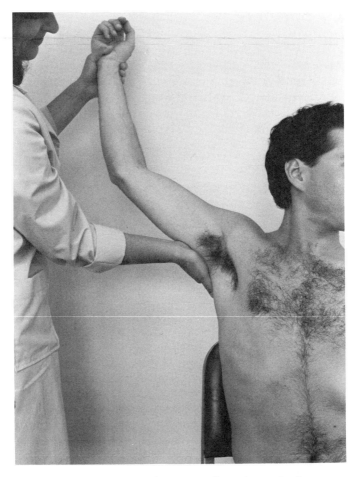

Fig. 12-11.   Stretch for pectoralis major and minor.

Pectoralis Minor

The pectoralis minor muscle refers pain primarily to the anterior shoulder[2,3] but also to the anterior chest[2,3] and sometimes down the ulnar side of the arm, forearm, and last three fingers.[2,3] Its pattern of referral is similar to that of the pectoralis major muscle.

The patient's complaints of pain are similar to the pain experienced from a pectoralis major trigger point, cardiac pain included. The shortened pectoralis minor may entrap the brachial plexus and cause a distribution of symptoms similar to thoracic outlet syndrome.

Examination of the patient usually reveals an increase in protraction of the shoulder girdle complex on the involved side. Passive movement of the shoulder into horizontal abduction and external rotation will be restricted and painful and may cause neurovascular symptoms into the upper extremity. Scapulothoracic mobility may also be restricted.

Trigger points are located near the muscle's attachment to the coracoid process and in the belly of the muscle.[3]

For stretch position, see Figure 12-11.

Coracobrachialis

The coracobrachialis muscle refers pain to the anterior deltoid region, the posterior aspect of the arm over the triceps, the dorsum of the forearm, and down to the dorsum of the hand.[3] The pain skips the elbow and wrist.

The patient complains of upper extremity pain, especially in the anterior shoulder and posterior arm. Reaching behind the body across the low back is painful and limited.[3] Reaching up in abduction and flexion at the shoulder may be painful.[3] Resistive shoulder flexion can be painful and weak, whereas passive extension of the shoulder may be painful and restricted.

The trigger point is located in the superior part of the muscle near its attachment to the coracoid process.[3]

For stretch position, see Figure 12-6.

Biceps Brachii

The biceps brachii muscle refers pain up over the muscle belly and into the anterior deltoid region of the shoulder.[3] The patient may also experience milder pain downward in the antecubetal space[3] and volar forearm and hand.[33]

The chief complaint is that of superficial anterior shoulder pain.[3] Weakness and pain may be present when the patient attempts to raise the hand above the head. Resisted elbow flexion with the wrist supinated will be painful and weak. Combined passive elbow and shoulder extension may be painful and restricted.

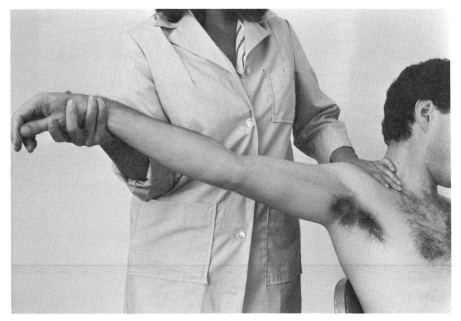

Fig. 12-12.   Stretch for biceps brachii.

The trigger points are located in the distal one third of the muscle.[3]
For stretch position, see Figure 12-12.

Triceps Brachii

The triceps brachii muscle has several variations of its referred pain pattern due to its three heads and subsequent trigger points. Areas of referred pain are as follows:[3] upward over the posterior arm to the back of the shoulder; the base of the neck in the upper trapezius region and sometimes down the dorsal forearm, skipping the elbow; the lateral epicondyle; the medial epicondyle; and the fourth and fifth digits.

With all of the possibilities of referred pain, the patient's complaint will be that of a hard-to-localize pain in the posterior shoulder region.[3] Extension of the elbow may be painful. Passive elbow flexion may be painful. Resisted elbow extension may be painful and weak.

Trigger points are located in each of the three heads and the referred pain pattern depends upon the location.[3]

For stretch position, see Figure 12-13.

ACKNOWLEDGMENTS

I would like to thank Joyce Klien, RN, CANP, for her assistance with the photography.

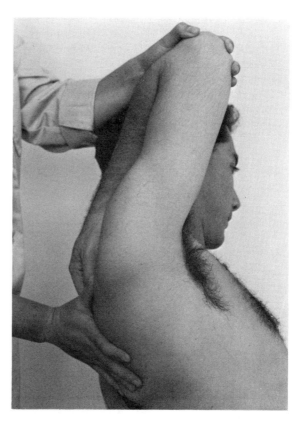

Fig. 12-13. Stretch for triceps brachii.

REFERENCES

1. Kellgren JH: Observations on referred pain arising from muscle. Clin Sci 3:175, 1938
2. Travell J, Rinzler SH: The myofascial genesis of pain. Postgrad Med 11:425, 1952
3. Travell J, Simons DG: Myofascial Pain and Dysfunction, The Trigger Point Manual. Williams & Wilkins, Baltimore, 1983
4. Berges PU: Myofascial pain syndromes. Postgrad Med 53:161, 1973
5. Bennett RM: Fibrositis: Misnomer for a common rheumatic disorder. West J Med 134:405, 1981
6. Kraft GH, Johnson EW, LeBan MM: The fibrositis syndrome. Arch Phys Med Rehabil 49:155, 1968
7. Albee FH: Myofascitis. A possible explanation of many apparently dissimilar conditions. Am J Surg 3:523, 1927
8. Jordan HH: Myogelosis: The significance of pathologic conditions of the musculature in disorders of posture and locomotion. Arch Phys Ther 36, 1942
9. Awad EA: Interstitial myofibrositis: hypothesis of the mechanism. Arch Phys Med Rehabil 54:449, 1973
10. Ibraham GA, Awad EA, Koltke FJ: Interstitial myofibrositis: serum and muscle enzymes and lactate dehydrogenase-isoenzymes. Arch Phys Med Rehabil 55:23, 1974

11. Copeman WSC, Ackerman WL: Edema or herniations of fat lobules as a cause of lumbar and gluteal "fibrositis". Arch Int Med 79:22, 1947
12. Travell J: Ethyl chloride spray for painful muscle spasm. Arch Phys Med 33:291, 1952
13. Long C: Myofascial pain syndromes: part II—syndromes of the head, neck, and shoulder-girdle. Henry Ford Hosp Med Bull 4:22, 1956
14. Travell J, Rinzler S, Herman M: Pain and disability of the shoulder and arm: treatment by intramuscular infiltration with procaine hydrochloride. JAMA 120:417, 1942
15. Brendstrup P, Jesperson K, Asboe-Hansen G: Morphological and chemical connective tissue changes in fibrositic muscles. Ann Rheum Dis 16:428, 1957
16. Miehlke K, Schuke G, Eger W: Clinical and experimental studies on the fibrositis syndrome. Rheumaforsch 19:310, 1960 (Ger)
17. Miehlke K, Schuke G: So-called muscular rheumatism. Internist 2:447, 1961 (Ger)
18. Schoen R, Miehlke K: Fibrositis or so-called muscle rheumatism. Med Klin 57:708, 1962 (Ger)
19. Henriksson KG, Bengtsson A, Larsson J, et al: Muscle biopsy findings of possible diagnostic importance in primary fibromyalgia (fibrositis, myofascial syndrome). Lancet 1395, Dec 1982
20. Hagberg M, Kvarnström S: Muscular endurance and electromyographic fatigue in myofascial shoulder pain. Arch Phys Med Rehabil 65:522, 1984
21. Simons DG, Stolov WC: Microscopic features and transient constriction of palpable bands in canine muscle. Am J Phys Med 55:65, 1966
22. Melzack R, Stillwell DM, Fox EJ: Trigger points and acupuncture points for pain: correlations and implications. Pain 3:3, 1977
23. Zohn DA, Mennell JM: Musculoskeletal Pain: Diagnosis and Physical Treatment. Little, Brown and Co, Boston, 1976
24. Williams HL, Elkins ED: Myalgia of the head. Arch Phys Ther 23:14, 1942
25. Lewit K, Simons DG: Myofascial pain: relief by postisometric relaxation. Arch Phys Med Rehabil 65:452, 1984
26. Gersten JW: Nonthermal neuromuscular effects of ultrasound. Am J Phys Med 37:235, 1958
27. Fischer E, White EA, Hendricks SL, et al: Effect of moderate and weak ultrasound exposures upon normal and denervated mammalian muscle. Am J Phys Med 37:284, 1958
28. Klemp P, Staberg B, Korsgrd J, et al: Reduced blood flow in fibromyotic muscles during ultrasound therapy. Scand J Rehab Med 15:21, 1982
29. Bonica JJ: Management of myofascial pain syndromes in general practice. JAMA 164:732, 1957
30. Kelly M: New light on the painful shoulder. Med J Aust 1:488, 1942
31. Sola AE, Williams RL: Myofascial pain syndromes. Neurol 6:91, 1956
32. Pace JB: Commonly overlooked pain syndromes responsive to simple therapy. Postgrad Med 58:107, 1975
33. Steinbrocker O, Isenberg SA, Silver M, et al: Observations on pain produced by injection of hypertonic saline into muscles and other supportive tissues. J Clin Invest 32:1045, 1953

13 | Medical Management of Myofascial Pain Dysfunction

Sanford E. Gruskin

Myofascial pain, as most pain dysfunction syndromes, has received myriad classifications. When connected with the head, neck, and shoulder girdle, it is most commonly referred to as tension, psychogenic, or nervous headache. Recently, these headaches have been classified under the heading of muscle contraction headaches and included with those of vascular origin.[1–6] Though Shaber refers to these as acute and chronic, he asks whether the disease process is genetic (intrinsic), acquired (extrinsic), or both.[7] Rather than further confuse the picture by interjecting new classifications, two states affecting myofascial pain are defined which directly relate to the mode of medical management of this malady. It will be unnecessary to go through a muscle-by-muscle diagnostic examination or to define the general characteristics of myofascial pain, as this has been covered elsewhere. The physical therapy aspects will also be referred to only in the most general terms since this too has been thoroughly covered.

The purpose of this chapter is to classify only where it has bearing on the specific medical management of these patients. In this regard, reference is made to only two general classes, those of extrinsic and intrinsic etiology. Extrinsic etiology implies that the specific traumatic force is extrinsic to the patient, namely an outside force directly traumatizing specific muscles. A psychogenic or tension-related muscle contraction is considered to be of intrinsic etiology. These terms are not to be confused with those of Shaber[7] [genetic (intrinsic); acquired (extrinsic)] but are related to the mitigating circumstances that precipitate the myofascial pain episode involving the neck and shoulder girdle. A diagnostic protocol will be developed whereby patients can be classified as primarily those with extrinsic or intrinsic etiologic factors that precipitate pain dysfunction. Once the patient is properly classified, proper medical management can easily be determined.

Extrinsic patients are those who have an active external force that directly precipitates their pain dysfunction. Among this group is the athlete who is constantly irritating the neck or shoulder girdle during physical workouts, the laborer who carries heavy loads and strains or injures specific muscle groups, and the secretary who cradles a phone on the shoulder, directly traumatizing the muscles. It may seem that these patients would be relatively easy to diagnose. As compared with those of intrinsic etiology they are, if not easier to diagnose, considerably easier from a management standpoint. These patients readily identify the active trigger point and admit to the episodes that precipitate pain. This group consists predominantly of males (in a ratio of 2 to 1). As obvious as the findings seem, it is still important to proceed with a thorough history and data base examination and to analyze the material in a logical, sequential manner to allow detection of a more serious problem which can otherwise be overlooked.

The second classification for myofascial pain is intrinsic, distinct from the previously mentioned extrinsic myofascial pain in that "intrinsic" is related to direct muscle contraction from tension. These patients are far more difficult to manage, as there is a tendency to treat the pain as a symptom and not as a total disease state. The intrinsic patients are usually middle-aged and may be defensive in nature. Headache is often the focus of pain that brings them in for examination.

It is important to question these patients thoroughly relative to their social and psychological profile. A specific data base is used for the history and examination, with questions designed to cover all aspects of social, occupational and physical history as well as guide the practitioner through a complete examination. Use of a specific data base serves several functions. Patients do not feel that they are being singled out for the psychological profile. The data base allows easy access into the psychological aspects of the disease and gives patients the impression that they are not alone with their problem. This group consists predominantly of women (in a ratio of 3 to 1) in their middle years. Usually, they have seen a multitude of practitioners, generally leaving with no specific diagnosis and the impression that the doctor thinks their pain is functional. To a practitioner taking a history, it is apparent that many of these patients have a round shouldered posture with a forward head position. They often actively contract their musculature during the history, most notably the masseter muscles in clenching their teeth.

On direct questioning, patients often deny having a psychological or tension problem. However, when specifically asked about their sleeping habits they admit to having difficulty maintaining sleep and awaken after only a short period, remaining restless throughout the night. Previous authors have discussed in detail the emotional state of these patients and agree that they exhibit a tense personality, having difficulty coping with daily activities and handling stress.[2,6,8,9] They may be emotionally unstable with a dependence on others.

Table 13-1. Profile of Patients Experiencing Pain Dysfunction from an Extrinsic versus an Intrinsic Factor

	Extrinsic	Intrinsic
Identifiable etiologic factor	Yes	No
Sex predilection	2:1 M	3:1 F
Age (yr)	20–39	30–59
Visible muscle contractions	No	Yes
Distribution	Unilateral	Bilateral
Sleep disorder	Falling asleep	Maintaining sleep
Associated headaches	No	Yes
Previous treatment	No	Yes
Emotional instability	No	Yes

The patients often use the myofascial pain to their benefit, allowing them to cope with the stresses and escape the responsibilities which they are unable to handle. The relationship between chronic pain and depression has been approached by several authors.[1,9,10] France et al discuss the possibility of two relationships existing between chronic pain and depression. They believe that one group of patients reacts to the chronic pain disorder by becoming depressed, whereas a second group develops chronic pain as a symptom of the depression.[9] The relationship may be somewhat more complicated than either author suggests. Other authors have found that the chronic intrinsic patient can be effectively managed with smaller doses of antidepressants than can the classic depressed patient.[1] As a first step in the medical management of myofascial pain, our patients were sent for an MMPI profile. However, this immediately built a barrier between patients and doctors because patients felt that we were implying that their problem was functional and not organic. The use of the MMPI has since been abandoned in favor of a psychological profile developed through careful questioning of the patient over several visits. Observance of posture and movements of a significant number of patients during the history taking has shown that they will elicit trigger point tenderness involving the upper trapezius muscle. A patient's confidence can be enhanced by predicting these trigger points at the initial examination. Before the specific trigger point is palpated, the patient is told that this will elicit referred pain to the area of their initial concern. In medical management of pain, it is important to gain the patient's confidence and trust. Patients who are antagonistic, challenging all aspects of the treatment, will remain an enigma. In summary, profiles have been developed of patients who experience pain dysfunction from an extrinsic versus an intrinsic factor (Table 13-1). The extrinsic patients are usually somewhat younger in age, predominantly male, and can usually point to a specific occurrence that causes their pain dysfunction. Their pain tends to be unilateral in distribution. They rarely admit to associated headaches. The psychological profile does not contribute anything of significance. In contrast, the intrinsic patients are somewhat older and are predominantly women. They usually cannot identify any specific factor that causes their dysfunction. The pain assumes a bilateral distribution with sides not necessarily equal in intensity. These patients usually have associated headaches. Thorough questioning may elicit significant emotional instability. They may admit to difficulty maintaining sleep. This, they may feel, causes not only the muscle pain, but precipitates many of the family emotional disorders. They may admit to a lack of ability to perform various obligations due to their pain dysfunction.

THE EXTRINSIC PATIENT

Patients with myofascial pain dysfunction of extrinsic etiology, if treated properly, will experience results that are complete and rapid. These patients should be approached with the full scope of treatment at onset to alleviate their pain dysfunction and return them to muscular harmony. After patients are classified into the extrinsic grouping, the mechanism of their pain is discussed. They are then placed on one of the nonsteroidal anti-inflammatory agents. These drugs provide significant analgesic as well as appropriate anti-inflammatory action. Patients must be placed on a sufficient dose of this medication. Our preferences are ibuprofen (Motrin) at a dose of 600 mg, four times a day; diflunisal (Dolobid) at a dose of 500 mg twice a day; or naproxen (Naprosyn) at a dose of 500 mg twice a day. These are highly effective medications and the choice depends on convenience of administration and previous drug therapy. A patient may have previously been given one of these drugs, but on an as-needed basis, which does not provide a sufficient constant blood level to obtain the appropriate anti-inflammatory effects. In such cases, that drug is avoided and another is used in its place. Patients then do not feel that they are being treated as they have previously been treated. The new medication, if it does not have any pharmacological advantages, at least possesses certain psychological advantages. The nonsteroidal anti-inflammatory agents are contraindicated in patients with a sensitivity to salicylates. These agents cause gastric irritation and are not to be used in patients with peptic ulcers or a history of gastrointestinal bleeding. They are also to be avoided in patients with impaired renal function. Platelet function is altered with these drugs, and anticoagulant therapy should be adjusted accordingly. The most common side effect from these agents is gastric irritation and nausea, which can be diminished to a large extent if patients take them with meals. If this is ineffective, switching from one nonsteroidal anti-inflammatory agent to another often alleviates the problem. Less frequent side effects include dizziness, headaches, nervousness, tinnitis, depression, insomnia, urticaria, neutropenia, agranulocytosis, aplastic anemia, thrombocytopenia, and acute renal failure. Aspirin should not be used in conjunction with the nonsteroidal anti-inflammatory agents as it has a tendency to increase the incidence of gastrointestinal problems and to diminish the anti-inflammatory activity.[11,12]

For those patients who have difficulty getting to sleep due to their extrinsic pain dysfunction, one of the benzodiazepines is prescribed. In this class, the choices are triazolam (Halcion) in a dose of 0.5 mg or tempazepam (Restoril) in a dose of 15 mg, 30 minutes prior to bedtime. These specific benzodiazepines are selected because of their short half-life ($+\frac{1}{2}$). Restoril has a $+\frac{1}{2}$ of 9 to 12 hours and Halcion has a $+\frac{1}{2}$ of 3 to 5 hours. These drugs allow the patients to reach a restful level of sleep rapidly, preventing further traumatization of the musculature and allowing them to awaken without the hangover of many hypnotic agents. These medications are prescribed for a short period of time for those patients whose pain dysfunction limits their sleeping. As are other benzodiazepines, they should be avoided in patients who are pregnant. In addition to the obvious effects of drowsiness, dizziness, and lethargy, these drugs produce nausea in a small percentage of patients. They can also contribute to mental confusion and memory impairment. A limited number of patients will complain of constipation, diarrhea, xerostomia, and altered taste. These drugs are not addictive; however, the patients may have some minor withdrawal symptoms and difficulty sleeping after prolonged use followed by discontinuation of the drug.[11,12] Following appropriate medication with the nonsteroidal anti-inflammatory drugs and the benzodiazepines, patients are instructed to undergo physical therapy. They are seen ~2 weeks later. If a patient's symptoms have improved, the benzodiazepines can be discontinued and the dosage of the nonsteroidal anti-inflammatory agent can be decreased. A patient who has shown no improvement during the 2-week period is maintained at the same level of medication and is scheduled for appropriate trigger point injections.

THE INTRINSIC PATIENT

Patients with intrinsic myofascial pain dysfunction cannot be approached as having a symptom-based problem. They have had their symptoms over a period of years and at times have used the dysfunction to manipulate those around them and, at best, have integrated the pain into their life style. To approach this as a symptom-oriented disease state will lead to failure. The patients cannot expect, nor can the practitioners anticipate, a rapid improvement of their symptomatology. It must be realized that certain patients cannot be managed. However, with a systematic, logical approach, many patients will return to normal function. Within this group, however, some patients will need the adjunctive care of a psychotherapist. At times, it is apparent that the patients are asking for psychological supportive care, although it is a rare patient that feels comfortable enough to voice problems. More often, after a number of visits as patients develop more trust in the pain management, they can appropriately be led into psychotherapy.

These patients, having seen multiple practitioners prior to their visit, will list a number of drugs they have previously and are presently taking. It is often difficult to convince the patients that they are on the appropriate drugs, but that they need more than the agents alone. They need a combination of medication, aggressive physical therapy, and the understanding of those who treat them.

As with the extrinsic patients, the pain and inflammatory aspects of the myofascial dysfunction of these patients are treated with nonsteroidal anti-inflammatory agents in the same dosage previously described. It is necessary to explain to these patients in considerable detail, the mechanism of action of these agents and the need to take them as directed without expecting immediate relief. Throughout the regimen, these patients should be constantly reminded to expect very gradual improvement in their symptoms.

The intrinsic patients with long-term tension-based pain dysfunction are approached as depressive patients. They frequently change their personalities to suit the circumstance. These people do not necessarily have difficulty getting to sleep but have difficulty in maintaining their level of sleep. The first line of medication is one of the benzodiazepines; however, rather than Restoril or Halcion an agent with a longer $+\frac{1}{2}$ that is more of a sedative, anti-depressant than a hypnotic is prescribed. Alprazolam (Xanax) 0.5 mg three times a day is used initially, with the dosage adjusted as needed. If patients become drowsy and have difficulty functioning, the dosage is decreased to 0.25 mg in the morning, at noon, in early evening, and 0.5 mg at bedtime. Those with mild anxiety and depression problems seem to respond very well to the use of Xanax. The contraindications and side effects from Xanax are similiar to those previously described with the other benzodiazepines. After the above medications are prescribed, an aggressive physical therapy program is maintained. Patients are seen for follow-up evaluation in ~2 weeks. After the 2-week interval, the patients are rarely symptom-free. If they report that they are symptom-free and able to function fully in their environment, it is doubtful they were placed in the appropriate category. Those that seem to be functioning better and have some diminution of their pain will be maintained on the same regimen and continue with the physical therapy.

Approximately 50 percent of these patients will have trigger point areas that are resistant to the usual physical therapy modalities and will require trigger point injections. The muscles that generally require trigger point injections are the upper trapezius, suboccipital, levator scapuli, and sternocleidomastoid muscles. Those patients who seem to make little or no progress with the Xanax and trigger-point therapy are withdrawn from Xanax and placed on cyclobenzaprine hydrochloride (Flexeril) at a dose of 10 mg three times a day. They are maintained on their nonsteroidal anti-inflammatory agents. Flexeril, like Xanax, is a benzodiazepine; however, it is closely related to the tricyclic antidepressants both from a structural and pharmacologic standpoint. Like the tricyclic drugs, many of the side effects include anticholinergic manifestations, namely drowsiness, xerostomia, tachycardia, and blurred vision. This drug should be avoided in patients with cardiac arrhythmias or heart block.[11,12] Patients should be maintained on Flexeril for 4 to 5 weeks. If there is no improvement with the combination of the nonsteroidal anti-inflammatory agents, Flexeril, physical therapy, appropriate trigger-point injections, as well as psychotherapy, tricyclic anti-depressants are considered.

Although many authors[1,2,6,9,13] discuss the use of the tricyclic antidepressant agents at an earlier stage of treatment, they should not be prescribed until the other chemotherapeutics have been tried and the patients have received a psychiatric consultation. The tricyclics used are imipramine, a dibenzazepine derivative, and amitriptyline, a dibenzocycloheptadiene derivative. These drugs have a high incidence of side effects most notably involving the anti-muscarinic effects of the drugs. There is also the risk of cerebral toxicity. As noted with Flexeril, these medications may cause cardiac toxicity which can result in hypotensive episodes and arrhythmias; they should be used with care in patients with cardiac disease. The tricyclics interact with numerous other medications; therefore, appropriate caution must be exercised. Side effects may include xerostomia, metallic taste, constipation, epigastric pain, dizziness, tachycardia, palpatation, blurred vision, and urinary retention.[11] The dosage should be 100 to 200 mg per day. Several authors refer to their use in a somewhat less than antidepressive dosage.[1,2,9] It is best to prescribe larger doses for short periods of time (3 to 5 weeks) and then decrease the dosage accordingly.

In a new approach recently tried with younger patients in good health who seem to have anxiety episodes related to the home or work environment, patients are placed on an exercise program involving daily runs, bicycling, or aerobic classes, starting at 20 minutes per day and working up to 1 hour per day, 6 days per week. The patients are placed on a diet consisting of 80 percent carbohydrates, 10 percent protein and 10 percent fat, which is supplemented with tryptophan twice a day, which promotes the release of beta-endorphin and helps nullify pain. The tryptophan also allows them increased relaxation and sleep. At this juncture, we are not certain that the exercise program itself is not causing a sufficient distraction for those patients in that their stress and tension are directed toward athletic endeavors and away from the muscle contraction associated with myofascial pain dysfunction.

TRIGGER POINT INJECTIONS

Credit must be given to Travell when we discuss trigger points and their treatment. She was years ahead of the rest of the profession in recognizing the role and treatment of trigger points.[6] Trigger point injection is now a recognized approach to myofascial pain dysfunction.[3,6,14] There is little question of the need for trigger point injections. The discussion centers on the subtleties of the technique and the agents used for the injection.

Agents or techniques advocated consist of dry needling, gammaglobulin, and sarapin, as well as the local anesthetics bupivacaine hydrochloride (Marcaine), procaine hydrochloride (Novacaine), lidocaine hydrochloride (Xylocaine), and mepivacain hydrochloride (Carbocaine).[3,6,14] Some authors advocate the addition of cortical steroids to the local anesthesia, whereas others use only isotonic saline solution.[6] Local anesthesia provides several immediate benefits. It provides a less painful injection procedure and allows for pain-free stretching of the patient by the physical therapist immediately after the injection. Furthermore, the patient's confidence is gained because of the immediate reversal of the positive trigger point findings. The stretching no longer produces pain, the range of motion is increased, palpation is pain-free, there is a decrease in the tenseness of the musculature, and muscle strength is increased.[6] Vasopressor agents are contraindicated not only because of the increased hazard of accidental intravenous injection and myotoxicity but also because the local anesthesic together with the vasopressor may increase muscle necrosis, compounding the problem.[6,15] Three percent Carbocaine supplied in 1.8-ml carpules is an effective and convenient agent for trigger point injections. The Carbocaine is prepackaged in carpules; the sterility chain is maintained because multiple entries into a vial are not necessary. Carbocaine is available without the addition of a vasopressor agent and conveniently fits in the syringes used in most dental and many medical facilities. A 27-gauge stainless steel needle (1½ in in length) is used. This length is sufficient to reach the designated trigger point and allows the tactile sense to determine when the trigger point is penetrated.

The injection procedure is considered a sterile procedure. The patient removes all binding clothes from the area of the injection and sterile drapes are provided. The operator wears sterile gloves and all materials are autoclaved or otherwise sterilized prior to use. The skin is prepared with a betadine solution covering the area of penetration and a sufficient adjacent area so that the operator on palpating the trigger point will not cross-contaminate the site of injection. The area of the trigger point is palpated and is identified by the operator both by feeling the tautness of the region and by precipitating the referred pain. The skin overlying this area is stretched by the practitioner who places the index finger and middle finger on either side of the skin overlying the trigger point, spreading these fingers to stretch the skin; with a sharp motion, the needle is inserted. A small amount of local anesthetic is injected as the trigger point is approached. Aspiration is always accomplished prior to any injections. As the operator contacts the trigger point, resistance can be felt and the local anesthesic is injected into the region. The injection technique requires a keen tactile sense to determine the exact moment at which the trigger point is penetrated. With an increasing number of injections, this becomes easier. Following the initial injection, the needle is withdrawn slightly and multiple injections are made in a circumferential pattern around the trigger point. The needle is then withdrawn, the area is gently massaged, and the additional trigger points are approached in a similiar manner.

The most common trigger point injections of the neck and shoulder are the upper trapezius, suboccipital, levator scapuli, and sternocleidomastoid muscles. The upper trapezius muscle is approached with the patient in a sitting position with the head tilted toward the affected side. The trigger point is identified on bimanual palpation; the overlying skin is stretched with the middle and index fingers with penetration between these fingers.

The suboccipital muscles, consisting of the recti capitis posteriores major and minor and the obliqui inferior and superior, are approached with the patient lying face down with the head extended over the edge of the table. These injections often involve the hairline, which during the period of preparation is thoroughly soaked in the betadine solution. The trigger points are identified on palpation, and the needle is inserted in a superior direction toward the base of the skull. Aspiration is accomplished before any anesthesic is administered because of the proximity of the vertebral artery.

The levator scapulae is approached from behind with the patient lying with the affected side upward. The trigger point is identified on manual palpation, and the index and middle finger are spread to stretch the skin as the needle is inserted. The needle should not penetrate deeply to assure that the thoracic cavity will not be entered.

The sternocleidomastoid muscle is approached with the patient in a sitting position with the operator above and behind the patient. The head is flexed toward the affected side and the operator grabs the muscle between the thumb and index finger, identifying the trigger points. Extreme care is necessary with this injection owing to the vital structures adjacent to muscle. The external jugular vein courses along the outer aspects of the sternocleidomastoid muscle. Aspiration during the injection is mandatory. Following the trigger point injections, the patients are immediately sent for physical therapy. They undergo active stretching after the trigger point injections, followed by moist heat application. After discharge from the physical therapist, the patients are instructed to maintain moist heat on the area for several hours.

CONCLUSIONS

It is imperative that a logical, sequential procedure be followed in medical management of myofascial pain dysfunction to the neck and shoulder. It cannot be overemphasized that these patients must be properly classified and then treated in a progressive manner. A haphazard approach to medical management of these patients will be frustrating at best. At times, these patients have seemed to be an integrated part of the practice; however, when their treatment can be brought a successful conclusion, it is most gratifying.

REFERENCES

1. Peter K: Headache–Diagnosis and effective management, West J Med 140:157, 1984
2. Martin M: Muscle-contraction (tension) headache. Psychosomatics 24:319, 1983
3. Rubin D: Myofascial trigger point syndromes: an approach to management. Arch Phys Med Rehabil 62:107, 1981
4. Nuechterlein K, Holroyd J: Biofeedback in the treatment of tension headache. Arch Gen Psychol 37:866, 1980
5. Ahles T, King A, Martin J: EMG biofeedback during dynamic movement as a treatment for tension headache. Headache 24:41, 1984
6. Travell J, Simons D: Myofascial Pain and Dysfunction. The Trigger Point Manual. Williams & Wilkins, Baltimore, 1983
7. Shaber P: Skeletal muscle: anatomy, physiology, and pathophysiology. Dental Clin North Am 27:435, 1983
8. Bell N, Abramowitz S, Folkins C, et al: Biofeedback, brief psychotherapy and tension headache. Headache 23:162, 1983
9. France R, Houpt J, Ellinwood E: Therapeutic effects of antidepressants in chronic pain. Gen Hosp Psychiatry 6:55, 1984

10. Carron H: Control of pain in the head and neck. Otolaryngol Clin North Am 14:631, 1981
11. Gilman A, Goodman L, Gilman A: The Pharmacological Basis of Therapeutics. 6th Ed. Macmillan, New York, 1983
12. Angel J: Physicians' Desk Reference. 38th Ed. Medical Economics, Oradell, New Jersey, 1984
13. Lance J: Headache. Ann Neurol 10:1, 1981
14. Rask M: The omohyoideus myofascial pain syndrome: report of four patients. J Craniomandibular Pract 2:256, 1984
15. Benoit P: Reversible skeletal muscle damage after administration of local anesthetics with and without epinephrine. J Oral Surg 36:198, 1978

14 | Total Shoulder Replacement

Larry F. Andrews
Carol Ann Gunnels

Although several prosthetic replacements for the upper part of the humerus, were introduced in the 1950s, reports of artificial shoulder joints appeared as early as 1894. When Pean reported the first artificial shoulder joint, it consisted of a constrained prosthesis whose humeral component was composed of an iridescent platinum. The humeral head was made of a hard rubber ball, crossed by two deep grooves placed at right angles to each other. Each groove contained two separate loops of metal, one joining the rubber ball to the platinum stem and the other holding the glenoid by screws. This was the first reported constrained or fixed fulcrum prosthesis; it lasted ~2 years.

Most of our present-day prostheses are really an extension of work previously done in the area of the hip. Prosthetic development in the shoulder occurred because less radical procedures such as resectional arthroplasties and arthrodesis had failed to produce satisfactory results. Although worthwhile, standard operations such as humeral head resection, reattachment of rotator cuffs to the proximal humerus, glenohumeral arthrodesis, and autogenous fibular graft replacements to the upper humerus had serious drawbacks. Humeral head resection and arthrodesis greatly limited glenohumeral motion and may not have totally eliminated shoulder discomfort. Similarly, autogenous fibular grafts decreased shoulder motion and were also subject to fracture. Therefore, to provide more motion and greater relief of pain, surgeons began to perform other arthroplastic procedures.

Hemi-replacements affecting the humeral head resulted in satisfactory outcomes for patients with uninvolved glenoids and shoulder muscles of good to normal strength. Materials such as acrylic and cobalt chrome were used to replace the proximal humerus. Some even combined fenestrations (as did the Austin-Moore prosthesis for the hip) within the prosthesis to allow for attachment of tendons and muscles surrounding the shoulder.

The problem, however, was often not confined to the humeral head alone. As the disease process advanced, it became necessary for replacement considerations of the glenoid as well as the humerus. Glenoid liners of metal or plastic were used initially. These early designs depended on strong shoulder muscles, especially the deltoid and rotator cuff.

Because of inadequate musculature surrounding the glenohumeral joint, surgeons turned toward fixed fulcrums. It was thought that these constrained prostheses could be used for irrevocably damaged glenohumeral joints with the added loss of stabilization resulting from a weakened rotator cuff. In a constrained prosthetic design, the main considerations were durability of parts and attachment of the prosthesis to the scapula (glenoid) without subsequent loosening.

To enhance the longevity of the fulcrum (or articulation process) in the constrained prosthesis, designs included two balls in opposition as in universal joints or reversed configurations using thin-walled, large cups with interarticulating large spheres extending from metal glenoids. To provide better deltoid leverage of the humerus, larger spheres were used in the fulcrum. It was thought that the larger radius enhanced not only strength but degrees of motion (Fig. 4-1).

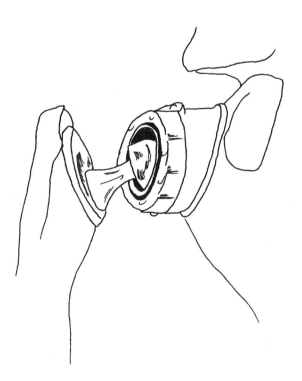

Fig. 14-1. The constrained prosthesis was designed to eliminate the need for rotator cuff muscles.

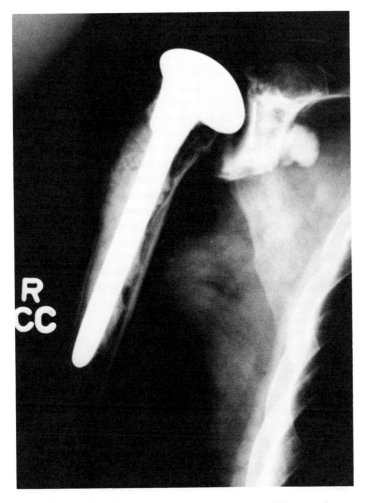

Fig. 14-2. The unconstrained prosthesis consists of a metal humeral component and a plastic glenoid as demonstrated by the metal clip.

Post felt that success with constrained prostheses depended more on protection of the scapular vault (bony configuration behind the glenoid) than on any ingenious design. Anything that destroys the thin cortical vault of the glenoid, its subcondylar plate, or cancellous bone mass increases the chances of loosening. Other complications have included dislocations and glenoid and prosthetic neck fractures.[1]

Neer found the active motion following the constrained prosthetic procedures disappointing. The fixed fulcrums failed to provide the power necessary for external rotation so essential for good function. He also felt that these prostheses invited mechanical failure.[2]

Cofield agreed and studied the unconstrained designs of Neer. Unconstrained implies that only the cartilage will be replaced. All other structures will be repaired. The major argument for an unconstrained over a constrained total shoulder replacement as presented by Cofield is that the failure rate of the unconstrained implants is less than that of the constrained. If the additional constraint can be offered by repair rather than arthroplasty, long-term results would be much more consistent and complications fewer.[3]

The early designs of prostheses were offered to treat simultaneous loss of articular cartilage and instability engendered by rotator cuff disease. However, as it became apparent that rotator cuff disease was not always present in these conditions, the trend toward the unconstrained prosthesis evolved. Together with this evolution, there was a trend toward better repair of surrounding soft tissues such as the rotator cuff. Partial anterior acromioectomies were performed to prevent impingement of soft tissue and overlying bone. Often, with rotator cuff injuries, all that was necessary was suture of torn edges to cancellous bone of the upper humerus; at times, transposition of subscapularis was used as an adjacent cuff closure. Thus, a larger percentage of rotator cuff tears were treated without resorting to unduly complex or uncertain surgical techniques.

The unconstrained replacement is not effective if there is a deficient deltoid muscle, and if there is poor closure of the rotator cuff in the face of a non-functioning cuff mechanism (Fig. 14-2).[4]

DIAGNOSTIC CATEGORIES REQUIRING TOTAL SHOULDER REPLACEMENT

Regardless of the diagnosis necessitating total shoulder replacement (TSR), one common feature was prevalent: cartilaginous erosion. Studies by Poppen and Walker offered one explanation for this destructive process. The excursion of the humeral head on its glenoid surface in the superior inferior plane was <1.5 mm in normal subjects. This occurred during each 30° of motion with a normal compressive force on the glenoid. The study demonstrated how increased excursion along varying centers of rotation resulted if the shear force directed upward or downward was excessive. This increase in excursion occurred when there was a muscle imbalance secondary to pain or a tear or functional loss of the rotator cuff. As the deltoid muscle pulled upward (shear) without the compressive counter-force provided by the rotator cuff, destruction of the cartilage resulted.[5] Each of the following diagnostic categories provides variations from the normal biomechanical function of the shoulder that lead to cartilaginous erosion and thus the need for TSR.

Osteoarthritis

"The lesion of primary glenohumeral osteoarthritis is remarkably constant and consistent." The areas of wear and sclerosis develop at the maximum point of joint reaction force: 90° of abduction.

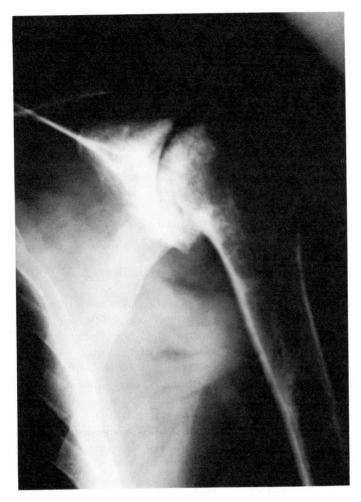

Fig. 14-3.   Shoulder x-ray depicting osteoarthritis.

The head becomes surrounded by marginal osteophytes which are more prominent inferiorly and posteriorly. In advanced cases, the glenoid becomes flattened and eroded posteriorly, as also occurs in the arthritis of recurrent dislocation and in the rheumatoid patient. The sloping glenoid may result in a posterior subluxation of the humeral head which in extreme cases resembles an old posterior dislocation.[2]

The forces necessary to generate this type of wear require the rotator cuff to be intact as was found to be the case in shoulders of patients who were treated surgically (Fig. 14-3).

Chronic Dislocation

A second classification of TSR candidates included those with histories of chronic dislocation. Years of recurrent dislocations and, in many cases, previous surgeries caused tightening of the joint capsule and produced a fixed subluxation in the opposite direction from the dislocation which leads to severe degenerative arthritis.

> Glenoid involvement was more severe than is usual in the shoulder with osteoarthritis. Some degree of erosion of the posterior part of the glenoid is characteristically present, making it necessary to lower the high side or elevate the low side when inserting the glenoid component.[2]

Bone grafts under the glenoid are required in some shoulders.[2]

Rheumatoid Arthritis

A large percentage of female TSR candidates have rheumatoid arthritis. Bilateral shoulder disability along with elbow disability is much more common in these patients than in other diagnostic categories. The presence of attenuated rotator cuffs, adherence of the long head of the biceps within the synovial sheath, and arthritis of the acromioclavicular joint has often been noted. There are, however, significant differences in the severity of the disease. Middle-aged women may have a mild form of rheumatoid arthritis. Although moderate to severe cases reveal a thinning of the rotator cuff, tears of complete thickness of the rotator cuff are often small and readily repaired. With the most severe degree of arthritis, massive disintegration of the rotator cuff is common, resulting in a softened rotator cuff that does not hold sutures and does not function. The exposed humeral head in these patients erodes deeply into the acromion, the outer aspect of the clavicle, and the coracoid.

To enhance the results of the TSR in the rheumatoid patient, excision of the acromioclavicular joint is done at the time of surgery. The prevention of shoulder stiffness and support of surrounding surgically repaired structures necessitates the need for an abduction splint.

Most of the rheumatoid patients with both elbow and shoulder complaints are first treated by TSR, as the relief usually has a beneficial effect on the elbow (Fig. 14-4).[2]

Trauma

Patients with trauma-induced total shoulders usually have had previous surgical procedures. They include those with displaced fractures and fracture-dislocations of the proximal end of the humerus of >6 month's duration. Muscle contracture and scarring, difficulty with bony union of the tuberosities, asso-

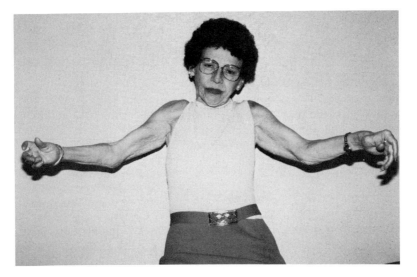

Fig. 14-4. Patient with rheumatoid arthritis demonstrating upper extremity involvement of shoulders, elbows, and hands.

ciated nerve injuries and shortening of the humeral shaft make treatment difficult; thus, the rehabilitation program proceeds at a slower rate. Neer found that the interval from injury to operation ranged from 7 months to 15 years and averaged >2 years.

Revision

The most difficult operative procedure of all is the prosthetic revision. Many prostheses had previously been inserted for fractures and were often anchored with acrylic cement. Other difficulties include massive rotator cuff defects, previously weakened deltoids, and >2 cm of bone loss at the proximal head of the humerus and glenoid. Finally, weakened deltoids often result from radical acromionectomies.

Miscellaneous

Other less frequently seen diagnoses necessitate total shoulder replacement. Shoulders with longstanding massive tears of the rotator cuff are characterized by attrition of the articular cartilage with thinning and a bumpy, so-called pebblestone appearance with decalcification and eventual collapse of the subchondral bone. With time, the humeral head becomes irregular. Without its smooth cartilaginous covering, it erodes into the acromion, clavicle, and coracoid process. Thus, surgical reconstruction is especially difficult in these shoulders. Some diagnoses such as chondrosarcoma may require long humeral components and grafts to maintain humeral length. To preserve this normal length, it is often important to fix the humeral component with methylmethacrylate. This is significant for assuring glenohumeral stability and preservation of length of the deltoid muscle for possible humeral elevation. It serves to remove strain from the bone graft shaft junction. However, it must be remembered that some patients with glenohumeral fusion who complain of loss of motion and generalized shoulder pain are treated by TSR on a limited basis—to regain rotation and reduce discomfort.[2]

PATIENT PROFILE

Patient selection depends on several factors, but pain is the primary factor that is considered when the decision regarding TSR is made. Patients being considered for TSR usually have such severe pain that their sleep is disturbed. Their pain has continued despite conservative treatment such as medications,

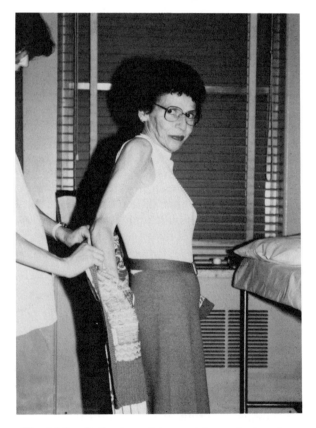

Fig. 14-5.   Patient requiring assistance in dressing.

physical therapy, and steroid injections. Many patients have undergone previous surgical procedures aimed at alleviating their pain.

Loss of motion and strength varies among patients presenting for TSR. The stage of their disease process and their presenting diagnosis seem to influence these two factors. Patients can often initially compensate for decreased glenohumeral motion by scapulothoracic motion. However, with progression of the disease, especially rheumatoid arthritis, the patient can no longer compensate in this manner and a significant loss of motion is noted. The increased incidence of rotator cuff tears in patients with rheumatoid arthritis influences the loss of strength with which the patient is initially seen.

As a result an increase in pain and a decrease in range of motion (ROM) and strength, the patient notes limitations in functional activities. Combing hair, washing the opposite axilla, using a back pocket, and dressing often become difficult is not impossible. Many patients compensate by changing hand dominance or, in the case of bilateral involvement, must seek assistance (Fig. 14-5).

Infection and extensive paralysis are contraindications to surgery. Patients who have weakness of the shoulder musculature can be considered candidates with the knowledge that their rehabilitation will be limited. All patients must be motivated and must cooperate fully in their postoperative rehabilitation if satisfactory results are to be achieved.

SURGICAL CONSIDERATIONS

A competent surgeon, skilled in all aspects of shoulder surgery, is the prime consideration in surgery. Preoperative consideration must be taken into account. A good physical therapy evaluation should be performed to determine the patient's loss of motion and strength. This evaluation may help the surgeon determine the need for a constrained or unconstrained prosthesis. A good medical consultation can help determine if there are any contraindications to the surgery.

Constrained TSRs are indicated in those patients who have constant pain or inaccurate rotator cuff function and in those who would not do as well with other standard operations. The surgeon must take into account the bone stock available in the scapula and the availability of shoulder girdle musculature. If there is severe osteoporosis from various causes such as tumor or surgical excavation of the glenoid vault, it would be prudent for the surgeon to avoid a constrained replacement since loosening may be the side effect. Post believed that there should also be a strong serratus anterior and trapezius to stabilize the scapula for a constrained prosthesis to be considered. A strong deltoid is also advisable except in cases in which passive motion is acceptable. In reality, patients, according to Post, do well with constrained prostheses even in the face of an inefficient deltoid if they understand the limitations of motion.[1]

The unconstrained total shoulder prosthesis probably is the more popular since the use of components (with satisfactory results) designed by Neer have been reported more in the literature. Fleming of Emory Clinic uses the Neer unconstrained shoulder prosthesis and feels that it can be used very well with an intact rotator cuff. He states that it is necessary to have the rotator cuff repaired with some type of graft material or to have the subscapularis transferred to the greater tuberosity. Fleming also states that the superior and inferior glenohumeral ligament complexes should be reattached very well as they are as important as the rotator cuff because they provide anterior stability. In making an approach to the shoulder initially, it is now thought to be very important not to take down any aspect of the deltoid but to make a deltoid pectoral approach. This makes rehabilitation much easier on the patient and provides for a greater possibility for elevation >90°. Fleming also discourages total acromionectomies, as do others, because of the effect that they have on the function of the deltoid. If there is a total acromionectomy, the humeral head may ride superiorly, thus defeating the force couple provided by the rotator cuff musculature and the deltoid. Therefore, in most cases, partial acromionectomy is performed, especially if impingement is found. This helps reduce pain in the arthritic acromioclavicular joint of the rheumatoid patient. The difficulty with the unconstrained prosthesis can occur if the anterior tissues are destroyed to such an extent that they cannot be closed over the prosthesis. This is often the case with radiation necessary for treatment of cancer and with trauma of the shoulder.

The importance of evaluating the postoperative results of various types of prostheses before attempting to use these designs is stressed. The wide use of the Neer total shoulder prosthesis can probably be attributed to the indepth studies available on the results of the shoulder surgery.

Early mobilization has been shown to decrease early postoperative pain. Use of continuous passive motion devices has been beneficial in cases in which the anterior aspect of the shoulder remains intact. Any repairs are protected for ~3 months before resistance is added to the exercise routine.

Complications may involve nerve paralysis, infections, and prosthetic loosening. Of particular note, most surgeons report radiolucent lines which in the weight-bearing extremities are thought to be related to prosthetic loosening. There is no general concensus on what the radiolucent line is, but it is agreed that the area is not filled with bone. With a non–weight-bearing prosthesis such as a total shoulder, the prosthesis is thought to hold up much longer. Possibly such designs as a porous coat will be used in the future and will discontinue the need for methylmethacrylate or other cements within the humerus, thus making revisions easier when necessary.

In final analysis, the surgical considerations depend on the patient's profile, i.e., their involvement of soft tissue extrinsic to the underlying bony defects, with the main goals of surgery for the patient being the loss of pain and an increase in daily functions.

POSTOPERATIVE MANAGEMENT

Following good surgical technique, the most important aspect for the total shoulder patient is postoperative management. The results of surgery would be unacceptable without maximum mobility of the joint provided by early and continued passive movement. Strengthening of the musculature around the shoulder, with emphasis on the rotator cuff and deltoid, must be continued throughout the life of the patient.

Post described an exercise program of passive and active assistive ROM exercises for patients following a constrained TSR. He emphasized that motion, especially external rotation, should never be forced beyond limits found at the time of surgery. The pendulum exercise was not recommended, nor was vigorous and heavy use of the shoulder (as in push-ups). These exercises could cause loosening of the prosthesis. He found that the severity of the disease process in most patients receiving TSR made active overhead motions impossible.

Neer has provided guidelines for postoperative management of the patient with an unconstrained shoulder.[6] Depending on the involvement of the patient's surrounding support structures, modifications for the rehabilitation can be determined. During the first 4 or 5 days, the patient is typically placed in a shoulder immobilizer. Recently, continuous passive motion machines have been used to provide earlier mobilization. Abduction braces are sometimes provided for patients with repairs of the rotator cuff. The healing of certain structures, such as a repaired rotator cuff, may require 6 to 12 weeks of protection from active motion. Pendulum exercises followed by over-the-door pulley exercises are then important for patient independence in passive mobility of the joint. Passive stretching should be included in the exercise program indefinitely to maintain motion (Fig. 14-6).

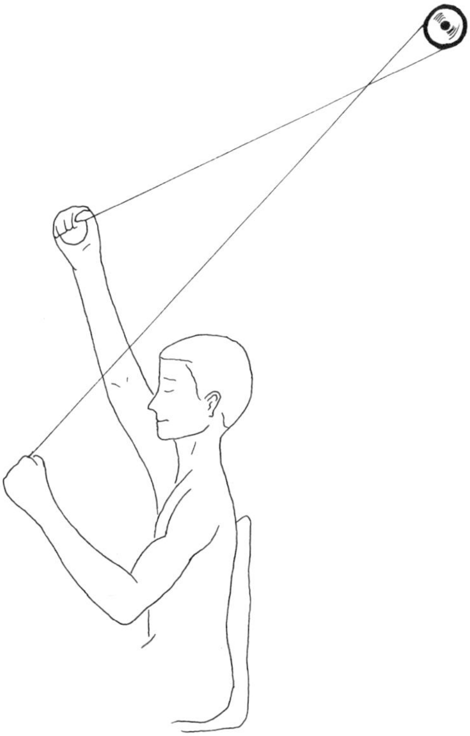

Fig. 14-6. Patient demonstrating the use of an over-the-door shoulder pulley for elevation >90°.

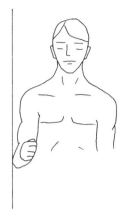

Fig. 14-7.   Middle deltoid strength-ening with isometric exercise.

   Mobilization of the joint in the trained hands of a therapist is often ben-eficial, especially for the severely involved shoulder. Isometrics may be ini-tiated early as long as they are performed correctly. Slow tension is important to minimize tissue stress and joint movement when performing the isometric exercises (Fig. 14-7).

   The main emphasis is on protection of the surgical repair. With initiation of resistive exercises, the elbow should remain flexed and by the side of the trunk. Rubber tubing is helpful to start early isometric exercises and for pro-gression of the program to active resistive exercises (Fig. 14-8).

   Following unconstrained TSR, Clayton reported improvement in shoulder function of >100 percent over preoperative ratings, while the ROM increased relatively little.[7] In his studies, Cofield found that patients typically regained approximately two-thirds of normal active motion with the best results being seen in patients with osteoarthritis.

   Each patient's program of rehabilitation should be individually designed, with goals modified according to the soft tissue constraints of both the involved shoulder and other joints such as the elbow and hands. Patients should un-derstand that once the early phases of rehabilitation have been completed, a maintenance program is to be followed. This allows for small gains in mobility and strength once progress has plateaued.

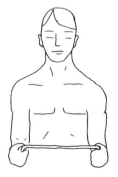

Fig. 14-8.   Isolation of exter-nal rotators with use of rubber tubing.

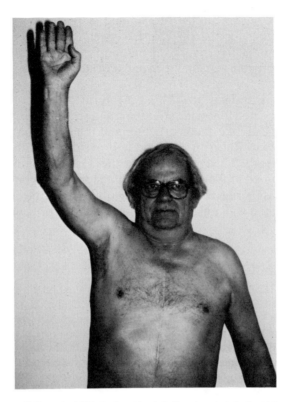

Fig. 14-9.   Successfully rehabilitated patient following total shoulder replacement with unconstrained prosthesis.

Short-term complications, which include excessive pain and swelling, require modifications of exercise schedules and external treatments of ice and heat. Long-term complication such as infection or prosthetic loosening can be addressed by the surgeon as they occur.

Total shoulder replacement is considered a success when the goals for relief of pain and increase in function are achieved. Expectations of a return to normal strength and motion may not be realistic. Finally, functional activities and life styles must be modified to the patient's benefit following surgery (Fig. 14-9).

SUMMARY

The two types of TSR prostheses currently in use are the constrained and unconstrained; the one predominantly used is the unconstrained prosthesis. Thorough evaluation of arm strength, functional needs, and patient expectations must be made prior to determination of prosthetic type for the patient's surgery. With the constrained prosthesis, preoperative muscle loss of the shoulder is usually more severe. Relief of pain and increases in function following surgery are gratifying for the patient. However, because of the increase in muscle involvement, active overhead motion is often not possible. Patients with constrained prostheses should avoid repeated stress of the shoulder to prevent loosening.

With the unconstrained prosthesis, a return to near-normal motion and function can be expected following stretching and strengthening exercises. With this type of prosthesis, the reconstruction and rehabilitation of the muscle is of utmost importance. Relief of pain and improvement of functional activities have been consistently achieved. Because the anatomy remains near normal with the unconstrained prosthesis, it is felt that motion, function, and prosthetic endurance will be superior to the constrained prosthetic device. This is probably the reason for the wider use of the unconstrained total shoulder prosthesis.

REFERENCES

1. Post M, Jablon M, Miller H, Singh M: Constrained total Shoulder joint replacement: a critical review. Clin Orthop 144:135, 1979
2. Neer CS, Watson LD, Stanton FJ: Recent experience in total shoulder replacement. J Bone Joint Surg 64-A:319, 1982
3. Cofield RH: Total joint arthroplasty: the shoulder. Mayo Clin Proc 54:500, 1979
4. Cofield RH: Unconstrained total shoulder prostheses. Clin Orthop 173:97, 1983
5. Poppen K, Walker N, Peter S: Normal and abnormal motion of the shoulder. J Bone Joint Surg 58-A:195
6. Neer CS: Arthroplasty of the shoulder: Neer technique. 3M, St. Paul
7. Clayton ML, Ferlic DC, Jeffers PD: Prosthetic arthroplasties of the shoulder. Clin Orthop 164:184, 1982

Index

Page numbers followed by *f* indicate figures; those followed by *t* indicate tables.